T0226736

Pediatric Rheumatology

Editor

ANDREAS REIFF

RHEUMATIC DISEASE CLINICS OF NORTH AMERICA

www.rheumatic.theclinics.com

Consulting Editor
MICHAEL H. WEISMAN

November 2013 • Volume 39 • Number 4

ELSEVIER

1600 John F. Kennedy Boulevard • Suite 1800 • Philadelphia, Pennsylvania, 19103-2899
http://www.theclinics.com

RHEUMATIC DISEASE CLINICS OF NORTH AMERICA Volume 39, Number 4
November 2013 ISSN 0889-857X, ISBN 13: 978-0-323-24235-6

Editor: Jennifer Flynn-Briggs

© **2013 Elsevier Inc. All rights reserved.**
This periodical and the individual contributions contained in it are protected under copyright by Elsevier, and the following terms and conditions apply to their use:

Photocopying
Single photocopies of single articles may be made for personal use as allowed by national copyright laws. Permission of the Publisher and payment of a fee is required for all other photocopying, including multiple or systematic copying, copying for advertising or promotional purposes, resale, and all forms of document delivery. Special rates are available for educational institutions that wish to make photocopies for non-profit educational classroom use. For information on how to seek permission visit www.elsevier.com/permissions or call: (+44) 1865 843830 (UK)/ (+1) 215 239 3804 (USA).

Derivative Works
Subscribers may reproduce tables of contents or prepare lists of articles including abstracts for internal circulation within their institutions. Permission of the Publisher is required for resale or distribution outside the institution. Permission of the Publisher is required for all other derivative works, including compilations and translations (please consult www.elsevier.com/permissions).

Electronic Storage or Usage
Permission of the Publisher is required to store or use electronically any material contained in this periodical, including any article or part of an article (please consult www.elsevier.com/permissions). Except as outlined above, no part of this publication may be reproduced, stored in a retrieval system or transmitted in any form or by any means, electronic, mechanical, photocopying, recording or otherwise, without prior written permission of the Publisher.

Notice
No responsibility is assumed by the Publisher for any injury and/or damage to persons or property as a matter of products liability, negligence or otherwise, or from any use or operation of any methods, products, instructions or ideas contained in the material herein. Because of rapid advances in the medical sciences, in particular, independent verification of diagnoses and drug dosages should be made.

Although all advertising material is expected to conform to ethical (medical) standards, inclusion in this publication does not constitute a guarantee or endorsement of the quality or value of such product or of the claims made of it by its manufacturer.

Rheumatic Disease Clinics of North America (ISSN 0889-857X) is published quarterly by Elsevier Inc., 360 Park Avenue South, New York, NY 10010-1710. Months of issue are February, May, August, and November. Business and editorial offices: 1600 John F. Kennedy Boulevard, Suite 1800, Philadelphia, PA 19103-2899. Periodicals postage paid at New York, NY and additional mailing offices. Subscription prices are USD 317.00 per year for US individuals, USD 555.00 per year for US institutions, USD 156.00 per year for US students and residents, USD 374.00 per year for Canadian individuals, USD 684.00 per year for Canadian institutions, USD 444.00 per year for international individuals, USD 684.00 per year for international institutions, and USD 218.00 per year for Canadian and foreign students/residents. To receive student/resident rate, orders must be accompanied by name of affiliated institution, date of term, and the *signature* of program/residency coordinator on institution letterhead. Orders will be billed at individual rate until proof of status received. Foreign air speed delivery is included in all *Clinics* subscription prices. All prices are subject to change without notice. **POSTMASTER:** Send address changes to *Rheumatic Disease Clinics of North America*, Elsevier Health Sciences Division, Subscription Customer Service, 3251 Riverport Lane, Maryland Heights, MO 63043. **Customer Service: 1-800-654-2452 (US and Canada). From outside of the US and Canada: 314-447-8871. Fax: 314-447-8029. For print support, e-mail: JournalsCustomerService-usa@elsevier.com. For online support, e-mail: JournalsOnline Support-usa@elsevier.com.**

Reprints. For copies of 100 or more of articles in this publication, please contact the Commercial Reprints Department, Elsevier Inc., 360 Park Avenue South, New York, New York, 10010-1710; Tel.: +1-212-633-3874, Fax: +1-212-633-3820, and E-mail: reprints@elsevier.com.

Rheumatic Disease Clinics of North America is covered in *MEDLINE/PubMed (Index Medicus), Current Contents/Clinical Medicine, Science Citation Index, ISI/BIOMED,* and *EMBASE/Excerpta Medica.*

Printed and bound by CPI Group (UK) Ltd, Croydon, CR0 4YY

Transferred to digital print 2012

Contributors

CONSULTING EDITOR

MICHAEL H. WEISMAN, MD
Division of Rheumatology, Cedars-Sinai Medical Center, Los Angeles, California

EDITOR

ANDREAS REIFF, MD
Division Head Rheumatology, Children's Hospital Los Angeles, Professor of Pediatrics, USC Keck School of Medicine, Los Angeles, California

AUTHORS

MICHAEL BENNETT, PhD
Assistant Research Professor of Pediatrics, Division of Nephrology and Hypertension, Cincinnati Children's Hospital Medical Center, University of Cincinnati, Cincinnati, Ohio

HERMINE I. BRUNNER, MD, MSc
Professor of Pediatrics, Division of Rheumatology, Cincinnati Children's Hospital Medical Center, University of Cincinnati, Cincinnati, Ohio

GLEICE CLEMENTE, MD
Assistant Doctor of Pediatric Rheumatology, Department of Pediatrics, Universidade Federal de São Paulo, São Paulo, Brazil

ROBERT A. COLBERT, MD, PhD
Senior Investigator, Chief, Pediatric Translational Research Branch, National Institute of Arthritis, Musculoskeletal and Skin Diseases (NIAMS), National Institutes of Health, Bethesda, Maryland

RANDY Q. CRON, MD, PhD
Professor, Department of Pediatrics, University of Alabama at Birmingham, Birmingham, Alabama

ADRIANA ALMEIDA DE JESUS, MD, PhD
Translational Autoinflammatory Disease Section, National Institute of Arthritis, Musculoskeletal and Skin Diseases (NIAMS), National Institutes of Health (NIH), Bethesda, Maryland

ESI MORGAN DEWITT, MD, MSCE
Associate Professor, Department of Pediatrics, College of Medicine, University of Cincinnati; Division of Rheumatology, James M. Anderson Center for Health Systems Excellence, Cincinnati Children's Hospital Medical Center, Cincinnati, Ohio

MARLA DUBINSKY, MD
Abe and Claire Levine Chair in Pediatric IBD Research, Associate Professor of Pediatrics, Director, Pediatric Inflammatory Bowel Disease Center, Cedars-Sinai Medical Center, Los Angeles, California

POLLY J. FERGUSON, MD
Associate Professor, Director, Division of Pediatric Rheumatology, Department of Pediatrics, Roy J. and Lucille A. Carver College of Medicine, University of Iowa, Iowa City, Iowa

IVAN FOELDVARI, MD
Hamburger Zentrum für Kinder- und Jugendrheumatologie, Hamburg, Germany

RAPHAELA GOLDBACH-MANSKY, MD, MHS
Translational Autoinflammatory Disease Section, National Institute of Arthritis, Musculoskeletal and Skin Diseases (NIAMS), National Institutes of Health (NIH), Bethesda, Maryland

OLCAY Y. JONES, MD, PhD
Chief, Division of Pediatric Rheumatology, Department of Pediatrics, Walter Reed National Military Medical Center, Bethesda, Maryland; Associate Clinical Professor, Myositis Center, Division of Rheumatology, Departments of Medicine, Anatomy and Regenerative Biology, George Washington University, Washington, DC

SIBEL KADAYIFCILAR, MD
Professor, Department of Ophthalmology, School of Medicine, Hacettepe University, Ankara, Turkey

JAMES D. KATZ, MD
Professor of Medicine, Director, Division of Rheumatology, Department of Medicine, and Director, Myositis Center, George Washington University, Washington, DC

GINA A. MONTEALEGRE SANCHEZ, MD, MS
Translational Autoinflammatory Disease Section, National Institute of Arthritis, Musculoskeletal and Skin Diseases (NIAMS), National Institutes of Health (NIH), Bethesda, Maryland

SEZA ÖZEN, MD
Professor, Department of Pediatrics, School of Medicine, Hacettepe University, Ankara, Turkey

SHERVIN RABIZADEH, MD, MBA
Assistant Professor of Pediatrics, Pediatric Inflammatory Bowel Disease Center, Cedars-Sinai Medical Center, Los Angeles, California

ANUSHA RAMANATHAN, MD
Assistant Professor of Pediatrics, Division of Rheumatology, Keck School of Medicine of USC, Children's Hospital of Los Angeles, Los Angeles, California

ANDREAS REIFF, MD
Division Head Rheumatology, Children's Hospital Los Angeles, Professor of Pediatrics, USC Keck School of Medicine, Los Angeles, California

LISA G. RIDER, MD
Deputy Chief, Environmental Autoimmunity Group, Program of Clinical Research, National Institute of Environmental Health Sciences, National Institutes of Health, Bethesda, Maryland; Clinical Professor of Medicine, Myositis Center, Division of Rheumatology, Department of Medicine, George Washington University, Washington, DC

HEMALATHA SRINIVASALU, MD
Assistant Professor of Pediatrics, Division of Rheumatology, Children's National Medical Center, George Washington University, Washington, DC

SARA M. STERN, MD
Assistant Professor, Division of Immunology, Rheumatology, and Allergy, Department of Pediatrics, University of Utah, Salt Lake City, Utah

MATTHEW L. STOLL, MD, PhD, MSCS
Assistant Professor, Department of Pediatrics, University of Alabama at Birmingham, Birmingham, Alabama

MARIA TERESA TERRERI, PhD, MD
Professor of Pediatrics and Head of Pediatric Rheumatology, Department of Pediatrics, Universidade Federal de São Paulo, São Paulo, Brazil

Contents

> The pathogenesis of monogenic autoinflammatory diseases converges on the presence of exaggerated immune responses that are triggered through activation of altered pattern recognition receptor (PRR) pathways and result in cytokine/chemokine amplification loops and the inflammatory clinical phenotype seen in autoinflammatory patients. The PRR response can be triggered by accumulation of metabolites, by mutations in sensors leading to their constitutive overactivation, or by mutations in mediator cytokine pathways that lead to amplification and/or inability to downregulate an inflammatory response in hematopoietic and/or nonhematopoietic cells. The study of the pathogenesis of sterile inflammation in patients with autoinflammatory syndromes continues to uncover novel inflammatory pathways.

> Autoinflammatory bone disease is a new branch of autoinflammatory diseases caused by seemingly unprovoked activation of the innate immune system leading to an osseous inflammatory process. The inflammatory bone lesions in these disorders are characterized by chronic inflammation that is typically culture negative with no demonstrable organism on histopathology. The most common autoinflammatory bone diseases in childhood include chronic nonbacterial osteomyelitis (CNO), synovitis, acne, pustulosis, hyperostosis, osteitis syndrome, Majeed syndrome, deficiency of interleukin-1 receptor antagonist, and cherubism. In this article, the authors focus on CNO and summarize the distinct genetic autoinflammatory bone syndromes.

> Before the biologic era, treatment of juvenile idiopathic arthritis (JIA) was often highly unsatisfactory, with children forced to endure the ill effects of lifelong disease, including pain and stiffness, disability, and even

biomarkers that are expected to improve the management of lupus nephritis in the future, and support the testing of novel medication regimens.

Childhood vasculitis is a complex and fascinating area in pediatric rheumatology that has experienced an unprecedented surge in research, leading to new knowledge over the past several years. Vasculitis is defined as the presence of inflammatory cell infiltration in blood vessel walls, usually with multisystemic involvement. The most frequent forms of vasculitis in childhood are the small-size vasculitides, of which Henoch-Schoenlein Purpura and other leucocytoclastic vasculitis are the best examples, followed by Kawasaki disease, a midsize vasculitis, and Takayasu arteritis, a large-size vasculitis, both of which are topics in this article.

This review updates recent trends in the classification of the juvenile idiopathic inflammatory myopathies (JIIM) and the emerging standard of treatment of the most common form of JIIM, juvenile dermatomyositis. The JIIM are rare, heterogeneous autoimmune diseases that share chronic muscle inflammation and weakness. A growing spectrum of clinicopathologic groups and serologic phenotypes defined by the presence of myositis autoantibodies are now recognized, each with differing demographics, clinical manifestations, laboratory findings, and prognoses. Although daily oral corticosteroids remain the backbone of treatment, disease-modifying anti-rheumatic drugs are almost always used adjunctively and biologic therapies may benefit patients with recalcitrant disease.

Juvenile localized scleroderma (jLS) and juvenile systemic sclerosis (jSS) are both orphan diseases, with jLS around 10 times more frequent than jSS. In recent years the time gap between the appearance of symptoms and diagnosis has become significantly shorter. This review focuses on the new classifications of jSS and jLS, and on the developments and adaptations of the outcome measures for certain organ involvements whereby progress has been made regarding pediatric patients.

This article provides an introduction to key aspects of outcomes research in pediatric rheumatology, focusing on arthritis. Patient-centered outcomes research addresses questions of interest to multiple stakeholders in order to guide the best health care decisions suited to a particular patient's circumstances and preferences. Discussion includes the importance of maintaining high-quality longitudinal patient registries and use of valid clinical and patient-reported outcome measures. Rapid, reliable translation of research on best practices into clinical care, as facilitated by quality improvement learning networks, leads to timely and meaningful improvement in patient outcomes.

RHEUMATIC DISEASE CLINICS OF NORTH AMERICA

**DOWNLOAD
Free App!**

Review Articles
THE CLINICS

NOW AVAILABLE FOR YOUR iPhone and iPad

Erratum

With regard to the article "**Ultrasound and Treatment Algorithms of RA and JIA**," by Sam R. Dalvi, MD, David W. Moser, DO, and Jonathan Samuels, MD, which appeared in *Rheumatic Disease Clinics of North America,* August 2013;39(3):669-688, the publisher would like to clarify that the affiliation for Sam R. Dalvi is incorrect. The correct affiliation for Sam R. Dalvi is: Assistant Professor of Medicine, Division of Rheumatology and Immunology, Duke University Medical Center, Durham, NC 27710, USA.

Rheum Dis Clin N Am 39 (2013) xiii
http://dx.doi.org/10.1016/j.rdc.2013.07.003
0889-857X/13/$ – see front matter © 2013 Elsevier Inc. All rights reserved.

rheumatic.theclinics.com

Foreword

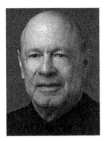

Michael H. Weisman, MD
Consulting Editor

Andreas Reiff has created a volume that addresses some of the most pressing issues facing pediatric rheumatology today. These issues are how to recognize and treat auto-inflammatory syndromes and how to take the advances in genetic identification of susceptibility and severity of pediatric rheumatic diseases and translate them into treatment approaches. Clearly the approach to myositis, scleroderma, and spondyloarthritis in the pediatric population requires a level of intensity and attention to new biomarkers and outcome measures that were not generally recognized 5 years ago, and this volume will be a very handy companion and support for the most modern and up-to-date approaches to individual patient care. In addition, Andreas has made it clear that he has given the next generation of clinical scholars the chance to learn how to synthesize the literature in a series of reviews that were highly mentored by experts in the field. It is gratifying to see how far, timely, and useful the *Rheumatic Disease Clinics of North America* have become over the years, and thanks to Andreas, this volume adds to the prestige and importance of continuing the series.

Michael H. Weisman, MD
Division of Rheumatology
Cedars-Sinai Medical Center
8700 Beverly Boulevard
Los Angeles, CA 90024, USA

E-mail address:
michael.weisman@cshs.org

Rheum Dis Clin N Am 39 (2013) xv
http://dx.doi.org/10.1016/j.rdc.2013.07.002
0889-857X/13/$ – see front matter © 2013 Published by Elsevier Inc.

rheumatic.theclinics.com

Preface

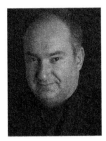

Andreas Reiff, MD
Editor

Dear Reader, Dear Colleagues,

It is a privilege and gives me great pleasure to present you the latest edition of Pediatric Rheumatology for the *Rheumatic Disease Clinics of North America* series. I am not sure that you are aware, but this little green book has a wide-reaching audience and is used as reference guide by many health care providers worldwide.

Since the publication of the last edition in 2007, our field is moving forward at an exhilarating pace and it is indeed an exciting time to practice and be involved with pediatric rheumatology. The concerted efforts of pediatric rheumatologists worldwide have resulted in unprecedented knowledge about new diseases, long-term outcomes, and new insights into treatment modalities. With the introduction of new data on the long-term use of biologic therapies, the once most therapeutically challenging diseases are now much better manageable and long-term outcomes for our patients seem to improve. In view of that, we have dedicated an article in this issue to outcomes research in pediatric rheumatology.

Unlike the previous versions, you will find that this new edition has three major innovations. First, it presents the reader with up-to-date information on the most relevant pediatric rheumatologic conditions, focusing on the science and new therapeutic accomplishments emerging over the past 5 years. You will find information about new biomarkers in SLE, newly discovered autoantibodies in dermatomyositis, new periodic fever syndromes, and new biologic treatment options in juvenile arthritis.

Second, we tried to dedicate the authorships of this edition to the future generation of pediatric rheumatologists. These will be our successors and the thought-leaders of tomorrow. For most articles, you will find junior faculty as lead authors assigned to senior and well-established authors in the field. We felt that this will allow the young generation to gain experience in comprehensively summarizing new information and establish themselves in the field of pediatric rheumatology.

Lastly, I have asked some of my colleagues in gastroenterology to contribute an article about the latest developments in the pathogenesis and treatment of inflammatory bowel disease. Since we frequently deal with gastroenterologic symptoms in our patients, I felt it might be helpful to take a look over the fence and understand the perspective of our gastroenterology colleagues in treating these diseases.

Rheum Dis Clin N Am 39 (2013) xvii–xviii
http://dx.doi.org/10.1016/j.rdc.2013.07.001
0889-857X/13/$ – see front matter © 2013 Published by Elsevier Inc.

rheumatic.theclinics.com

We understand that we may not have been able to cover the entire spectrum of all the innovations that are occurring in the field of pediatric rheumatology, but we hope that this issue will serve you as a valuable tool to learn new information and your patients to receive better care and a better chance to overcome their challenging chronic diseases.

It was a privilege for me to serve as guest editor for this issue and I want to express my heartfelt gratitude to all of my national and international colleagues for their outstanding contributions. Special thanks to Pamela Hetherington at Elsevier for her dedication and patience in bringing this effort to fruition and to my wife, Diann, for allowing me the time away from home to finish this book.

Andreas Reiff, MD
Children's Hospital Los Angeles
USC Keck School of Medicine
Los Angeles, CA, USA

E-mail address:
areiff@chla.usc.edu

Monogenic Autoinflammatory Diseases
Disorders of Amplified Danger Sensing and Cytokine Dysregulation

Gina A. Montealegre Sanchez, MD, MS,
Adriana Almeida de Jesus, MD, PhD,
Raphaela Goldbach-Mansky, MD, MHS*

KEYWORDS

- Cryopyrin-associated periodic syndrome (CAPS)
- Neonatal-onset multisystem inflammatory disease (NOMID)
- Proteasome-associated autoinflammatory syndrome (PRAAS)
- Chronic atypical neutrophilic dermatosis with lipodystrophy and elevated temperature (CANDLE) • Deficiency of the IL-1 receptor antagonist (DIRA)
- Inflammasome • Autoinflammatory diseases
- Intracellular pattern recognition receptors (PRR)

KEY POINTS

- Monogenic autoinflammatory diseases are caused by single-gene defects in innate immune regulatory pathways. They present in childhood with sterile inflammation and can mimic infections.
- Gain-of-function mutations in *NLRP3/CIAS1*, encoding the first intracellular danger sensor identified in humans, cause the clinical spectrum of the cryopyrinopathies and link danger recognition to the activation of the proinflammatory alarm cytokine interleukin (IL)-1.
- The pivotal role of IL-1 in the cryopyrinopathies was confirmed in clinical studies using IL-1 blocking therapies and encouraged their use in the classic periodic fever syndromes, familial Mediterranean fever, tumor necrosis factor receptor–associated periodic syndrome, and hyperimmunoglobulinemia D with periodic fever syndrome.
- Novel autoinflammatory conditions with poor responses to IL-1 blocking therapies include the proteasome-associated autoinflammatory syndromes (PRAAS), deficiency of IL-36 receptor antagonist, CARD14-mediated psoriasis and early-onset inflammatory bowel disease, and suggest a role of cytokine dysregulation beyond IL-1.

Continued

Translational Autoinflammatory Disease Section, National Institute of Arthritis and Musculoskeletal and Skin Diseases (NIAMS), National Institutes of Health (NIH), Building 10, Room 6D47-B, 10 Center Drive, Bethesda, MD 20892, USA
* Corresponding author.
E-mail address: goldbacr@mail.nih.gov

Rheum Dis Clin N Am 39 (2013) 701–734
http://dx.doi.org/10.1016/j.rdc.2013.08.001
0889-857X/13/$ – see front matter Published by Elsevier Inc.

Continued

- Early diagnosis of these syndromes is essential because effective therapies, particularly for the IL-1–mediated conditions, can change patients' lives and disease outcomes.
- An emerging theme in our understanding of the pathogenesis of exaggerated sterile inflammatory responses in autoinflammatory syndromes converges on dysregulation in intracellular innate immune sensing, and on the amplification of proinflammatory cytokine circuits that cannot be downregulated.

OLD AND EMERGING NEW CONCEPTS

Monogenic autoinflammatory diseases can be defined as a group of immune dysregulatory conditions marked by excessive inflammation that is predominantly mediated by increased responses to known and unknown triggers by cells and molecules of the innate immune system (**Table 1**).[1] These illnesses typically present in childhood and can mimic infections or hematologic malignancies, but the inflammatory lesions are aseptic and nonmalignant. The discovery of single-gene defects in the interleukin (IL)-1 pathway that cause the spectrum of the cryopyrinopathies or cryopyrin-associated periodic syndromes (CAPS) and the rare condition, deficiency of the IL-1 receptor antagonist (DIRA), pointed to the pivotal role of IL-1 and provided deeper insights into the molecular bases that drive the inflammatory phenotypes. These findings translated into therapeutic approaches using IL-1 blocking agents, which have become standard of care for the cryopyrinopathies and DIRA, and their use has been expanded to other monogenic disorders, the periodic fever syndromes, and to disorders with unidentified genetic causes, including aphthous stomatitis, pharyngitis and adenitis (PFAPA) syndrome, systemic-onset juvenile idiopathic arthritis (SJIA), adult-onset Still disease (AOSD), and Behçet disease, that share clinical similarities with monogenic autoinflammatory diseases.

The journey of deciphering inflammatory phenotypes started in 1997 with the discovery of the genetic cause of familial Mediterranean fever (FMF), the most prevalent autoinflammatory disease worldwide,[2,3] followed by the discovery of the genetic cause of 2 other periodic fever syndromes, tumor necrosis factor (TNF) receptor–associated periodic syndrome (TRAPS)[4] and hyperimmunoglobulinemia D with periodic fever syndrome (HIDS).[5–7] These 3 syndromes share the episodic nature of fever and periods of remission and can be grouped as classic hereditary periodic fever syndromes. The cryopyrinopathies, comprising familial cold autoinflammatory syndrome (FCAS), Muckle-Wells syndrome (MWS), and neonatal-onset multisystem inflammatory disease (NOMID), also known as chronic infantile neurologic cutaneous and articular (CINCA) syndrome; and DIRA are caused by single-gene mutations in loci regulating IL-1 processing, secretion, and signaling. Therapeutic interventions blocking IL-1 in an autoinflammatory bone disease with clinical similarities to DIRA, namely Majeed syndrome, confirmed a prominent role for IL-1 in this condition as well.

A group of recently described autoinflammatory syndromes that are unresponsive to IL-1 blocking therapy include the proteasome-associated autoinflammatory syndromes (PRAAS) or chronic atypical neutrophilic dermatosis with lipodystrophy and elevated temperature (CANDLE), an autoinflammatory condition presenting with lipodystrophy and myositis; deficiency of IL-36 receptor antagonist (DITRA) and CARD14-mediated psoriasis (CAMPS), 2 conditions presenting with pustular skin disease; and early-onset inflammatory bowel disease (IBD). Other newly discovered conditions that present with inflammatory dysregulation only partially involving IL-1 include disorders caused by mutations in PLCγ2[8,9] and pyogenic arthritis pioderma gangrenosum and

Table 1
Demographic, genetic and clinical features of the monogenic autoinflammatory diseases (AID)

		Inheritance/Ethic Distribution	Gene/Protein	Clinical Manifestations							Treatment
				Skin	CNS	Eye	Inner Ear	MSK	Systemic Inflammation		
IL-1-Mediated Diseases	Cryopyrin-opathies										Anti-IL1 agents: anakinra, canakinumab, rilonacept
	FCAS	AD/Primarily European	*NLRP3* (1q44)/ Cryopyrin (NLRP3)	Cold-induced neutrophilic urticaria	Headache	Conjunctivitis	None	Myalgia, arthralgia	Fever, ↑ acute phase reactants *Complications:* Amyloidosis is uncommon (~2%)		
	MWS	AD/Northern European	*NLRP3* (1q44)/ Cryopyrin (NLRP3)	Neutrophilic urticaria	Headache	Conjunctivitis episcleritis, optic disk edema *Complications:* corneal opacification	Cochlear edema *Complications:* SNHL hearing loss	Myalgia, arthralgia, oligo-arthritis	Fever, ↑ acute phase reactants, occasional lymphadenopathy Pericarditis, pleuritis and peritonitis are rare *Complications:* Amyloidosis is observed in ~25% of cases. Peritoneal adhesions		
	NOMID	AD, sporadic/Any ethnicity	*NLRP3* (1q44)/ Cryopyrin (NLRP3)	Neutrophilic urticaria	Headache, chronic aseptic meningitis *Complications:* Developmental delay	Conjunctivitis Uveitis *Complications:* Papilledema, progressive vision loss, corneal opacification	Cochlear edema *Complications:* SNHL hearing loss	Arthralgia and chronic arthritis *Complications:* Epiphyseal overgrowth, joint contractures	Fever, ↑ acute phase reactants, occasional lymphadenopathy hepatosplenomegaly Pericarditis, pleuritis and peritonitis are rare. *Complications:* Amyloidosis in untreated patients who achieve adulthood		

(continued on next page)

Table 1 (*continued*)

		Inheritance/Ethnic Distribution	Gene/Protein	Clinical Manifestations						Treatment
				Skin	CNS	Eye	Inner Ear	MSK	Systemic Inflammation	
Classic Periodic Fever Syndromes	FMF	AR or AD/Jewish, Arab, Armenian, Turkish, Italian	*MEFV* (16p13.3)/ Pyrin	Erysipelas-like erythema (ELE)	Aseptic meningitis (rare)	Uncommon	None	Exercise-induced myalgia, protracted febrile myalgia, arthritis *Complications:* sacroiliitis, joint arthrosis, hip arthritis & erosions	Fever and ↑ acute phase reactants Serositis: peritonitis, pleuritis, pericarditis, epididymitis *Complications:* Peritoneal adhesions Amyloidosis risk varies according with genotype and environment.	Daily oral colchicine, anti-IL1 agents (anakinra, rilonacept and canakinumab
	TRAPS	AD/Broad ethnic distribution Originally Irish/ Scottish	*TNFRSF1A* (12p13)/ 55kDaTNF receptor	Migratory erythema often associated myalgia; ELE	Headache; aseptic meningitis (rare)	Periorbital edema, conjunctivitis Uveitis	None	Migratory myalgia, arthralgia, non-erosive arthritis	Fever, ↑ acute phase reactants and occasional lymphadenopathy Serositis: peritonitis, pleuritis, pericarditis, scrotal pain *Complications:* Amyloidosis is observed in ~14% of cases. Peritoneal adhesions	Etanercept, anti-IL1 agents (anakinra)

	Disease	Inheritance/Ethnicity	Gene (locus)/Protein	Skin	CNS	Eye		Musculoskeletal	Systemic	Treatment
	HIDS	AR/Dutch, Northern European	MVK (12q24)/Mevalonate kinase	Maculo-papular purpuric exanthema, apthous oral ulcers	Uncommon	Uncommon	None	Arthralgia, non-erosive acute polyarthritis; myalgia (rare)	Fever, ↑ acute phase reactants, cervical lymphadenopathy, hepatosplenomegaly. Peritonitis is uncommon. Pericarditis is rare. *Complications:* Amyloidosis risk is unknown.	NSAIDs, CS, simvastatin, anti-IL1 (anakinra, canakinumab)
Autoinflammatory Bone Diseases	DIRA	AR/ Newfoundland, Puerto Rican, Brazilian, Dutch, Palestinian	IL1RN (2q14.2)/IL1RA	Pustular dermatitis	Rare CNS vasculitis *Complications:* Rare encephalo-malacia	Conjunctivitis is rare	None	Recurrent multifocal aseptic osteomyelitis Periostetis *Complications:* Vertebral and odontoid destruction	Occasional fever in few patients and increased acute phase reactants *Complications:*	Anti-IL1 agents (anakinra, rilonacept in clinical trial)
	Majeed	AR/Originally Jordanian	LPIN2 (18p11.31)/Lipin2	Pustular dermatoses	Uncommon	Uncommon	Uncommon	Recurrent multifocal aseptic osteomyelitis *Complications:* Contractures joint deformities	Hematologic manifestations: dyserythropoietic anemia	CS, anti-TNF agents, anti-IL-1 agents- anakinra and canakinumab
IFN-Mediated Diseases	PRAAS CANDLE	AR/Originally Japan Any race or ethnicity	PSMB8 (6p21.3)/	Nodular exanthema, panniculitis, lipodystrophy, periorbital erythema	Aseptic meningitis *Complications:* Basal ganglia calcification	Conjunctivitis	None	Arthralgias, arthritis, myalgias, myositis *Complications:* Joint contractures	Fever, dyslipidemia, growth delay, intra-abdominal fat deposition, pancreatic abnormalities, microcytic anemia, cytopenias *Complications:* Lipodystrophy, failure to thrive	CS, JAK inhibition in clinical trial (baricitinib)

(continued on next page)

Table 1 (*continued*)

		Inheritance/Ethic Distribution	Gene/Protein	Clinical Manifestations						Treatment
				Skin	CNS	Eye	Inner Ear	MSK	Systemic Inflammation	
NF–κB Mediated Diseases	CAMPS	AD	CARD14/CARD14	Plaque or pustular psoriasis	Uncommon	Uncommon	None	Arthritis in 30% of patients	Fever can be present with super-infections of the skin	MTX, CsA, anti-TNF agents, psoriasis medications
	DITRA	AR/Originally Tunisia-England	IL36RN (2q14)/IL36RA	Generalized pustular psoriasis Oral mucosa involvement	Uncommon	Uncommon	None	Uncommon	Fever, asthenia, elevated acute phase reactants and leucocytosis	CS, CsA, retinoids, anti-TNF agents
Other Pathogenesis Pathways	PAPA	AD/Originally Caucasian; any ethnicity	PSTPIP1 (12q24-q25.1)/PSTPIP1	Pyoderma gangrenosum pathergy, skin abscesses, cystic acne, hidradenitis	Uncommon	Uncommon	None	Deforming aseptic pyogenic arthritis Complications: Joint destruction Impaired QOL related to physical disability	Occasional lymphadenopathy, splenomegaly, thrombocytopenia.	CS, anti-TNF agents, anti-IL1 agents
	PGA	AD, sporadic/Originally Caucasian but other ethnicities also seen	NOD2/CARD15 (16q12.1-13)	Icthyosis-like exanthema non-caseating granulomata	Rare, central neuropathy, stroke, and hearing loss	Chronic uveitis, cataract, glaucoma, blindness. Complications: Blindness	None	Polyarthritis, hypertrophic tenosynovitis	Fever is rare. Elevated acute phase reactants	CS, methotrexate, azathioprine, cyclosporine, anti-TNF agents
	EO-IBD	AR/Originally Lebanese and Turkish	IL10 (1q31-q32); IL10RA (11q23); IL10RB (21q22.11)/IL-10; IL-10RA/IL-10RB	Folliculitis	Uncommon	Uncommon	None	Arthritis	Fever, severe colitis: bloody diarrhea, abscesses, perianal fistula, oral aphtous lesions	CS, CsA, AZA, mesalamine, mercaptopurine, MTX, TAC, anti-TNF agents, allogenic HSCT

PLCγ2-associated diseases	AD/Ashkenazi Jewish and European	PLCG2 (16q23.3)	None	PLAID: cold-induced urticaria and granulomatous skin rash. APLAID: blistering skin lesions and cellulitis	None	PLAID: none APLAID: corneal blisters evolving to corneal erosions, ulcerations, intraocular hypertension and cataracts.	None	PLAID: seronegative inflammatory arthritis (rare) APLAID: arthralgia	PLAID: Positive autoantibodies and autoimmune manifestations, recurrent and/or severe infections APLAID: interstitial lung disease, mild immunodeficiency, ulcerative colitis	PLAID: IVIG for immuno-deficiency APLAID: high dose corticosteroids and anti-IL-1 agent (partial response).

Abbreviations: AD, autosomal dominant; APLAID, autoinflammation and PLCγ2-associated antibody deficiency and immune dysregulation; AR, autosomal recessive; AZA, azathioprine; CAMPS, CARD14 mediated psoriasis; CAPS, cryopyrin associated periodic syndrome; CNS, central nervous system; CS, corticosteroids; CsA, cyclosporine; DIRA, deficiency of interleukin 1 receptor antagonist; DITRA, deficiency of interleukin 36 receptor antagonist; EO-IBD, early-onset inflammatory bowel disease; FCAS, familial cold autoinflammatory syndrome; FMF, familial Mediterranean fever; HIDS, hyperimmunoglobulinemia D syndrome with periodic fever; HSCT, hematopoietic stem cell transplantation; IVIG, intravenous immunoglobulin; JAK, Janus Kinase; MSK, musculoskeletal; MTX, methotrexate; MWS, Muckle-Wells syndrome; NOMID, neonatal-onset multisystem inflammatory disease; NSAIDs, non-steroidal anti-inflammatory drugs; PAPA, pyogenic arthritis, pyoderma gangrenosum and acne syndrome; PGA, pediatric granulomatous arthritis; PLAID, PLCγ2-associated antibody deficiency and immune dysregulation; PRAAS, proteasome associated autoinflammatory syndromes; SNHL, sensorineural hearing loss; TAC, tacrolimus; TNF, tumor necrosis factor; TRAPS, TNF receptor associated periodic syndrome.

acne (PAPA) syndrome.[10] Studies of the disease pathogenesis of other disorders point to a role of cytokine dysregulation in pathways involving interferon (IFN), NF-κB/IL-17 and IL-10 signaling pathways. The complex clinical and laboratory features, which, in some novel conditions, can overlap with those seen in patients with autoimmune diseases, illustrate that innate and adaptive immune responses can be dysregulated in some conditions and need to be viewed as coexisting consequences of mutations in adaptive and innate immunity cells. Mutant protein in CAMPS and DITRA is mainly expressed in keratinocytes, which points to a role of primary keratinocyte dysregulation in pustular, neutrophilic dermatitis, and provides us with clues to tissue-specific factors that lead to organ-specific disease manifestations.

Summary of Implications on our Understanding of Disease Pathogenesis

Novel conditions add evidence to the hypothesis that autoinflammatory syndromes are caused by exaggerated/increased sensing of extracellular and intracellular danger
The genetic defect in many autoinflammatory disorders is in components of cytosolic innate pattern recognition receptors (PRRs) (NLRP3, NOD2, pyrin) pathways, affecting their function directly, or by affecting molecules involved in coordinating cytokine responses (**Fig. 2, Table 2**).[11]

Innate immune response evolved to protect organisms from exogenous and endogenous dangers that threaten harm/destroy the organism. The ultimate purpose of the immune response is to remove or sequester the source of the disturbance, and to restore functionality and tissue homeostasis.[12] To do that, the innate immune system uses a finite number of germline-encoded PRRs that recognize exogenous nonself molecules and endogenous self molecules. The first PRRs identified and characterized were the toll-like receptors (TLRs) and later others including RIG-I-like helicase receptors (RLR) and the C-type lectin receptors (CLRs), which mainly sense exogenous pathogen-associated molecular patterns (PAMPs).[13] More recently, PRRs that also recognize endogenous cytoplasmic damage-associated molecular patterns (DAMPs) have been discovered. A generic immune response to extracellular and intracellular triggers has the following components: a trigger that is recognized by a molecular sensor that elicits mediators that lead to cytokine and chemokine production with the goal of recruiting immune cells into the tissue and coordinating a tissue defense. The immune response is tissue specific (**Fig. 1**).[12]

The discovery that mutations in the NLRP3 inflammasome, the first intracellular PRR identified in humans,[14,15] cause the disease spectrum of CAPS, provided a molecular mechanism that links intracellular stress recognition with the initiation of a cytokine response (inflammatory mediator). This response occurs through caspase-1–mediated IL-1 and IL-18 activation and thus provides a conceptual framework to understand the episodic inflammatory events that underlie autoinflammation.[16] Since the discovery of cryopyrin/NLRP3, 23 structurally similar NOD-like receptors (NLRs) have been found in humans.[17] Pediatric granulomatous arthritis (PGA) is caused by autosomal dominant gain-of-function mutations in the NACHT domain (exon 4) of 1 of these NLRs, *NOD2/CARD15*, but the inflammatory cytokine responses induced by the triggers to NOD2 are more complex, not clearly tied to IL-1 release, and involve nuclear factor kappa B (NFκB) activation.

Recently, an increasing number of sensors that are triggered not only by viral DNA and RNA but also by self DNA and RNA, has been found to be coupled to the transcription of type I interferons (IFN type I) and the induction of interferon response genes.[18] An increasing number of inflammatory conditions, including the autoimmune condition systemic lupus erythematosus (SLE)[19] and the monogenic condition

Aicardi-Goutieres syndrome (AGS), which is caused by mutations in enzymes associated with the digestion of single-stranded or mispaired dsDNA, RNA/DNA hybrids, and deoxynucleotide triphosphates,[20] present with an increase in IFN response genes and raise the question whether novel autoinflammatory conditions presenting with induction of interferon response genes are associated with dysregulation in these IFN type I–coupled sensor pathways.

The inability to downregulate unopposed cytokine signaling leads to the development of vicious cytokine cycles that amplify and perpetuate inflammatory responses

The absence of functional receptor antagonists of 2 IL-1 receptor family members, *IL1RN* and *IL1F5/IL36RN,* generates cytokine amplification loops in response to triggered events that cannot be downregulated and can escalate to a systemic inflammatory response syndrome and death. The clinical consequences of the absence of a negative regulator counteracting cytokine signaling on the IL-1 and IL-36 receptor are illustrated in the disease expression of DIRA and DITRA, respectively.

Primary dysregulation of keratinocyte activation can initiate the recruitment of hematopoietic cells into the tissue and initiate inflammatory amplification loops that lead to pustular dermatoses

The proteins encoded by mutated *CARD14* in CAMPS, and mutated *IL36RN/IL1F5* in DITRA, CARD14 and the IL-36 receptor antagonist, respectively, are both mainly expressed in keratinocytes, and the fact that these diseases can present with generalized pustulosis, fever, and/or systemic inflammation point to dysregulated keratinocyte responses as the instigator of an inflammatory immune response localized to the skin.

The molecular targets mutated in existing and emerging new autoinflammatory syndromes suggest a unifying hypothesis that the increased systemic and tissue-specific inflammatory response seen in these patients may constitute a heightened immune response to extracellular and/or intracellular triggers, either because of enhanced sensor function, accumulation of triggers/inducers, or increased production of mediates, all contributing to the development of amplification loops of proinflammatory cytokine production and signaling.

IL-1–MEDIATED AUTOINFLAMMATORY DISEASES

The clinical disease manifestations of the cryopyrinopathies (FCAS, MWS, and NOMID/CINCA), the classic autoinflammatory syndromes (FMF, TRAPS, HIDS), and the monogenic autoinflammatory bone diseases (DIRA and Majeed syndrome) significantly respond to IL-1 blocking therapies, suggesting a key pathogenic role of IL-1 in the disease pathogenesis. As our understanding of the disease pathogenesis in most of these disorders is centered around IL-1β activation by the NLRP3 inflammasome, their pathogenesis is discussed together.

Pathogenesis Considerations in IL-1–Mediated Conditions

The NLRP3 inflammasome integrates sensing of a trigger and IL-1 maturation and secretion (see **Fig. 2**). The *NLRP3* gene encodes the protein cryopyrin, which together with the adapter proteins, ASC (apoptosis-associated speck-like protein containing a CARD) and CARDINAL, and 2 procaspase-1 molecules forms the NLRP3 inflammasome, a caspase-1/IL-1β activating platform. On stimulation, the NLRP3 inflammasome activates the proteolytic enzyme caspase-1, which cleaves inactive pro-IL-1β and pro-IL-18 into their active forms (see **Fig. 2**).[21–23] Inflammasome activation requires a priming (first) signal, through for example a TLR, that leads to the transcription

Table 2
Known and putative proinflammatory mechanisms

Disease Gene/Protein	Trigger	Sensor	Mediator pathway/ Cytokine Amplification Loop	Target Organ	Therapeutic Targets
CAPS *NLRP3*/Cryopyrin	TLR stimulants (PAMPs), NLR stimulants (DAMPs), Cold in FCAS pts.	**Constitutive *NLRP3* inflammasome activation**	IL-1β secretion is increased	Skin, CNS, eye, inner ear, joints and bone	IL-1, IL-1β, (future targets caspase-1, Inflammasome activity)
FMF *MEFV*/Pyrin	Stress (DAMPs), Infection (PAMPs)	**Increased/constitutive pyrin inflammasome function, decreased NLRP3 inhibition**	IL-1β secretion is increased, neutrophil activation	Skin, joints, muscles, serositis, CNS, and eye	IL-1
TRAPS *TNFRSF1A*/55kDaTNF receptor	Stress (DAMPs), Infections (PAMPs)	TLRs, NLRs, other	**Increase ROS production due to trapped mutant TNFR and MAPK activation (p-p38, p-JNK)**	Skin, eye, joints, serositis, CNS	IL-1 and TNF
HIDS *MVK*/Mevalonate kinase	**Possible accumulation of non isoprenylated protein?,** vaccinations, infections, stress	NLRP3 inflammasome?	Increase in NLRP3 dependent IL-1 production (largely unknown mechanisms)	Skin, joints, muscle, GI, CNS, eye	IL-1
DIRA *IL1RN*/IL1RA	Stress (DAMPs), Infections (PAMPs), mechanical stress on skin	TLRs, NLRs, other?	**Unopposed IL-1α, β signaling**	Skin, bone, CNS, and eye	IL-1
Majeed *LPIN2*/Lipin2	**Accumulation of fatty acids that may trigger NLRP3 inflammasome?**	NLRP3 inflammasome?	Increased IL-1 production?	Skin, bone, and bone marrow	IL-1 (?)

Disease / Gene	Trigger	Sensing	Signaling	Affected tissues	Pathway
CANDLE *PSMB8/β5i*	**Accumulation of polyubiquitinated proteins, other?**	Intracellular receptor coupled to IFN response gene stimulation?	IFN mediated and other including pERK	Skin, joints, muscle, GI, eye, adipose tissue, CNS, and bone marrow	IFN + unknown pathways
CAMPS *CARD14/CARD14-CARMA2*	PAMPs, mechanical irritation, infection	TLRs, RIG-I-like, other?	**Constitutive NFKB activation in keratinocytes**	Skin and joints	NF-κB + IL-17 + IL-12/IL-23
DITRA *IL36RN/IL36RA*	Infections (PAMPs), Stress (DAMPs)	TLR, NLR, other	**Unopposed IL-36 signaling**	Skin	(Future target IL-36) + unknown pathways
PAPA *PSTPIP1/PSTPIP1*	Skin puncture, acne lesion, unknown	TLRs, NLRs, other	NLRP3 dependent IL-1 release and unknown	Skin, joints	IL-1 (arthritis) + unknown pathways
PGA *NOD2/CARD15*	Stress (DAMPs), Infections (PAMPs)	**Constitutive NOD2 and NFkB activation**	RIP2 kinase mediated NFkB activation	Skin, eye, joints, CNS	NF-κB + unknown pathways
EO-IBD *IL10RA, IL10RB, IL10/ IL10RA, IL10RB, IL10*	Commensal bacteria	TLRs, NLRs in colon, other	**Decreased antiinflammatory signaling through IL-10 receptor**	GI tract, colon, skin	Reconstitute IL-10 signaling
PLCγ2-associated diseases *PLCG2*	Cold-induced	NF-kB activation, other	**PLCγ2-mediated NF-kB activation + other (?)**	Skin, eye, lungs, immune system	IL-1 + unknown

In bold are the primary defects induced by the genetic mutation.

Abbreviations: CAMPS, CARD14 mediated psoriasis; CANDLE, chronic atypical neutrophilic dermatosis with lipodystrophy and elevated temperature syndrome; CAPS, cryopyrin associated periodic syndromes; CNS, central nervous system; DAMPs, damage associated molecular patterns; DIRA, deficiency of the interleukin-1 receptor antagonist; DITRA, deficiency of the interleukin-36 receptor antagonist; ERK, extracellular signal-regulated kinases; FMF, familial Mediterranean fever; GI, gastrointestinal tract; HIDS, hyperimmunoglobulinemia D with periodic fever syndrome; IFN, interferon; IL-1, interleukin 1α and β; IL-1β, interleukin 1β; IL-1Ra, interleukin 1 receptor antagonist; IL-36, interleukin 36; MAPK, mitogen-activated protein kinase; NLRs, nucleotide oligomerization domain (NOD)-like receptors; p-JNK, phosphorylated-JNK; PAMPs, pathogen associated molecular patterns; PAPA, pyogenic sterile arthritis, pyoderma gangrenosum and acne syndrome; PGA, pediatric granulomatous arthritis; RIG-i-like, retinoic acid-inducible gene 1; RIP2, receptor interacting protein kinase 2; ROS, reactive oxygen species; TLR, toll-like receptor; TNF, tumor necrosis factor; TNFR, tumor necrosis factor receptor; TRAPS, TNF receptor-associated periodic syndrome.

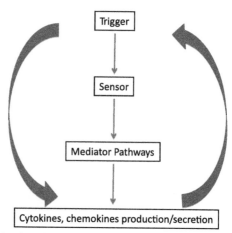

Other (not discussed): i.e cell growth, differentiation, cell cycle/death

Fig. 1. Components of an inflammatory response. An immune response is triggered by exogenous or endogenous triggers that are sensed by a molecular sensor, a pattern recognition receptor (PRR) that can be located on the cell surface or in the cytoplasm. A triggering event is linked to the activation of mediators that lead to the stimulation and secretion of cytokines and chemokines, which lead to the recruitment of immune cells into the tissue and the coordination of an immune response. The immune response is often tissue specific and may explain the difference in organ manifestations in autoinflammatory diseases. Some mutations that lead to cytokine dysregulation also influence cell growth and differentiation and/or cell death, often in a cell-specific manner.

and translation of pro-IL-1β; and a second signal that leads to inflammasome and caspase-1 activation. Signal 1 is delivered through exogenous triggers that include whole pathogens (such as *Staphylococcus aureus*, *Listeria monocytogenes*, and *Candida albicans*), PAMPs, such as lipopolysaccharide (LPS; viral), nucleic acids, muramyl dipeptide (MDP), and bacterial toxins. Caspase-1 activation in response to bacterial infections also induces a rapid proinflammatory cell death termed pyroptosis.[24]

Endogenous triggers released during cellular injury or death (ie, extracellular ATP and hyaluronan), as well as indicators of metabolic stress (ie, glucose, monosodium urate [MSU], calcium pyrophosphate dehydrate [CPPD] crystals, amyloid-β fibrils, cholesterol crystals) and phagocytosed environmental, large, insoluble, inorganic crystalline structures likely provide signal 2. These chemically diverse triggers cannot possibly bind directly to the inflammasome, which spurred on the search for a common NLRP3 inflammasome-activating final pathway.

Potential mechanisms of inflammasome activation may involve production of mitochondrial reactive oxygen species (ROS); ion fluxes such as K^+ efflux from the cell and Ca^{2+} release from the endoplasmic reticulum (ER); and protein kinase activation (recently reviewed by Haneklaus and colleagues[25]). Two molecules that directly bind to the NLRP3 inflammasome have been described so far: the oxidized mitochondrial (oxi-mito) DNA that is released by dysfunctional mitochondria and cyclic AMP (cAMP). Both are attractive candidates for a converging mechanism and whereas binding of oxi-mito DNA activates the inflammasome,[26] cAMP binding is inhibitory.[27] *NLRP3* mutations affect binding of the negative regulator cAMP to the NACHT domain,[27] which leaves mutant NLRP3 inflammasomes more amenable to activation and may help to explain the constitutive activation of the mutant NLRP3 inflammasome in patients with *CAPS*.

Many factors contribute to the activation and function of the NLRP3 inflammasome and mutations in the 3 genes causing the hereditary fever syndromes are believed to affect factors that enhance/influence NLRP3 inflammasome-mediated IL-1 activation and secretion.

MEFV, the *FMF* gene, encodes pyrin, which can bind to the ASC adapter protein.[28] One hypothesis is that the interaction between the wildtype pyrin and ASC may inhibit the NLRP3 inflammasome assembly.[28] Mutant pyrin is believed to be a less effective inhibitor, which may lead to increased inflammasome activity. This is consistent with data from animal models whereby pyrin knockout mice or mice expressing a truncated protein have increased caspase-1 activation, increased IL-1β maturation, and a defect in macrophage apoptosis.[23] Data from a knock-in mouse model also suggest that pyrin can form an NLRP3-independent pyrin inflammasome that activates IL-1.[29] How these models integrate in vivo in patients remains to be sorted out in the future.

Mutations in mevalonate kinase cause *HIDS* and constitute an enzymatic block that leads to a shortage of isoprenoids, which are products of the cholesterol biosynthesis pathway, that subsequently leads to a decrease in posttranslational prenylation.[30] In vitro data from patients with HIDS suggest that farnesol or geranylgeraniol compounds can reverse accentuated IL-1β secretion, and that inhibitors of sterol biosynthesis, which favor nonsterol isoprenoid biosynthesis, also reduce IL-1β secretion by HIDS leukocytes,[31] thus suggesting that patients with HIDS with a shortage of isoprenoids have increased IL-1β secretion. However, the search for molecular mechanisms that link a shortage of isoprenoids to IL-1 production and secretion is an area of ongoing research.

Mechanistic studies in *TRAPS* have recently shifted the focus from TNF as the pivotal cytokine to intracellular mechanisms ultimately leading to an increase of multiple cytokines including IL-1 production. Mutant TNFR1 receptors fail to bind to TNF and are not transported to the cell surface but remain trapped in the ER of the cells, where they accumulate to 10-fold higher than wildtype levels, whereas cell surface receptor levels of wildtype and mutant protein are greatly reduced.[32,33] Cells from patients with TRAPS mutations spontaneously activate JNK and p38 MAP kinases (MAPKs); which may also lead to an ROS-dependent increase in IL-1 production or provide a first signal for IL-1 transcription and promote the presence of pro-IL-1β.

Although NLRP3 mutations in patients with *CAPS* lead to overproduction and secretion of active IL-1β on stimulation, the mutations in *DIRA* reflect the effects of an inability to block and terminate IL-1 signaling. The IL-1 receptor antagonist (IL-1Ra), which is absent or nonfunctional in DIRA, usually competes with the proinflammatory cytokines IL-1α and IL-1β for binding to the IL-1 type I receptor (IL-1RI). Stimulation of patients' cells with IL-1α or β, or LPS leads to increased production of several proinflammatory cytokines and chemokines including IL-6, IL-8, MIP-1α, and TNF, suggesting that IL-1 signaling cannot be blocked in these patients and remains hyperactive (see **Fig. 2**).[34,35]

Majeed syndrome is a rare condition that has only once been reported outside of Jordan; however, the disease pathogenesis may tie in with inflammasome activation. Mutations in *LPIN2* cause loss of function of the Mg^{2+}-dependent phosphatidate phosphatase activity of the enzyme, lipin-2, which is involved in the phospholipid biosynthesis pathway. Lipin-2 associates with the nuclear/ER membrane and catalyzes the conversion of phosphatidate to diacylglycerol, a precursor for the production of phospholipids that are components of cell membranes, essential for the

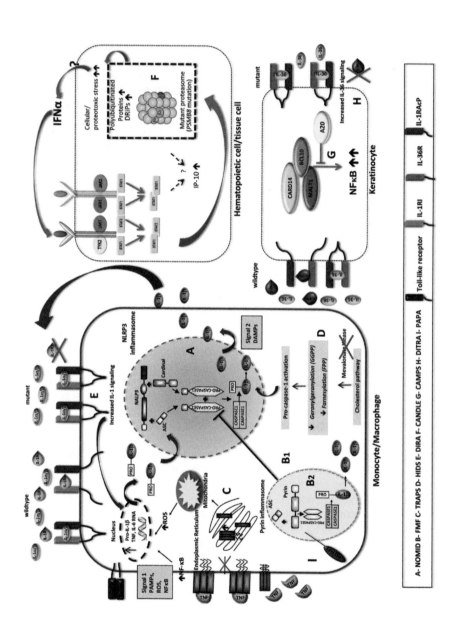

absorption, transport, and storage of lipids, and serve as a reservoir for signaling molecules. The Majeed mutation, S734L, in human lipin-2 alters a highly conserved serine residue in the C-LIP domain that leads to loss of lipin-2 phosphatidate phosphatase activity.[36,37] The effect of mutant lipin-2 might be compensated for in tissues with high expression of lipin-1 and lipin-3 (in liver and fat), but not in monocytes where lipin-2 is most highly expressed. Lipin-2 dampens the proinflammatory signaling that is produced by macrophages when exposed to excessive saturated fatty acids[38]; the accumulation of free fatty acids in monocytes and macrophages may

◄───

Fig. 2. Proposed mechanisms of activation of proinflammatory signaling pathways in autoinflammatory diseases: (A) cryopyrinopathies (CAPS). Unlike wildtype NLRP3, mutated NLRP3 (which causes CAPS) is constitutively activated and believed to oligomerize and bind to adapter molecules apoptotic speck protein (ASC) and CARDINAL to form an active catalytic complex with 2 pro–caspase-1 molecules. Via autocatalysis, this complex generates active caspase-1, which cleaves inactive pro–interleukin (IL)-1β into its active form, IL-1β. (B) FMF. (B$_1$) Wildtype pyrin can inhibit inflammasome activation by direct binding to caspase-1. Mutated pyrin cannot exert its inhibitory effect on the inflammasome, leading to unopposed inflammasome activation. (B$_2$) Wildtype pyrin can also interact directly with ASC forming the pyrin inflammasome, which is activated in the presence of FMF-causing mutations. (C) TRAPS. TNFR1 molecules are transported from the ER to the Golgi and then to the cell surface. Wildtype TNFR1 complexes are bound to extracellular TNF, leading to NFκB activation. Receptor cleavage from the cell surface abrogates receptor signaling and the soluble receptor can buffer soluble TNF. Mutated TNFR1 (which causes TRAPS) is misfolded and cannot be transported to the cell surface. Misfolded TNFR1 is sequestered in the ER, where it may lead to abnormal signaling through increased mitochondrial reactive oxygen species (ROS) production. (D) HIDS. Mevalonate kinase, a critical enzyme in the biosynthesis of sterol and nonsterol isoprenoids, catalyzes the conversion of mevalonate to mevalonate phosphate. In HIDS, activity of this enzyme is reduced, resulting in a decreased concentration of mevalonate phosphate, geranylgeranyl pyrophosphate (GGPP), and farnesyl pyrophosphate (FPP), leading to decreased activity of geranylgeranyltransferase and impaired geranylgeranylation of several proteins. Through an unknown mechanism, the reduced geranylgeranylation would lead to an increased pro–caspase-1 activation and consequent caspase-1 activation with resulting overproduction of IL-1β. (E) DIRA. Deficiency of IL-1Ra leads to unopposed IL-1α and IL-1β signaling. (F) CANDLE. Proteasomes are an ATP-dependent protein degradation system that targets intracellular polyubiquitinated proteins derived from self structures or foreign structures for proteolytic destruction. Patients who are homozygous for *PSMB8* mutations show various assembly defects, with impaired proteolytic activity which is proposed to lead to an increase in, ie, polyubiquitination of DRiPs, which might accumulate in tissues from these patients and induce an increased inflammatory response. Serum cytokine analysis in CANDLE and gene expression profiling identified the IFN signaling pathway as the most differentially regulated cytokine pathway. (G) CAMPS. Mutated CARD14 protein is mainly expressed in keratinocytes and leads to NFκB activation and increased chemokine production. (H) DITRA. Deficiency of IL-36Ra in the keratinocyte leads to unopposed IL-36 signaling. (I) PAPA. Wildtype PSTPIP1, a regulatory molecule of the NLRP3 inflammasome, binds to pyrin. Mutated PSTPIP1 is proposed to not dissociate from its binding to pyrin, leading to uninhibited inflammasome and pyrin inflammasome activities. ASC, apoptotic speck protein; BCL10, B-cell lymphoma/leukemia 10; CARD14, caspase recruitment domain-containing protein 14; DAMPs, damage-associated molecular patterns; IFN, interferon; IP-10, IFNγ-inducible protein 10; IL-1α/β, interleukin-1α/β; IL-1β, interleukin-1β; IL-1Ra, interleukin-1 receptor antagonist; IL-6, interleukin-6; IL-36, interleukin-36; IL36Ra, interleukin-36 receptor antagonist; JAK1, Janus kinase 1; JAK2, Janus kinase 2; MALT1, mucosa-associated lymphoid tissue lymphoma translocation protein 1; MAPK, mitogen-activated protein kinase; PAMPs, pathogen-associated molecular patterns; p-JNK, phosphorylated-JNK; ROS, reactive oxygen species; STAT1, signal transducer and activator of transcription 1; TNF, tumor necrosis factor; TNFR, tumor necrosis factor receptor; TYK2, tyrosine kinase 2.

lead to activation of the NLRP3 inflammasome, a possible mechanism that needs further exploration.

A case report of a rapid and complete response to IL-1 blockade with anakinra and canakinumab in 2 patients with Majeed syndrome strongly suggests an IL-1β–mediated pathology and may link another dysregulated lipid biosynthesis pathway (HIDS being the other) to IL-1 possibly through NLRP3 inflammasome activation.

Clinical Features and Therapeutic Considerations for IL-1–Mediated Conditions

The cryopyrinopathies or CAPS (including FCAS, MWS, and NOMID)

The term cryopyrinopathies or CAPS encompasses 3 diseases described historically: FCAS, MWS, and NOMID/CINCA, all caused by autosomal dominant gain-of-function mutations in *NLRP3/CIAS1*. Although FCAS is at the mild end of the clinical spectrum, NOMID is at the most severe end.

Genetics and epidemiology Of the 130 disease-causing mutations in *NLRP3/CIAS1*, 90% are located in exon 3.[15,39] The inheritance pattern in FCAS and MWS is usually familial,[15] and the sporadic nature in patients with NOMID/CINCA[40,41] is attributed to the severe phenotype of untreated patients, which results in their inability to reproduce. The face of NOMID has dramatically changed with IL-1 blocking therapy, so that more familial cases of NOMID will likely be seen in the future. Although genetic testing is confirmatory, the diagnosis needs to be made on clinical grounds. Approximately 50% of patients with NOMID/CINCA and a much smaller percentage of patients with FCAS and MWS do not have germline mutations in *NLRP3* detected by Sanger sequencing, a technique used to search for mutations in clinical assays. Of those patients who do not have mutations on Sanger sequencing, about 70% have evidence of somatic mosaicism,[42] which currently can only be detected by cell cloning and deep sequencing in research settings.

A rapid and complete clinical response to a treatment trial with an IL-1 blocking agent in patients with suspected CAPS can help to confirm the clinical diagnosis.

Based on estimates by centers treating these patients, the prevalence of CAPS is 1 to 2 patients per 1,000,000 people in Europe and the United States.

Clinical manifestations In general, all patients with CAPS present with episodes of fever, neutrophilic urticaria, conjunctivitis, arthralgia, and increased levels of acute phase reactants.[43] Onset, frequency, severity of overlapping symptoms, as well as degree of multiorgan involvement, long-term morbidity, and mortality differ among patients with FCAS, MWS, and NOMID/CINCA.

In FCAS, the febrile attacks are triggered by exposure to cold. Attacks often start within 2 hours of cold exposure, peak at 2 to 6 hours, and last for 12 to 48 hours. FCAS symptoms typically present in early childhood, but first presentations later in life are also seen. In FCAS, permanent organ damage is rare and secondary amyloidosis may occur in less than 2% of patients.[44]

MWS is of intermediate severity. In patients with MWS, the febrile attacks are usually more frequent and can persist at a low-grade level with exacerbations.[45] In addition to conjunctivitis, eye inflammation can involve the sclera (episcleritis) and anterior chamber (uveitis). During severe attacks, patients often complain of headache and present with aseptic meningitis or papilledema. In MWS, the most concerning disability is sensorineural hearing loss that typically develops in the second to third decade of life as a consequence of chronic inner ear inflammation, which leads to damage of the Corti organ.[46,47] Secondary amyloidosis is frequently observed in patients living in Europe where it is found in 25% to 33% of untreated patients.[48]

The percentage of patients developing amyloidosis is lower in the United States for all amyloidosis conditions in general, suggesting that environmental factors can contribute to the risk of disease independently of the genetics.

In NOMID, systemic and organ inflammation is constant and low-grade fevers, rashes, aseptic meningitis, and arthropathy often start in the first weeks of life, with frequent exacerbations (**Fig. 3**A–E).[49] Older children present with persistent low-grade fever, neutrophilic urticaria, arthropathy, and aseptic meningitis, which leads to headaches and increased intracranial pressure, with early-morning nausea and vomiting. These symptoms can undulate in severity but acute phase reactants never normalize and the disease is poorly responsive to steroids and disease-modifying anti-rheumatic drugs.

Patients with untreated NOMID develop permanent organ damage early in life.[50] Chronic aseptic neutrophilic meningitis that presents as irritability, headaches, and seizures, leads to the development of increased intracranial pressure, hydrocephalus and papilledema, brain atrophy, and cognitive impairment. Ongoing cochlear inflammation seen as cochlear enhancement on magnetic resonance imaging (MRI), leads to sensorineural hearing loss within the first years of life. Chronic papilledema results in optic nerve atrophy and progressive vision loss usually in the third decade of life, but anterior and rarely posterior uveitis can also contribute to the blindness.[49] Cognitive delay is multifactorial as a result of perinatal insult and the degree of central nervous system (CNS) inflammation.

About 50% to 70% of patients with NOMID present with a deforming arthropathy that results in abnormal epiphyseal calcification, cartilage overgrowth, and joint deformities. Premature patellar ossification and patellar overgrowth is a typical finding in NOMID.[51]

Treatment of CAPS Despite clinical heterogeneity, all patients with FCAS, MWS, and NOMID respond dramatically and invariably to IL-1 blockade. The rapid improvement in clinical and laboratory parameters and safety data in all patients with CAPS led to the approval of 3 anti-IL-1 agents for the treatment of CAPS by the US Food and Drug Administration: the long-acting IL-1 inhibitors rilonacept[52,53] and canakinumab,[54] and the short-acting IL-1 receptor antagonist anakinra[50] in the United States; rilonacept and canakinumab are approved by the European Medicines Agency in Europe.

Although preventing exposure to cold improves the cold-induced symptoms, optimal treatment with IL-1 blockage leads to complete resolution of symptoms in most cases and is the treatment of choice in patients with FCAS.[54,55] In patients with MWS and NOMID, optimal IL-1 inhibiting therapy needs to be initiated early to prevent the development and progression of organ damage.[50] Careful monitoring of CNS disease and inner ear inflammation is required to establish optimal treatment doses.

Sustained responses to IL-1 blocking therapies such as rilonacept[53] and canakinumab[56] are seen; treatment with anakinra may require some dose adjustment with prolonged use.[50,57]

The classic periodic fever syndromes (FMF, TRAPS, HIDS)

FMF

Genetics and epidemiology FMF is caused by autosomal recessive mutations in the *MEFV* gene.[2,3] However, the description of patients with clinical FMF and only 1 single *MEFV* mutation suggests the possibility that a dominant inheritance is possible.[58] The most common missense mutations detected in patients with FMF are M694V, M680I, M694I, and E726,[2,39] and almost half of the disease-causing mutations described so far are located in exon 10.

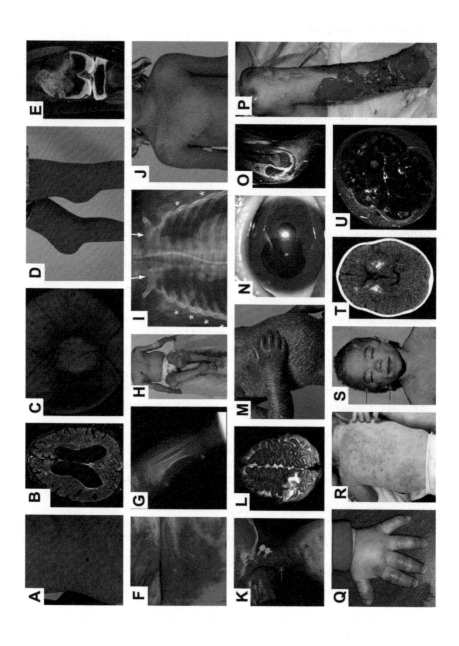

FMF is the most prevalent monogenic autoinflammatory disease, affecting more than 100,000 individuals worldwide,[59] primarily eastern Mediterranean populations, including Sephardic Jews, Armenian, Arabian, and Turkish descendants.

Clinical manifestations Most patients have disease onset before the third decade of life. FMF attacks typically last 1 to 3 days and flares recur periodically from once a week to once every few years, with symptom-free intervals between flares.[60,61]

Acute attacks of FMF are characterized by recurrent episodes of fever, abdominal pain secondary to an acute generalized peritonitis, arthritis (mainly nonerosive oligoarthritis) and skin rash (erysipelas-like erythema). Episodes of abdominal pain can mimic an acute abdomen often leading to appendectomy or cholecystectomy. In a small percentage of patients, episodes of myalgias can be prolonged (up to 6 weeks), debilitating, associated with fever, increased erythrocyte sedimentation rate (ESR) but normal creatinine kinase level.[62] This protracted febrile myalgia in patients with FMF is believed to be caused by vasculitis.[62] Other symptoms are serosal inflammation presenting as pleuritis, pericarditis, and scrotal pain, and rarely aseptic meningitis.[63] Patients with FMF may have an increased risk of sacroiliitis, irrespective of HLA-B27 status or colchicine prophylaxis.

Type AA secondary amyloidosis is the most frequent complication of FMF, occurring in 13% of Turkish patients.[64] Frequency of amyloidosis differs between countries and, in a multicenter study, the country of recruitment was the most important risk factor for the occurrence of renal amyloidosis.[65] Kidneys are the most affected organs and patients present with progressive proteinuria, nephrotic syndrome, and chronic renal failure.[64] Secondary AA amyloidosis is caused by persistently increased serum amyloid A (SAA) levels. The development of AA amyloidosis is unlikely with low serum concentrations of this protein (<4 mg/L).[66] All patients with FMF should be screened regularly for amyloidosis by urinalysis.

Treatment Since 1972, when colchicine was introduced as a treatment option, it has remained the standard of care for prophylaxis of attacks and prevention of amyloidosis. Doses of 1 to 2 mg per day of colchicine prevent the acute inflammatory attacks and the development of systemic amyloidosis.[67] Given the cytokine profile reported in FMF, and the interactions of IL-1β and pyrin, IL-1 inhibition needs to be considered for those patients who have severe side effects or are unresponsive to colchicine.[68] A recent randomized placebo-controlled trial has suggested rilonacept,

◄

Fig. 3. (*A*) Urticarial rash in a patient with CAPS, Muckle-Wells syndrome. (*B*) Severe hydrocephalus and cerebral atrophy in NOMID. (*C*) Papilledema in NOMID. (*D*) Patellar overgrowth in NOMID. (*E*) Knee MRI showing cartilaginous proliferation (*red arrow*) and widening of the growth plate of the distal femur in a patient with CAPS NOMID. (*F*) Pustulosis in DIRA. (*G*) Metaphyseal osteolytic lesions in distal and proximal tibia (*red arrowheads*) in a very young patient with DIRA; periosteal elevation is also seen. (*H*) Bony overgrowth in a patient with DIRA (rare). (*I*) Widening of multiple ribs (*asterisk*) and clavicles (*arrows*) in DIRA osteomyelitis. (*J*) Chest deformities in DIRA. (*K*) Block vertebral formation (*red arrow*) following osteolytic vertebral lesions in DIRA. (*L*) Enhancement in the right postcentral and precentral gyrus in a patient with vasculitis in DIRA. (*M*) Generalized psoriasis in CAMPS. (*N*) Anterior synechiae and cataract with chronic uveitis in a patient with Blau syndrome. (*O*) Sagittal image of a fat-suppressed T2-weighted sequence showing synovial thickening and enhancement with moderate fluid (*red arrow*) in the right elbow joint in pyogenic arthritis. (*P*) Extensive pyoderma gangrenosum lesion in a patient with PAPA syndrome. (*Q*) Finger swelling in CANDLE syndrome. (*R*) Erythematous annular and nodular rash in CANDLE syndrome. (*S*) Characteristic facial lipodystrophy (*red arrows*) in CANDLE syndrome. (*T*) Basal ganglia calcifications in CANDLE syndrome. (*U*) Myositis in CANDLE syndrome.

a long-acting IL-1 inhibitor, as a treatment option for patients who are refractory or intolerant to colchicine. In this study, enrolling 14 patients with FMF during 12 months, rilonacept reduced the frequency of FMF attacks more significantly than placebo.[69] Case series and case reports have also described the efficacy of the other IL-1 inhibitors, anakinra[70,71] and canakinumab,[70,72] for FMF treatment. There are also anecdotal data supporting the use of TNF inhibitors in this disease.[73,74]

TRAPS

Genetics and epidemiology TRAPS is caused by autosomal dominant mutations in the *TNFRSF1A* gene, which encodes the TNF receptor type 1 (TNFR1). More than 100 mutations have been found to cause TRAPS.[39]

Clinical manifestations and diagnosis Clinical manifestations usually present in childhood and adolescence, but in about 20% of patients they appear first in adulthood. The mean length of the fever episodes is around 14 days but can last from 1 to 4 weeks.

Patients with TRAPS usually present with recurrent fever, abdominal pain, pleuritis, myalgias, arthralgias, and periorbital edema or conjunctivitis. Myalgias are frequently associated with an overlying tender erythematous skin rash that migrates from proximal to distal accompanying the myalgia pain. MRI shows segmental muscle edema, and on biopsy, a monocytic fasciitis is present.[75] Periorbital edema is more common in TRAPS than in the other periodic fever syndromes and recurrent conjunctivitis or anterior uveitis can be present in up to half of the patients.[76] Neurologic manifestations are rare and include headaches, aseptic meningitis, optic neuritis, and behavioral alterations.

Amyloidosis is the most serious long-term complication of TRAPS and develops in 14% to 24% of patients.[77] Given the overlap in symptoms with other autoinflammatory diseases, a definite diagnosis of TRAPS can only be made in the presence of a mutation in *TNFSRF1A*.

Treatment TNF inhibition is effective in some cases. In a prospective study, etanercept reduced but did not completely normalize the frequency and severity of the attacks and abnormal inflammatory markers.[78] There are other studies that suggest that etanercept efficacy diminishes over time. In some centers, anakinra and canakinumab have become the treatment of choice.[79,80] However, individual cases of anakinra failure have been reported.[81]

HIDS/mevalonate kinase deficiency

Genetics and epidemiology HIDS is caused by autosomal recessive mutations in the *MVK* gene (mevalonate kinase gene).[6,7] Currently, about 30 disease-causing variants have been identified and most patients with mutation-positive HIDS have at least 1 copy of the substitution V377I.[82] The substitution I268T is the second most common variant[82] in patients with HIDS in western Europe.[39]

Clinical manifestations and diagnosis Typically, HIDS presents early in life, usually before 1 year of age. HIDS episodes last 3 to 7 days and occur every 4 to 6 weeks. Patients with HIDS present with recurrent episodes of fever that is often preceded by malaise and chills. Polyarthralgia or arthritis (nonerosive arthritis of large joints), as well as marked bilateral, tender, cervical lymphadenopathy are seen. Other symptoms include abdominal pain, vomiting, diarrhea, splenomegaly, and a variety of skin lesions, including maculopapular, urticarial, nodular, or purpuric rashes. Childhood vaccinations can precipitate an attack; other provocative factors include trauma, surgery, emotional stress, and infections.[83]

During febrile episodes, patients may present with increased levels of acute phase reactants (ESR and C-reactive protein [CRP]), increased urinary mevalonic acid levels and increased IgD and IgA levels. However, IgD concentrations are nonspecific and should not be used to make a diagnosis, especially in children less than 3 years of age. IgD levels can also be increased in other inflammatory conditions, such as FMF and TRAPS.[84] Genetic testing in children less than 5 years of age with recurrent fevers may be indicated. Amyloidosis is uncommon in patients with HIDS.

Treatment Initial suggestions to use simvastatin proved ineffective.[85–87] However, there are reports of patients responding to etanercept[88] and the IL-1 blocking agents anakinra[89,90] and canakinumab.[90]

The monogenic autoinflammatory bone diseases (DIRA, Majeed syndrome)

DIRA and Majeed syndrome are 2 monogenic autoinflammatory disorders caused by loss of function mutations in the IL-1 receptor antagonist, *IL1RN*, in DIRA, and *LPIN2* in Majeed syndrome.[91] Both conditions present early in life with sterile bone inflammation involving the ribs, long bones, and proximal femur (see **Fig. 3**G–K). In DIRA, rarely CNS vasculitis can been seen (see **Fig. 3**L). Patients with DIRA typically have pustular skin lesions (see **Fig. 3**F),[34,35] whereas, in Majeed syndrome, the skin lesions are more variable and seem to be less prominent.[92,93] Founder mutations causing DIRA are seen in Newfoundland, the Netherlands, Lebanon, northern Puerto Rico, Brazil[94] and, most recently, Turkey; disease-causing mutations in Majeed syndrome have, with 1 exception, only been seen in Jordanian patients.

Treatment Treatment of DIRA is IL-1 blockade with anakinra; other IL-1 blocking therapies have not been evaluated. In Majeed syndrome, IL-1 inhibition was used successfully in 2 patients but more data are needed to determine if this should be the treatment of choice.[95]

The monogenic inflammatory bone diseases are discussed in detail elsewhere in this issue by Ferguson and colleagues.

AUTOINFLAMMATORY SYNDROMES WITH VARIABLE RESPONSES TO IL-1 BLOCKAGE
Clinical and Therapeutic Considerations

Blau syndrome/early-onset sarcoidosis (PGA)

Epidemiology and genetics PGA is caused by autosomal dominant gain-of-function mutations in the NACHT domain (exon 4) of *NOD2/CARD15*, but the inflammatory cytokines responses are more complex, involve NFκB activation, and are not clearly tied to IL-1 release.[96,97]

PGA can be inherited in an autosomal dominant pattern and familial cases have traditionally been called Blau syndrome. However, mutations can occur sporadically and, in these instances, the disease has historically been referred to as early-onset sarcoidosis.[98,99] The identification of overlapping mutations led to the recognition that these 2 disorders are the same disease. So far, 12 disease-causing mutations in *NOD2* gene have been reported to cause PGA. PGA symptoms include granulomatous inflammation of the eyes, joints, and skin, leading to an early-onset (before 4 years of age) classic triad of disease manifestations comprising chronic uveitis, arthritis, and dermatitis.

Clinical presentation and diagnosis Chronic arthritis is the most consistent finding and mainly manifests as polyarthritis (95%). A symmetric hypertrophic tenosynovitis is often observed. Most patients have chronic, persistent eye involvement that can be limited to the anterior part of the eye (anterior uveitis), but in the majority of patients presents as panuveitis.[100] Cataract and synechiae (see **Fig. 3**N) represent damage from chronic inflammation and steroid treatment,[99] and up to 40% of untreated patients develop irreversible blindness.[100] Most patients develop ichthyosis-like exanthema during some of their flares.[98,99] Less commonly observed findings include fever, camptodactyly, and central neuropathy.[98]

Laboratory examinations demonstrate persistent leukocytosis, thrombocytosis, and increased ESR and CRP. Synovial, skin, and liver biopsies may show noncaseating granulomas, even though a definitive diagnosis is only achieved with DNA sequencing showing *NOD2/CARD15* mutations.[100]

Treatment Optimal therapy for PGA has not been established. Nonsteroidal antiinflammatory drugs (NSAIDs) can be used for mild clinical manifestations, whereas severe symptoms are treated with systemic corticosteroids. Immunosuppressant (methotrexate and cyclosporine) and biologics targeting TNF and IL-1 (etanercept, infliximab, and anakinra) have been reported to result in clinical benefit, especially in patients with refractory uveitis.[99,100]

Pyogenic sterile arthritis, pyoderma gangrenosum, and acne syndrome

Genetics and epidemiology Pyogenic sterile arthritis, pyoderma gangrenosum, and acne (PAPA) syndrome is caused by autosomal dominant mutations in *PTSPIP1*.[10] The disease is rare, with less than 10 families identified so far.

Pathogenesis The pathogenesis of PAPA is not well understood. *PSTPIP1* encodes CD2-binding protein-1, a cytoskeletal protein that is designated proline-serine-threonine-phosphatase interacting protein-1 (PSTPIP1). PSTPIP1 is an adaptor protein that interacts with PEST-type protein tyrosine phosphatases (PEST-PTPs), Wiskott-Aldrich syndrome protein (WASP), and pyrin, the protein encoded by *MEFV*, the FMF gene.[101,102] Disease-causing *PSTPIP1* mutations are believed to diminish the interactions with PEST-type protein, which results in increased phosphorylation of mutated PSTPIP1 and increased interaction with pyrin.[102] Four disease-causing variants have been described in *PTSPIP1*. It is suggested that PSTPIP1 mutants increase activation of the pyrin inflammasome–associated IL-1β activation,[103] even though PSTPIP1 does not seem to be an essential regulator of the NLRP3, AIM2 or NLRC4 IL-1β–activating inflammasomes in a mouse model.[104] Additional studies are needed to provide clues to better therapies because IL-1 inhibiting approaches are only partially effective (ie, for the treatment of pyogenic arthritis but less for severe skin disease).

Clinical manifestations PAPA syndrome is a pyogenic autoinflammatory disease that presents with pyogenic arthritis (see **Fig. 3**O), pyoderma gangrenosum (see **Fig. 3**P), and severe cystic acne. Patients with PAPA present with early-onset episodes of painful sterile and deforming arthritis, cutaneous ulcers (pyoderma gangrenosum), and pathergy; cystic lesions or skin abscesses are seen at needle injection sites.[10] Cystic acne and hidradenitis suppurativa of the axilla and groin can develop around puberty. Fever is rarely observed in these patients. Symptoms usually persist into adulthood with significant joint destruction and impaired quality of life related to physical disability.[105] Other clinical findings/complications from disease and treatment in patients with PAPA include osteomyelitis, recurrent otitis, lymphadenopathy, splenomegaly, thrombocytopenia, hemolytic anemia, pharyngeal papillomatosis, and large granular T-cell lymphocytosis.[105]

Treatment Treatment of PAPA syndrome is challenging and corticosteroids, thalidomide, cyclosporine, dapsone, tacrolimus, and intravenous immunoglobulin have been used with variable responses.[105] Several case reports indicate positive responses to TNF inhibition with etanercept, infliximab, and adalimumab in 2 patients and to IL-1 inhibition with anakinra in 1 case[105] but poor responses to anakinra, infliximab, and etanercept have also been seen.[105] In general, monoclonal anti-TNF antibodies (infliximab and adalimumab) were considered more effective in treating skin manifestations of PAPA syndrome, whereas IL-1 inhibition seems to be more effective for joint disease.[105]

NON-IL-1–MEDIATED AUTOINFLAMMATORY SYNDROMES
Pathogenesis Considerations for non-IL-1–Mediated Conditions, PRAAS/CANDLE

The finding that mutations in *PSMB8* cause a severe inflammatory phenotype in humans, *PRAAS/CANDLE*, was unexpected given that *psmb8/lmp7* knockout mice lack spontaneous development of systemic symptoms, muscle inflammation, or lipodystrophy.[106] Proteasomes are ATP-dependent protein degradation systems that target intracellular polyubiquitinated proteins derived from self structures or foreign structures for proteolytic destruction.[107,108] Proteasome cleavage of proteins leads to the production of peptides for antigen presentation, but failure of mutant proteasome to clear immature proteins can lead to an increased inflammatory response (see **Fig. 2**).[109] In patients homozygous for *PSMB8* mutations, the assembly of the inducible proteasome complex is defective[110–112] and polyubiquitinated proteins accumulate in tissues from these patients. Serum cytokine analysis in patients with Nakajo-Nishimura syndrome (NNS) and CANDLE showed an increase in IL-6, IFNγ-inducible protein 10 (IP-10, also called CXCL10), monocyte chemoattractant protein (MCP)-1 (CCL2), and IL-1 receptor antagonist.[111,113] Gene expression profiling using whole-blood microarray identified the IFN pathway as the most differentially regulated pathway in patients with CANDLE,[113] and signal transducers and activators of transcription (STAT)-1, a downstream mediator of IFN type I and type II signaling, showed higher constitutive phosphorylation and was more highly induced on IFNγ stimulation in patients' monocytes compared with healthy controls. Inhibition with the Janus kinase (JAK) inhibitor tofacitinib decreased the STAT-1 phosphorylation and IFNγ-induced IP-10.[113] Increased p38 MAPK responses have also been observed in PRAAS.[111,112] These observations suggest that a putative intracellular stress response might lead to an IFN response signature, which is similar to the IFN response signature seen in SLE. The IFN response signature has also been seen in patients with AGS, who present with a noninfectious, viral encephalitis-like disease resulting in rapid demyelination often within the first years of life and basal ganglia calcifications.[114] Whether targeting IFN signaling constitutes a therapeutic strategy in patients with PRAAS/CANDLE is currently being assessed (clinical trials identifier NCT01724580). We suggest that a transient increase in defective ribosomal products (DRiPs) and polyubiquitinated proteins accumulate and trigger a proteotoxic response through yet unknown sensors that are possibly IFN type 1 induced (see **Fig. 2**). Alternatively, similarly to AGS, in which loss of function mutations in the exonuclease *TREX1* and other enzymes associated with the digestion of single-stranded or mispaired dsDNA, RNA/DNA hybrids, and deoxynucleotide triphosphates lead to a self nucleotide-induced type I IFN-associated signature,[20] the interferon signature in CANDLE may also be induced by yet unknown triggers.

PRAAS/CANDLE
Genetics and epidemiology The first description of Japanese patients presenting with "nodular erythema, elongated and thickened fingers and emaciation" dates back to a report from Nakajo in 1939.[115] Nishimura and colleagues[116] reported 3 similar patients in 1950 and the disease was later named Nakajo-Nishimura syndrome (NNS) in Japan.

The first reports of non-Japanese patients were on a Palestinian patient reported by Megarbane and colleagues,[117] and 2 Mexican siblings and 1 Portuguese patient reported by Garg and colleagues.[118] The presence of joint contractures, muscular atrophy, microcytic anemia, and panniculitis-induced lipodystrophy led to the term JMP syndrome for joint contractures, muscular atrophy, microcytic anemia, and panniculitis-induced lipodystrophy.

In 2010, Torrelo and colleagues[119] proposed the acronym CANDLE.

In 2011, several studies showed that JMP syndrome,[110] NNS,[111] Japanese autoinflammatory syndrome with lipodystrophy (JASL),[112] and CANDLE[113] are all caused by autosomal recessive mutations in the proteasome subunit β type 8 (*PSMB8*) gene, indicating that these disorders are phenotypes along the same disease spectrum.[113,119] Currently, 4 mutations in *PSMB8* (T75M, A92T, C135X, and G201V) have been described, but genetic heterogeneity is present.[113]

Clinical manifestations Common clinical features seen in PRAAS/CANDLE include high fevers, violaceous skin rashes varying from small nodules to violaceous plaques, also described as pernio-like lesions covering the trunk and extremities, facial rashes leading to various degrees of edema, mimicking heliotrope rashes in some patients, drumstick-like widening of the distal fingers tips, arthritis with variable degrees of joint contractures, and progressive lipodystrophy initially affecting the face and extremities but can be generalized (see **Fig. 3**Q–U). Other common clinical findings are myositis, hepatosplenomegaly, basal ganglia calcification, microcytic anemia, and increased acute phase reactants (ESR and CRP). More variable symptoms include muscle atrophy, dyspnea, seizures, lymphadenopathy, low weight and height, and metabolic abnormalities including truncal obesity and hyperlipidemias, insulin resistance, and acanthosis nigricans.[113,118] They seem to be exaggerated in patients on steroids.[111,112] Severe inflammatory attacks are more pronounced in childhood than later in life. They can escalate in a systemic inflammatory syndrome resulting in organ failure and sudden death. The spectrum of organ damage that can be observed includes severe lipodystrophy, calcifications in vessels and soft tissues, and rarely cardiomyopathy and cardiac arrhythmias.[118]

Treatment In 9 patients we studied, most clinical symptoms partially responded to high doses of steroids (1–2 mg/kg/d)[113]; NSAIDs, colchicine, dapsone, methotrexate, tacrolimus, and azathioprine were not effective in most of the patients.[113] A variable response was observed to anti-TNF, anti–IL-1, and anti-IL-6 agents, but complete disease remission was not achieved with any of the therapies described.[113] Lipodystrophy progressed in all patients despite immunosuppressive and cytokine targeted therapy.[113] The increase in STAT-1 phosphorylation and the strong IFN response suggest that interference with IFN signaling may be a therapeutic strategy for the treatment of CANDLE/PRAAS.

Pathogenesis Considerations for Non- IL-1–Mediated Conditions, DITRA, CAMPS

Two pustular psoriasis-like conditions were recently shown to be caused by monogenic defects, including the autosomal recessive loss of function mutations in the IL-36 receptor antagonist causing *DITRA*, and the autosomal dominant gain-of-function mutations in *CARD14* causing *CAMPS*.

In both instances, the mutated protein is highly expressed in keratinocytes. *IL36RN* encodes the IL-36 receptor antagonist (IL-36Ra), which binds to IL-36 receptor, and completely blocks binding by IL-36α, IL-36β, and IL-36γ, and further downstream prevents NFκB activation in response to TLR agonist stimulation.[120,121] The absence of the IL-36 receptor antagonist in patients with DITRA leads to constitutively enhanced

IL-36 receptor signaling in keratinocytes and hematopoietic cells. In patients with *CARD14* mutations, hematopoietic cells do not even express CARD14. Transfection of mutant *CARD14* into a keratinocyte cell line leads to increased NFκB activation, and a gene expression profile showing induction of chemokines similar to those found in psoriasis biopsies. Overall, these conditions suggest that keratinocyte dysregulation may drive the recruitment of hematopoietic cells into the skin and a pustular/psoriasis-like phenotype.[122,123]

DITRA

Genetics and epidemiology Recently 16 family members of 9 Tunisian families with generalized pustular psoriasis and fever flares were found to be homozygous for a mutation in the *IL36RN* gene, L27P, indicating a founder mutation in Tunisia leading to this disease.[120] Additionally, 3 unrelated English patients with a similar phenotype presented with mutations in *IL36RN*.[121]

Clinical manifestations and diagnosis More than 70% of the patients described developed the disease during childhood (between 7 days and 11 years of age).[120] Patients with DITRA present with recurrent and sudden-onset generalized erythematous and pustular skin rashes, associated with high fevers up to 40°C to 42°C, asthenia, increased CRP, and leucocytosis.[120,121] Secondary skin infections and sepsis may also occur.[120] In all patients, the disease flares were believed to be triggered by viral or bacterial infections (14/16 patients), withdrawal of retinoid therapy (n = 7), menstruation (n = 6), and pregnancy in (n = 4).[120,121]

Treatment Definitive treatment of this disease has not been established yet. Acitretin was used as treatment in 12 of the 19 patients described so far.[120,121] Other therapeutic regimens tried with variable individual responses included oral steroids in 4 patients, methotrexate in 3 patients, cyclosporine in 3 patients, adalimumab in 2 patients, infliximab in 2, and etanercept in 1.[120,121] Topical steroids were used in 3 patients.[120] IL-1 blocking therapy has not been reported in these patients. However, data from a transgenic mouse model expressing IL-36β leads to a psoriasis-like phenotype; knocking out the IL-1 receptor in this model does not improve the disease in the mice thus suggesting that IL-36–mediated keratinocyte activation does not require IL-1 signaling.[124]

CAMPS

Genetics and epidemiology Autosomal dominant gain-of-function mutations in the *CARD14* gene cause a spectrum of more localized plaque psoriasis or more generalized pustular psoriasis in 2 large kindreds, and severe generalized pustular psoriasis in an unrelated child who had a sporadic de novo mutation in *CARD14*.[123] Mutations in *CARD14* were also shown to cause a familial syndrome described as pityriasis rubra pilaris in 15 members of 3 families.[122]

Clinical manifestations The skin lesions in patients with *CARD14* mutations range from typical localized plaque psoriasis to generalized disease, involving 100% of the body surface area (see **Fig. 3**M).[122,123] Fever and other systemic manifestations are generally not present but can occur with superinfections of the skin in patients with CAMPS. The fact that CARD14 mutations provoke a disease spectrum from localized plaque psoriasis to generalized pityriasis rubra pilaris and pustular psoriasis, indicates that this disease at different levels of severity can be induced by a common pathogenic pathway.

Treatment The therapeutic approach in CAMPS is similar to the treatment of moderate to severe psoriasis using methotrexate, cyclosporine, and anti-TNF agents.

Familial pityriasis rubra pilaris is considered refractory to the standard therapies and a partial response has been described with retinoids, cyclosporine, and etanercept.[122,125] The similarities in gene expression studies in CAMPS and nonallelic psoriasis suggests that newer drugs targeting IL-12/23 and likely IL-17 may be of benefit, which was recently confirmed by treating a child with severe CAMPS using ustekinumab.[126]

Pathogenesis Considerations for non-IL-1–Mediated Conditions, Early-Onset IBD

The loss of IL-10 signaling in mouse models and humans leads to an early-onset inflammatory bowel phenotype as the main organ manifestation with severe systemic inflammation, EO-IBD. These lack of function mutations result in the loss of IL-10 signaling, as demonstrated by deficient STAT-3 phosphorylation after stimulation with IL-10 and proves that loss of signaling of the antiinflammatory cytokine IL-10 is sufficient to cause enterocolitis as the main clinical feature. Levels of TNFα and other inflammatory cytokines, including IL-1α, IL-1β, and IL-6, are also increased in these patients. These data suggest a major role for IL-10 in counteracting commensal bacterial activation of the gut mucosa.

Early-onset IBD

Epidemiology and genetics Infantile IBD is caused by autosomal recessive mutations in IL-10R and IL-10 encoding genes.[127] Four of 9 patients with severe IBD presented with symptoms in the first year of life.[127] In 2010, an autosomal recessive mutation in the *IL-10* gene in 2 unrelated patients with refractory early-onset IBD was found. Six disease-causing mutations in each of the IL-10 receptor genes (*IL10RA* and *IL10RB*) and 2 mutations in the IL-10 gene have been described.

Clinical presentation and diagnosis Symptoms in patients with early-onset IBD usually start in the first year of life, before 3 months of age, and include severe enterocolitis, characterized by bloody diarrhea, colonic abscesses, perianal fistulas, oral ulcers, failure to thrive, and recurrent fever.[127,128] Musculoskeletal manifestations include acute recurrent arthritis of large joints, especially affecting the knees.[128] Remarkably, recurrent folliculitis has been observed in 75% of patients.[128] Recurrent infections, such as otitis media, bronchitis, pneumonia, septic arthritis, and renal abscesses may indicate immunodeficiency in patients with early-onset IBD.[127,128]

Treatment Because early-onset IBD is a severe disease and frequently refractory to standard immunosuppressants, hematopoietic stem cell transplantation (HSCT) has been proposed as a curative treatment.[129] HSCT was performed in 9 of 29 patients with IL-10 deficiency and complete clinical remission was achieved in all but 1 of the patients.[128,129]

Many of the primary immunodeficiencies present with infections and with features of autoimmunity or autoinflammation. Recently, conditions with prominent fever episodes that also present with immunodeficiencies were described, thus illustrating that an immune defect may have different effects in different cell types.[9,130]

SUMMARY

An underlying theme in the pathogenesis of monogenic autoinflammatory diseases converges on the presence of exaggerated immune responses that are triggered through activation of altered PRR pathways and result in cytokine/chemokine amplification loops and the inflammatory clinical phenotype seen in patients with autoinflammatory diseases. The excessive/increased extracellular or intracellular PRR responses are caused by monogenic defects that: (1) Can lead to abnormally increased metabolites that accumulate in the cells/tissue and trigger PRP responses (ie, CANDLE, and possibly Majeed and HIDS), or (2) are caused by mutations in sensors leading to their constitutive overactivation (as in CAPS and PGA), or (3) insitage alterations in the PRP associated mediator pathways that lead to cytokine amplification (TRAPS) and/or the inability to downregulate an inflammatory disease pathway (as in DIRA and DITRA). The altered PRP response can occur in hematopoietic cells but also in nonhematopoietic cells. Gain-of-function mutations affecting NFkB-mediated signaling in keratinocytes lead to chronic pustular skin lesions and to the subsequent recruitment of hematopoietic cells to the site. Thus, dysregulation in inflammatory pathways affecting hematopoietic but also nonhematopoietic cells may further our understanding of the organ specific inflammation that clinically often distinguishes the different syndromes. The study of molecular pathways of sterile inflammation in patients with autoinflammatory syndromes has pointed to specific dysregulated PRP/cytokine pathways and led to the use of IL-1 blocking therapies. The identification of novel autoinflammatory syndromes continues to uncover novel targets for therapeutic interventions.

REFERENCES

1. Kastner DL, Aksentijevich I, Goldbach-Mansky R. Autoinflammatory disease reloaded: a clinical perspective. Cell 2010;140:784–90.
2. Consortium FF. A candidate gene for familial Mediterranean fever. Nat Genet 1997;17:25–31.
3. Consortium TI. Ancient missense mutations in a new member of the RoRet gene family are likely to cause familial Mediterranean fever. Cell 1997;90:797–807.
4. McDermott MF, Aksentijevich I, Galon J, et al. Germline mutations in the extracellular domains of the 55 kDa TNF receptor, TNFR1, define a family of dominantly inherited autoinflammatory syndromes. Cell 1999;97:133–44.
5. Drenth JP, Cuisset L, Grateau G, et al. Mutations in the gene encoding mevalonate kinase cause hyper-IgD and periodic fever syndrome. International Hyper-IgD Study Group. Nat Genet 1999;22:178–81.
6. Frenkel J, Houten SM, Waterham HR, et al. Mevalonate kinase deficiency and Dutch type periodic fever. Clin Exp Rheumatol 2000;18:525–32.
7. Houten SM, Kuis W, Duran M, et al. Mutations in MVK, encoding mevalonate kinase, cause hyperimmunoglobulinaemia D and periodic fever syndrome. Nat Genet 1999;22:175–7.
8. Ombrello MJ, Remmers EF, Sun G, et al. Cold urticaria, immunodeficiency and autoimmunity related to PLCG2 deletions. N Engl J Med 2012;366(4):330–8.
9. Zhou Q, Lee GS, Brady J, et al. A hypermorphic missense mutation in PLCG2, encoding phospholipase Cgamma2, causes a dominantly inherited autoinflammatory disease with immunodeficiency. Am J Hum Genet 2012;91:713–20.
10. Wise CA, Gillum JD, Seidman CE, et al. Mutations in CD2BP1 disrupt binding to PTP PEST and are responsible for PAPA syndrome, an autoinflammatory disorder. Hum Mol Genet 2002;11:961–9.
11. Henderson C, Goldbach-Mansky R. Monogenic autoinflammatory diseases: new insights into clinical aspects and pathogenesis. Curr Opin Rheumatol 2010;22:567–78.
12. Medzhitov R. Origin and physiological roles of inflammation. Nature 2008;454:428–35.

13. Janeway CA Jr, Medzhitov R. Innate immune recognition. Annu Rev Immunol 2002;20:197–216.

14. Martinon F, Tschopp J. Inflammatory caspases: linking an intracellular innate immune system to autoinflammatory diseases. Cell 2004;117:561–74.

15. Hoffman HM, Mueller JL, Broide DH, et al. Mutation of a new gene encoding a putative pyrin-like protein causes familial cold autoinflammatory syndrome and Muckle-Wells syndrome. Nat Genet 2001;29:301–5.

16. Dinarello CA. Immunological and inflammatory functions of the interleukin-1 family. Annu Rev Immunol 2009;27:519–50.

17. Ting JP, Williams KL. The CATERPILLER family: an ancient family of immune/apoptotic proteins. Clin Immunol 2005;115:33–7.

18. Atianand MK, Fitzgerald KA. Molecular basis of DNA recognition in the immune system. J Immunol 2013;190:1911–8.

19. Bennett L, Palucka AK, Arce E, et al. Interferon and granulopoiesis signatures in systemic lupus erythematosus blood. J Exp Med 2003;197:711–23.

20. Crow YJ. Type I interferonopathies: a novel set of inborn errors of immunity. Ann N Y Acad Sci 2011;1238:91–8.

21. Mariathasan S, Newton K, Monack DM, et al. Differential activation of the inflammasome by caspase-1 adaptors ASC and Ipaf. Nature 2004;430:213–8.

22. Martinon F, Burns K, Tschopp J. The inflammasome: a molecular platform triggering activation of inflammatory caspases and processing of proIL-beta. Mol Cell 2002;10:417–26.

23. Chae JJ, Komarow HD, Cheng J, et al. Targeted disruption of pyrin, the FMF protein, causes heightened sensitivity to endotoxin and a defect in macrophage apoptosis. Mol Cell 2003;11:591–604.

24. Bergsbaken T, Fink SL, Cookson BT. Pyroptosis: host cell death and inflammation. Nat Rev Microbiol 2009;7:99–109.

25. Haneklaus M, O'Neill LA, Coll RC. Modulatory mechanisms controlling the NLRP3 inflammasome in inflammation: recent developments. Curr Opin Immunol 2013;25:40–5.

26. Shimada K, Crother TR, Karlin J, et al. Oxidized mitochondrial DNA activates the NLRP3 inflammasome during apoptosis. Immunity 2012;36:401–14.

27. Lee GS, Subramanian N, Kim AI, et al. The calcium-sensing receptor regulates the NLRP3 inflammasome through Ca^{2+} and cAMP. Nature 2012;492:123–7.

28. Richards N, Schaner P, Diaz A, et al. Interaction between pyrin and the apoptotic speck protein (ASC) modulates ASC-induced apoptosis. J Biol Chem 2001;276:39320–9.

29. Chae JJ, Cho YH, Lee GS, et al. Gain-of-function Pyrin mutations induce NLRP3 protein-independent interleukin-1beta activation and severe autoinflammation in mice. Immunity 2011;34:755–68.

30. Kuijk LM, Beekman JM, Koster J, et al. HMG-CoA reductase inhibition induces IL-1beta release through Rac1/PI3K/PKB-dependent caspase-1 activation. Blood 2008;112:3563–73.

31. Mandey SH, Kuijk LM, Frenkel J, et al. A role for geranylgeranylation in interleukin-1beta secretion. Arthritis Rheum 2006;54:3690–5.

32. Lobito AA, Kimberley FC, Muppidi JR, et al. Abnormal disulfide-linked oligomerization results in ER retention and altered signaling by TNFR1 mutants in TNFR1-associated periodic fever syndrome (TRAPS). Blood 2006;108:1320–7.

33. Simon A, Park H, Maddipati R, et al. Concerted action of wild-type and mutant TNF receptors enhances inflammation in TNF receptor 1-associated periodic fever syndrome. Proc Natl Acad Sci U S A 2010;107:9801–6.

34. Aksentijevich I, Masters SL, Ferguson PJ, et al. An autoinflammatory disease with deficiency of the interleukin-1-receptor antagonist. N Engl J Med 2009; 360:2426–37.
35. Reddy S, Jia S, Geoffrey R, et al. An autoinflammatory disease due to homozygous deletion of the IL1RN locus. N Engl J Med 2009;360:2438–44.
36. Donkor J, Zhang P, Wong S, et al. A conserved serine residue is required for the phosphatidate phosphatase activity but not the transcriptional coactivator functions of lipin-1 and lipin-2. J Biol Chem 2009;284:29968–78.
37. Fakas S, Qiu Y, Dixon JL, et al. Phosphatidate phosphatase activity plays key role in protection against fatty acid-induced toxicity in yeast. J Biol Chem 2011;286:29074–85.
38. Valdearcos M, Esquinas E, Meana C, et al. Lipin-2 reduces proinflammatory signaling induced by saturated fatty acids in macrophages. J Biol Chem 2012;287:10894–904.
39. Infevers: an online database for autoinflammatory mutations. Available at: http://fmf.igh.cnrs.fr/ISSAID/infevers/. Accessed May 20, 2013.
40. Aksentijevich I, Nowak M, Mallah M, et al. De novo CIAS1 mutations, cytokine activation, and evidence for genetic heterogeneity in patients with neonatal-onset multisystem inflammatory disease (NOMID): a new member of the expanding family of pyrin-associated autoinflammatory diseases. Arthritis Rheum 2002;46:3340–8.
41. Feldmann J, Prieur AM, Quartier P, et al. Chronic infantile neurological cutaneous and articular syndrome is caused by mutations in CIAS1, a gene highly expressed in polymorphonuclear cells and chondrocytes. Am J Hum Genet 2002;71:198–203.
42. Tanaka N, Izawa K, Saito MK, et al. High incidence of NLRP3 somatic mosaicism in patients with chronic infantile neurologic, cutaneous, articular syndrome: results of an International Multicenter Collaborative Study. Arthritis Rheum 2011;63:3625–32.
43. Arostegui JI, Aldea A, Modesto C, et al. Clinical and genetic heterogeneity among Spanish patients with recurrent autoinflammatory syndromes associated with the CIAS1/PYPAF1/NALP3 gene. Arthritis Rheum 2004;50:4045–50.
44. Stych B, Dobrovolny D. Familial cold auto-inflammatory syndrome (FCAS): characterization of symptomatology and impact on patients' lives. Curr Med Res Opin 2008;24:1577–82.
45. Dode C, Le Du N, Cuisset L, et al. New mutations of CIAS1 that are responsible for Muckle-Wells syndrome and familial cold urticaria: a novel mutation underlies both syndromes. Am J Hum Genet 2002;70:1498–506.
46. Hawkins PN, Lachmann HJ, Aganna E, et al. Spectrum of clinical features in Muckle-Wells syndrome and response to anakinra. Arthritis Rheum 2004;50:607–12.
47. Muckle TJ, Well SM. Urticaria, deafness, and amyloidosis: a new heredo-familial syndrome. Q J Med 1962;31:235–48.
48. Aganna E, Martinon F, Hawkins PN, et al. Association of mutations in the NALP3/CIAS1/PYPAF1 gene with a broad phenotype including recurrent fever, cold sensitivity, sensorineural deafness, and AA amyloidosis. Arthritis Rheum 2002; 46:2445–52.
49. Goldbach-Mansky R, Dailey NJ, Canna SW, et al. Neonatal-onset multisystem inflammatory disease responsive to interleukin-1beta inhibition. N Engl J Med 2006;355:581–92.
50. Sibley CH, Plass N, Snow J, et al. Sustained response and prevention of damage progression in patients with neonatal-onset multisystem inflammatory

disease treated with anakinra: a cohort study to determine three- and five-year outcomes. Arthritis Rheum 2012;64:2375–86.

51. Hill SC, Namde M, Dwyer A, et al. Arthropathy of neonatal onset multisystem inflammatory disease (NOMID/CINCA). Pediatr Radiol 2007;37:145–52.

52. Hoffman HM, Throne ML, Amar NJ, et al. Long-term efficacy and safety profile of rilonacept in the treatment of cryopryin-associated periodic syndromes: results of a 72-week open-label extension study. Clin Ther 2012;34:2091–103.

53. Goldbach-Mansky R, Shroff SD, Wilson M, et al. A pilot study to evaluate the safety and efficacy of the long-acting interleukin-1 inhibitor rilonacept (interleukin-1 Trap) in patients with familial cold autoinflammatory syndrome. Arthritis Rheum 2008;58:2432–42.

54. Lachmann HJ, Kone-Paut I, Kuemmerle-Deschner JB, et al. Use of canakinumab in the cryopyrin-associated periodic syndrome. N Engl J Med 2009;360:2416–25.

55. Hoffman HM, Throne ML, Amar NJ, et al. Efficacy and safety of rilonacept (interleukin-1 Trap) in patients with cryopyrin-associated periodic syndromes: results from two sequential placebo-controlled studies. Arthritis Rheum 2008;58:2443–52.

56. Kuemmerle-Deschner JB, Hachulla E, Cartwright R, et al. Two-year results from an open-label, multicentre, phase III study evaluating the safety and efficacy of canakinumab in patients with cryopyrin-associated periodic syndrome across different severity phenotypes. Ann Rheum Dis 2011;70:2095–102.

57. Neven B, Marvillet I, Terrada C, et al. Long-term efficacy of the interleukin-1 receptor antagonist anakinra in ten patients with neonatal-onset multisystem inflammatory disease/chronic infantile neurologic, cutaneous, articular syndrome. Arthritis Rheum 2010;62:258–67.

58. Stoffels M, Szperl A, Simon A, et al. MEFV mutations affecting pyrin amino acid 577 cause autosomal dominant autoinflammatory disease. Ann Rheum Dis 2013. [Epub ahead of print].

59. Heller H, Sohar E, Pras M. Ethnic distribution and amyloidosis in familial Mediterranean fever (FMF). Pathol Microbiol (Basel) 1961;24:718–23.

60. Ben-Chetrit E, Levy M. Familial Mediterranean fever. Lancet 1998;351:659–64.

61. Chae JJ, Aksentijevich I, Kastner DL. Advances in the understanding of familial Mediterranean fever and possibilities for targeted therapy. Br J Haematol 2009;146:467–78.

62. Langevitz P, Zemer D, Livneh A, et al. Protracted febrile myalgia in patients with familial Mediterranean fever. J Rheumatol 1994;21:1708–9.

63. Gedalia A, Zamir S. Neurologic manifestations in familial Mediterranean fever. Pediatr Neurol 1993;9:301–2.

64. Tunca M, Akar S, Onen F, et al. Familial Mediterranean fever (FMF) in Turkey: results of a nationwide multicenter study. Medicine (Baltimore) 2005;84:1–11.

65. Touitou I, Sarkisian T, Medlej-Hashim M, et al. Country as the primary risk factor for renal amyloidosis in familial Mediterranean fever. Arthritis Rheum 2007;56:1706–12.

66. Lachmann HJ, Goodman HJ, Gilbertson JA, et al. Natural history and outcome in systemic AA amyloidosis. N Engl J Med 2007;356:2361–71.

67. Zemer D, Pras M, Sohar E, et al. Colchicine in the prevention and treatment of the amyloidosis of familial Mediterranean fever. N Engl J Med 1986;314:1001–5.

68. Moser C, Pohl G, Haslinger I, et al. Successful treatment of familial Mediterranean fever with Anakinra and outcome after renal transplantation. Nephrol Dial Transplant 2009;24:676–8.

69. Hashkes PJ, Spalding SJ, Giannini EH, et al. Rilonacept for colchicine-resistant or -intolerant familial Mediterranean fever: a randomized trial. Ann Intern Med 2012;157:533–41.
70. Meinzer U, Quartier P, Alexandra JF, et al. Interleukin-1 targeting drugs in familial Mediterranean fever: a case series and a review of the literature. Semin Arthritis Rheum 2011;41:265–71.
71. Ozen S, Bilginer Y, Aktay Ayaz N, et al. Anti-interleukin 1 treatment for patients with familial Mediterranean fever resistant to colchicine. J Rheumatol 2011;38:516–8.
72. Mitroulis I, Skendros P, Oikonomou A, et al. The efficacy of canakinumab in the treatment of a patient with familial Mediterranean fever and longstanding destructive arthritis. Ann Rheum Dis 2011;70:1347–8.
73. Seyahi E, Ozdogan H, Celik S, et al. Treatment options in colchicine resistant familial Mediterranean fever patients: thalidomide and etanercept as adjunctive agents. Clin Exp Rheumatol 2006;24:S99–103.
74. Ozcakar ZB, Yuksel S, Ekim M, et al. Infliximab therapy for familial Mediterranean fever-related amyloidosis: case series with long term follow-up. Clin Rheumatol 2012;31:1267–71.
75. Hull KM, Drewe E, Aksentijevich I, et al. The TNF receptor-associated periodic syndrome (TRAPS): emerging concepts of an autoinflammatory disorder. Medicine (Baltimore) 2002;81:349–68.
76. Jesus AA, Oliveira JB, Aksentijevich I, et al. TNF receptor-associated periodic syndrome (TRAPS): description of a novel TNFRSF1A mutation and response to etanercept. Eur J Pediatr 2008;167:1421–5.
77. Aksentijevich I, Galon J, Soares M, et al. The tumor-necrosis-factor receptor-associated periodic syndrome: new mutations in TNFRSF1A, ancestral origins, genotype-phenotype studies, and evidence for further genetic heterogeneity of periodic fevers. Am J Hum Genet 2001;69:301–14.
78. Bulua AC, Mogul DB, Aksentijevich I, et al. Efficacy of etanercept in the tumor necrosis factor receptor-associated periodic syndrome: a prospective, open-label, dose-escalation study. Arthritis Rheum 2012;64:908–13.
79. Gattorno M, Pelagatti MA, Meini A, et al. Persistent efficacy of anakinra in patients with tumor necrosis factor receptor-associated periodic syndrome. Arthritis Rheum 2008;58:1516–20.
80. Sacre K, Brihaye B, Lidove O, et al. Dramatic improvement following interleukin 1beta blockade in tumor necrosis factor receptor-1-associated syndrome (TRAPS) resistant to anti-TNF-alpha therapy. J Rheumatol 2008;35:357–8.
81. Quillinan N, Mannion G, Mohammad A, et al. Failure of sustained response to etanercept and refractoriness to anakinra in patients with T50M TNF-receptor-associated periodic syndrome. Ann Rheum Dis 2011;70:1692–3.
82. Cuisset L, Drenth JP, Simon A, et al. Molecular analysis of MVK mutations and enzymatic activity in hyper-IgD and periodic fever syndrome. Eur J Hum Genet 2001;9:260–6.
83. Drenth JP, Haagsma CJ, van der Meer JW. Hyperimmunoglobulinemia D and periodic fever syndrome. The clinical spectrum in a series of 50 patients. International Hyper-IgD Study Group. Medicine (Baltimore) 1994;73:133–44.
84. Ammouri W, Cuisset L, Rouaghe S, et al. Diagnostic value of serum immunoglobulinaemia D level in patients with a clinical suspicion of hyper IgD syndrome. Rheumatology (Oxford) 2007;46:1597–600.
85. Simon A, Drewe E, van der Meer JW, et al. Simvastatin treatment for inflammatory attacks of the hyperimmunoglobulinemia D and periodic fever syndrome. Clin Pharmacol Ther 2004;75:476–83.

86. Bader-Meunier B, Florkin B, Sibilia J, et al. Mevalonate kinase deficiency: a survey of 50 patients. Pediatrics 2011;128:e152–9.
87. van der Hilst JC, Bodar EJ, Barron KS, et al. Long-term follow-up, clinical features, and quality of life in a series of 103 patients with hyperimmunoglobulinemia D syndrome. Medicine (Baltimore) 2008;87:301–10.
88. Takada K, Aksentijevich I, Mahadevan V, et al. Favorable preliminary experience with etanercept in two patients with the hyperimmunoglobulinemia D and periodic fever syndrome. Arthritis Rheum 2003;48:2645–51.
89. Rigante D, Ansuini V, Bertoni B, et al. Treatment with anakinra in the hyperimmunoglobulinemia D/periodic fever syndrome. Rheumatol Int 2006;27:97–100.
90. Galeotti C, Meinzer U, Quartier P, et al. Efficacy of interleukin-1-targeting drugs in mevalonate kinase deficiency. Rheumatology (Oxford) 2012;51:1855–9.
91. Ferguson PJ, Chen S, Tayeh MK, et al. Homozygous mutations in LPIN2 are responsible for the syndrome of chronic recurrent multifocal osteomyelitis and congenital dyserythropoietic anaemia (Majeed syndrome). J Med Genet 2005; 42:551–7.
92. Majeed HA, Kalaawi M, Mohanty D, et al. Congenital dyserythropoietic anemia and chronic recurrent multifocal osteomyelitis in three related children and the association with Sweet syndrome in two siblings. J Pediatr 1989;115:730–4.
93. Ferguson PJ, El-Shanti HI. Autoinflammatory bone disorders. Curr Opin Rheumatol 2007;19:492–8.
94. Jesus AA, Osman M, Silva CA, et al. A novel mutation of IL1RN in the deficiency of interleukin-1 receptor antagonist syndrome: description of two unrelated cases from Brazil. Arthritis Rheum 2011;63:4007–17.
95. Herlin T, Fiirgaard B, Bjerre M, et al. Efficacy of anti-IL-1 treatment in Majeed syndrome. Ann Rheum Dis 2013;72(3):410–3.
96. Miceli-Richard C, Lesage S, Rybojad M, et al. CARD15 mutations in Blau syndrome. Nat Genet 2001;29:19–20.
97. Kanazawa N, Okafuji I, Kambe N, et al. Early-onset sarcoidosis and CARD15 mutations with constitutive nuclear factor-kappaB activation: common genetic etiology with Blau syndrome. Blood 2005;105:1195–7.
98. Rose CD, Arostegui JI, Martin TM, et al. NOD2-associated pediatric granulomatous arthritis, an expanding phenotype: study of an international registry and a national cohort in Spain. Arthritis Rheum 2009;60:1797–803.
99. Rose CD, Martin TM, Wouters CH. Blau syndrome revisited. Curr Opin Rheumatol 2011;23:411–8.
100. Arostegui JI, Arnal C, Merino R, et al. NOD2 gene-associated pediatric granulomatous arthritis: clinical diversity, novel and recurrent mutations, and evidence of clinical improvement with interleukin-1 blockade in a Spanish cohort. Arthritis Rheum 2007;56:3805–13.
101. Wu Y, Spencer SD, Lasky LA. Tyrosine phosphorylation regulates the SH3-mediated binding of the Wiskott-Aldrich syndrome protein to PSTPIP, a cytoskeletal-associated protein. J Biol Chem 1998;273:5765–70.
102. Shoham NG, Centola M, Mansfield E, et al. Pyrin binds the PSTPIP1/CD2BP1 protein, defining familial Mediterranean fever and PAPA syndrome as disorders in the same pathway. Proc Natl Acad Sci U S A 2003;100:13501–6.
103. Yu JW, Fernandes-Alnemri T, Datta P, et al. Pyrin activates the ASC pyroptosome in response to engagement by autoinflammatory PSTPIP1 mutants. Mol Cell 2007;28:214–27.
104. Wang D, Hoing S, Patterson HC, et al. Inflammation in mice ectopically expressing human Pyogenic Arthritis, Pyoderma Gangrenosum, and Acne (PAPA)

Syndrome-associated PSTPIP1 A230T mutant proteins. J Biol Chem 2013;288: 4594–601.

105. Demidowich AP, Freeman AF, Kuhns DB, et al. Brief report: genotype, phenotype, and clinical course in five patients with PAPA syndrome (pyogenic sterile arthritis, pyoderma gangrenosum, and acne). Arthritis Rheum 2012;64:2022–7.

106. Stohwasser R, Kuckelkorn U, Kraft R, et al. 20S proteasome from LMP7 knock out mice reveals altered proteolytic activities and cleavage site preferences. FEBS Lett 1996;383:109–13.

107. Ciechanover A. Intracellular protein degradation: from a vague idea through the lysosome and the ubiquitin-proteasome system and onto human diseases and drug targeting. Neurodegener Dis 2012;10:7–22.

108. Goldberg AL. Functions of the proteasome: from protein degradation and immune surveillance to cancer therapy. Biochem Soc Trans 2007;35:12–7.

109. Seifert U, Bialy LP, Ebstein F, et al. Immunoproteasomes preserve protein homeostasis upon interferon-induced oxidative stress. Cell 2010;142:613–24.

110. Agarwal AK, Xing C, DeMartino GN, et al. PSMB8 encoding the beta5i proteasome subunit is mutated in joint contractures, muscle atrophy, microcytic anemia, and panniculitis-induced lipodystrophy syndrome. Am J Hum Genet 2010;87:866–72.

111. Arima K, Kinoshita A, Mishima H, et al. Proteasome assembly defect due to a proteasome subunit beta type 8 (PSMB8) mutation causes the autoinflammatory disorder, Nakajo-Nishimura syndrome. Proc Natl Acad Sci U S A 2011;108: 14914–9.

112. Kitamura A, Maekawa Y, Uehara H, et al. A mutation in the immunoproteasome subunit PSMB8 causes autoinflammation and lipodystrophy in humans. J Clin Invest 2011;121:4150–60.

113. Liu Y, Ramot Y, Torrelo A, et al. Mutations in proteasome subunit beta type 8 cause chronic atypical neutrophilic dermatosis with lipodystrophy and elevated temperature with evidence of genetic and phenotypic heterogeneity. Arthritis Rheum 2012;64:895–907.

114. Livingston JH, Stivaros S, van der Knaap MS, et al. Recognizable phenotypes associated with intracranial calcification. Dev Med Child Neurol 2013;55:46–57.

115. Nakajo A. Secondary hypertrophic osteoperiostosis with pernio. J Derm Urol 1939;45:77–86.

116. Nishimura N, Deki T, Kato S. Hypertrophic pulmonary osteo-arthropathy with pernio-like eruption in the two families: report of the three cases. Jpn J Derm Venereol 1950;60:136–41.

117. Megarbane A, Sanders A, Chouery E, et al. An unknown autoinflammatory syndrome associated with short stature and dysmorphic features in a young boy. J Rheumatol 2002;29:1084–7.

118. Garg A, Hernandez MD, Sousa AB, et al. An autosomal recessive syndrome of joint contractures, muscular atrophy, microcytic anemia, and panniculitis-associated lipodystrophy. J Clin Endocrinol Metab 2010;95:E58–63.

119. Torrelo A, Patel S, Colmenero I, et al. Chronic atypical neutrophilic dermatosis with lipodystrophy and elevated temperature (CANDLE) syndrome. J Am Acad Dermatol 2010;62:489–95.

120. Marrakchi S, Guigue P, Renshaw BR, et al. Interleukin-36-receptor antagonist deficiency and generalized pustular psoriasis. N Engl J Med 2011;365:620–8.

121. Onoufriadis A, Simpson MA, Pink AE, et al. Mutations in IL36RN/IL1F5 are associated with the severe episodic inflammatory skin disease known as generalized pustular psoriasis. Am J Hum Genet 2011;89:432–7.

122. Fuchs-Telem D, Sarig O, van Steensel MA, et al. Familial pityriasis rubra pilaris is caused by mutations in CARD14. Am J Hum Genet 2012;91:163–70.

123. Jordan CT, Cao L, Roberson ED, et al. PSORS2 is due to mutations in CARD14. Am J Hum Genet 2012;90:784–95.

124. Blumberg H, Dinh H, Trueblood ES, et al. Opposing activities of two novel members of the IL-1 ligand family regulate skin inflammation. J Exp Med 2007;204:2603–14.

125. Medlej-Hashim M, Delague V, Chouery E, et al. Amyloidosis in familial Mediterranean fever patients: correlation with MEFV genotype and SAA1 and MICA polymorphisms effects. BMC Med Genet 2004;5:4.

126. Habal N, Chen Y, Jordan C, et al. Pathogenesis Study of Infantile-Onset, Severe Pustular Psoriasis Reveals a De Novo Mutation in CARD14 Causing Psoriasis Which Responds Clinically to IL-12/23 Blocking Treatment with Ustekinumab. [abstract]. Arthritis Rheum 2011;63(Suppl 10):310.

127. Glocker EO, Kotlarz D, Boztug K, et al. Inflammatory bowel disease and mutations affecting the interleukin-10 receptor. N Engl J Med 2009;361:2033–45.

128. Kotlarz D, Beier R, Murugan D, et al. Loss of interleukin-10 signaling and infantile inflammatory bowel disease: implications for diagnosis and therapy. Gastroenterology 2012;143:347–55.

129. Engelhardt KR, Shah N, Faizura-Yeop I, et al. Clinical outcome in IL-10- and IL-10 receptor-deficient patients with or without hematopoietic stem cell transplantation. J Allergy Clin Immunol 2013;131(3):825–30.

130. Boisson B, Laplantine E, Prando C, et al. Immunodeficiency, autoinflammation and amylopectinosis in humans with inherited HOIL-1 and LUBAC deficiency. Nat Immunol 2012;13:1178–86.

Autoinflammatory Bone Diseases

Sara M. Stern, MD[a],*, Polly J. Ferguson, MD[b]

KEYWORDS

- Chronic nonbacterial osteomyelitis • Autoinflammatory bone diseases
- Majeed syndrome • DIRA • SAPHO syndrome • CRMO • Cherubism

KEY POINTS

- Chronic nonbacterial osteomyelitis (CNO), synovitis, acne, pustulosis, hyperostosis, osteitis syndrome, Majeed syndrome, deficiency of interleukin-1 receptor antagonist (DIRA), cherubism, and juvenile mandibular chronic osteomyelitis are autoinflammatory bone diseases.
- Autoinflammatory bone diseases are innate immune system activation disorders.
- The bone inflammation in these syndromes is characterized by a subacute or chronic inflammation that is culture negative and has no demonstrable organism on histopathology.
- Antiinflammatory medications are typically used as first-line therapies in CNO. Recently bisphosphonates and tumor necrosis factor-α antagonists have been used for second-line therapies to prevent pathologic fractures, pain, and disease relapse.
- Majeed syndrome, DIRA, and cherubism are distinct genetic autoinflammatory bone syndromes.

OVERVIEW

Autoinflammatory bone disease is a new branch of autoinflammatory diseases caused by seemingly unprovoked activation of the innate immune system leading to an osseous inflammatory process.[1] The inflammatory bone lesions in these disorders are characterized by chronic inflammation that is typically culture negative with no demonstrable organism on histopathology.[2–6] The most common autoinflammatory bone diseases in childhood include chronic nonbacterial osteomyelitis (CNO), synovitis, acne, pustulosis, hyperostosis, osteitis (SAPHO) syndrome, Majeed syndrome, deficiency of interleukin-1 receptor antagonist (DIRA), and cherubism. In this article, the authors focus on CNO and summarize the distinct genetic autoinflammatory bone syndromes (**Table 1**).

Disclosure: PJF is supported by the National Institute of Arthritis and Musculoskeletal and Skin Diseases at the National Institutes of Health [1R01AR059703-01A1].
[a] Division of Immunology, Rheumatology, and Allergy, Department of Pediatrics, University of Utah, PO Box 581289, Salt Lake City, UT 84158, USA; [b] Division of Pediatric Rheumatology, Department of Pediatrics, Roy J. and Lucille A. Carver College of Medicine, University of Iowa, Iowa City, IA, USA
* Corresponding author.
E-mail address: Sara.Stern@hsc.utah.edu

Table 1
Autoinflammatory bone diseases summary chart

	CNO	Majeed Syndrome	DIRA	Cherubism	Childhood SAPHO
Clinical Manifestations					
Fever	Not typical	Common	Uncommon	No	Not typical
Common CNO sites	Femur, tibia, pelvis, calcaneus, ankle, vertebrae, & clavicle	Similar to CNO	Long bones (especially proximal femur), vertebral bodies, ribs, & clavicle	Maxilla and mandible	Similar to CNO
Area of long bone affected	75% around metaphyses	Metaphyses predominance	Metaphyses predominance	Long bones rarely affected	Similar to CNO
Extraosseous manifestations	Skin, joints, gastrointestinal tract, and lungs	Congenital dyserythropoietic anemia, inflammatory dermatosis, growth failure, hepatomegaly, joint contractures	Generalized pustulosis, osteitis, periostitis, systemic organ involvement	Cervical lymphadenopathy	Palmoplantar pustulosis, severe acne, or psoriasis
Inflammatory markers	Normal to mildly elevated	Elevated	Elevated	Normal to mildly elevated	Normal to mildly elevated
Genetics					
Inheritance	Unknown	Autosomal recessive	Autosomal recessive	Autosomal dominant	Unknown
Gene defect	Unknown	LPIN2	IL1RN	SH3BP2	Unknown
Protein name	Unknown	Lipin2	IL-1Ra	SH3BP2	Unknown
Ethnicity	Worldwide distribution	Arabic, Turkish	Puerto Rican, European, Lebanese	Worldwide distribution	Likely similar to CNO

CNO
Introduction

In 1972, Giedion and colleagues[7] first described CNO as a subacute and chronic symmetric osteomyelitis. In the past 40 years, our understanding of CNO has become more sophisticated because of numerous breakthroughs. The recent advances in imaging technology have led to the enhanced ability to diagnose inflammatory bone lesions. Multiple breakthroughs in immunology have led to a more sophisticated appreciation of the function of the innate immune system. This understanding enabled the characterization of autoinflammatory diseases and, therefore, autoinflammatory bone diseases. There have been many discoveries of the genetic associations of autoinflammatory syndromes. Finally, the use of the tumor necrosis factor α (TNFα) antagonist and bisphosphonates enabled more effective treatments in nonsteroidal antiinflammatory drug (NSAID)–resistant disease. These breakthroughs have enabled the rheumatology community to have a more advanced understanding of CNO.

Nomenclature and Disease Pattern

The terminology for CNO has changed multiple times in the past 40 years. It was first called *subacute* and *chronic symmetric osteomyelitis*.[7] However, since that time, it has most commonly been called *chronic recurrent multifocal osteomyelitis* (CRMO). The term *CRMO* was coined by Probst and colleagues[8] in 1978 and is characterized as a chronic inflammatory bone disorder that had multifocal bone lesions and had multiple recurrences. However, not all patients have multifocal bone lesions or numerous recurrences. Therefore, the term *chronic nonbacterial osteomyelitis* has been used as an umbrella term and is inclusive of all the varied presentations of this disease.[2]

There are 3 disease patterns for CNO: a course that resolves within 6 months, a persistent course, and a course characterized by multifocal bone lesions and multiple recurrences.[2,9,10] The multifocal recurrent disease pattern is most consistent with CRMO and SAPHO (Synovitis, Acne, Pustulosis, Hyperostosis, and Osteitis) syndrome.[11]

Cause and Pathogenesis of CNO

By definition, the bone lesions seen in CNO are culture negative and have no demonstrable organism on histopathology.[2–6] Antibiotic therapy should not cause resolution of symptoms. In a small case series, azithromycin was shown to improve radiological and clinical signs and symptoms of CNO.[12] This effect may be mediated through the antiinflammatory properties of azithromycin instead of its antimicrobial properties. Although there have been many proposed pathogens causing CNO, there has been no definitive evidence that microbes trigger CNO. *Propionibacterium acnes* has been recently proposed as a cause for CNO. This pathogen has been cultured in adults with palmoplantar pustulosis, a common skin manifestation seen in SAPHO and CNO. Rarely was this bacteria cultured when the pustules of patients with palmoplantar pustulosis and SAPHO or CNO were analyzed for *P acnes*.[13] In one series of adult patients with SAPHO, *P acnes* was cultured from the bone from 7 of the 15 patients tested.[13] However, in most patients with SAPHO and CNO, cultures of the bone are negative or when positive are thought to be a contaminant.

The chronic inflammation seen with CNO seems to be caused by activation in the innate immune system as typically seen in autoinflammatory diseases.[1] This seemingly unprovoked activation may lead to an imbalance of proinflammatory and antiinflammatory cytokines and, therefore, disruption in immune homeostasis. Currently, the cause and pathophysiology of CNO are not firmly established in nonsyndromic forms of the disease. However, there have been several developments in the possible pathophysiology mechanisms and genetic associations for this disease.

There is evidence that links the interleukin-10 (IL-10) pathway to the development of CNO. Hofmann and colleagues[14] reported that peripheral blood monocytes stimulated with the toll-like receptor 4 agonist lipopolysaccharide (LPS) secreted significantly less IL-10 compared with healthy control monocytes. This outcome occurred independently of IL-10 promoter polymorphisms because an association with CNO and the high IL-10 expressing -1082G>A alleles and the GCC haplotype[14] was found. Because LPS-stimulated CNO monocytes have a decreased production of IL-10, this is the opposite of what would be expected with the high expressing allele, suggesting other mechanisms are involved.

Next, these investigators demonstrated that the decrease in IL-10 secretion from LPS-stimulated CNO monocytes is associated with attenuated extracellular-signal regulated kinase (ERK)1/2 activity.[15] This decrement in ERK1/2 signaling then results in reduced levels of the transcription factor Sp-1, a transcription factor that drives IL-10 gene expression in monocytes.[15,16] They showed that Sp-1 recruitment to the IL-10.636 Sp-1 element is reduced in LPS-stimulated CNO monocytes. In addition, they found that histone H3 serine-10 phosphorylation (H3S10p), an activating marker, is decreased around the IL-10-636 element of the IL-10 promoter.[15,16] The attenuation of Sp-1 and reduced H3S10p suggest that epigenetic factors play a role in the decreased gene expression of IL-10 seen in CNO.[15,16] A unified hypothesis has been proposed to explain these separate pathophysiology mechanisms in CNO. The investigators concluded that impaired mitogen-activated protein kinase signaling, decreased H3S10p, and attenuated Sp-1 recruitment to the IL-10 promoter results in impaired gene expression of IL-10 with subsequent disruption of the proinflammatory and antiinflammatory cytokine balance. This disruption in immune homeostasis might explain part of the clinical presentation of CNO.[16]

There is increasing evidence for the theory that CNO is genetically driven. The two strongest pieces of evidence are that two similar diseases with autoinflammatory bone lesions are genetically driven and animal models with genetic defects have a similar phenotype. Majeed syndrome and DIRA are genetically linked diseases with features that include autoinflammatory bone lesions. Majeed syndrome is caused by mutations in LPIN2 and DIRA with mutations in IL1RN.[17–19]

There have been many animal models with genetic defects leading to autoinflammatory bone lesions. Currently, there are reports of autoinflammatory bone lesions seen in mice, lemurs, and dogs. Two murine models have developed CNO, the cmo mice and the Lupo mice.[20,21] Both of these murine models have a mutation in pstpip2 and present with similar clinical features as seen in humans. The cmo mice generally develop a clinically severe presentation.[20] Pstpip2 acts in the cytosol as an F-actin–associated phosphoprotein, interacts with PEST-type protein tyrosine phosphatases, and is involved in cytoskeletal organization.[22,23] Murine pstpip2 is similar to human PSTPIP1 and PSTPIP2. PSTPIP1 regulates the NLRP3 inflammasome through binding to pyrin and is the genetic defect seen in the autosomal-dominant autoinflammatory syndrome pyogenic arthritis pyoderma gangrenosum acne syndrome.[24]

There is a possible genetic association locus at chromosome 18q21.3-18q22 and CRMO.[25] This genetic association is not yet linked to the pathophysiological development of CNO. There have been cases of families with multiple affected members with CNO and cases with first- and second-degree relatives with inflammatory bowel disease, psoriasis, and other chronic inflammatory conditions. This finding provides additional evidence of a genetic association.[2,5,6] Genetic mutations in PSTPIP1, PSTPIP2,

CARD15/NOD2, and *IL1RN* have been examined in small series and do not seem to be the causative genetic feature in CNO.[2,26,27]

Epidemiology

CNO is primarily a disease of childhood. It has many similarities to SAPHO syndrome, which is a disorder primarily seen in adults. The incidence and prevalence of CNO is unknown. Although a diversity of ethnicities and populations throughout the world is affected by CNO, most reports are from Scandinavia, Europe, Australia, and North America. There is a female predominance, and the mean age of disease onset is around 10 years old.[2,5,6]

Clinical Presentation

CNO is a diagnosis of exclusion and is established by the clinical presentation, imaging studies, and a culture-negative bone biopsy. Pain with or without swelling at the site of the bony lesion is the typical presenting symptom. Bone lesions tend to cluster around the metaphysis; can occur at atypical locations for bacterial osteomyelitis, such as the clavicle; and when multifocal, often have a symmetric distribution.[3,28] Seventy-five percent of bone lesions are perimetaphyseal.[29] Appendicular and axial skeletal lesions are also seen. The most common CNO sites are the femur, tibia, pelvis, calcaneus, ankle, vertebrae, and clavicle.[2,3,5,6] CNO is the most common disease cause to affect the medial third of the clavicle in all age groups.[28] A unifocal pattern of disease occurs in 10% to 20% of patients.[5,6]

CNO is a systemic disease that can affect the skin, joints, gastrointestinal tract, and lungs. Patients with CNO frequently have other coexisting chronic inflammatory diseases.[2,5,6,27] In one study, 20% to 50% of patients had or developed another autoimmune/inflammatory disease.[2,5] The most frequent associated autoimmune and/or inflammatory diseases included arthritis, psoriasis, inflammatory bowel disease, vasculitis, myositis/fasciitis, and parotitis. Typically, these patients have more bony lesions than patients without a comorbid inflammatory disease.[5]

Patients with CNO tend to have normal, mild, or moderately elevated inflammatory laboratory changes. Markers of inflammation, including erythrocyte sedimentation rate, C-reactive protein, white blood cell count and platelet count, can be moderately increased or completely normal.[2–6,30] Inflammatory markers are typically higher in patients with comorbid autoimmune diseases.[5]

Imaging Studies

Radiographs, technetium bone scans, and/or magnetic resonance imaging (MRI) are generally used to detect the lesions and screen for multifocality.[28,31,32] Computerized tomography can detect lesions but exposes children to significant levels of radiation, so it is generally not recommended. Typical radiographic findings include a lytic lesion at or around the metaphysis that progresses to sclerosis or hyperostosis.[28] Recently whole-body MRI imaging has been studied as a radiation-free method of imaging.[31,33] Whole-body MRI imaging is a useful method to detect asymptomatic lesions without radiation exposure. The lesions are best seen on short tau inversion recovery sequences and can be used to identify subclinical spinal involvement, synovitis of adjacent joints, and sacroiliitis. Whole-body MRI tends to poorly detect lesions in the small joints of the hands and feet, ribs, and sternoclavicular and costovertebral joint junctions. There has never been a study to compare bone scintigraphy and whole-body MRI. Whole-body MRI should be considered in working up indeterminate cases of CNO and as an imaging technique used to monitor disease activity and response to therapy.

Histopathology

A bone biopsy is often needed to confirm a diagnosis of CNO.[2,4] This biopsy is especially necessary in isolated bone lesions because bone malignancies can mimic CNO. In children who present with multifocal disease for many months in duration, the need for a confirmatory bone biopsy is debatable.[4,30] The presence of clavicular involvement with palmar-plantar pustulosis or psoriasis vulgaris is very strong evidence of CNO. However, caution should be used in the absence of strong supporting evidence of CNO because serious disorders, such as intraosseous lymphoma and other forms of neoplasia, can mimic CNO.[34] A classification criteria and clinical algorithm has been proposed to aid the clinician in the diagnosis of CNO.[2,4]

CNO is characterized by subacute or chronic inflammation, with a lymphocytic or mixed inflammatory infiltrate, and often marrow fibrosis.[3,9] By definition, the biopsy is culture negative and has no demonstrable organism on histopathology.

Treatment

NSAIDs are the gold standard initial therapy for CNO.[2,26,27,35] However, there is a discrepancy in the literature regarding the efficacy of NSAIDs in the treatment of CNO. In 2 published studies from Germany, Beck and colleagues[26] demonstrated a complete response to naproxen in 43% of the patients, whereas Girschick and colleagues[9] noted that although 100% of patients with a nonrelapsing course responded to naproxen, only 42% of patients with a relapsing course responded. Indomethacin might be more effective than naproxen but is associated with more side effects.[36] Case studies and small case series have been published addressing the treatment of CNO with various medications, including corticosteroids and disease-modifying antirheumatic drugs (methotrexate [MTX] and sulfasalazine).[37] Because of the small numbers, there is no conclusion about the efficacy of these agents.

TNFα seems to be an important cytokine in CNO. This cytokine plays an important role in the activation of osteoclasts in CNO.[2,14] There have been several case reports, small retrospective series, and a few larger series on TNFα antagonist treatment in CNO.[5,38,39] In a larger series involving 11 patients on TNFα antagonists, 10 of the 11 responded to the therapy, and there was a 46% remission rate.[5] Smaller case series have also showed a favorable response to TNFα antagonists in the treatment of CNO. Eleftheriou and colleagues[38] evaluated 3 pediatric patients treated with TNFα blocking agents with CRMO or SAPHO and all 3 showed a clinical improvement. However, 1 patient stopped therapy prematurely because of an invasive fungal infection. Catalano-Pons and colleagues[6] published the results from a French cohort of 40 pediatric cases of which 2 had used TNFα antagonists, although the treatment response was not thoroughly detailed. Other biologic medications have been used in case reports that include interferon (INF)-α, INF-γ, and anakinra. The case report on anakinra initially showed a response, but the response was not sustained.[38]

Pamidronate has also been recently used for the treatment of CNO.[40–44] This therapy is hypothesized to treat CNO by inactivating osteoclasts, decreasing pain, and possibly through an antiinflammatory mechanism. In one study, all 9 patients treated responded to pamidronate.[43] The clinical response typically occurred in the first 3 days. Four patients experienced a recurrence in their CNO 12 to 18 months after their first pamidronate course. All 4 patients responded to a repeat course of pamidronate. In another study evaluating the response to pamidronate, 4 of the 5 patients showed clinical improvement.[41] In a third study, 6 of the 7 patients improved with pamidronate. However, synovial joint disease was unresponsive to the therapy.[42] Pamidronate therapy may be particular beneficial in spinal lesions and vertebral fractures by improving vertebral shape and decreasing the kyphotic angle.[42,44] Hospach and colleagues[44] reported on patients with axial disease and found that all 7 had an improvement in spinal lesions after pamidronate therapy. Urinary N-telopeptide/urine creatinine (uNTX/uCr), a marker of collagen-I breakdown, has been proposed as a marker for disease flare after bisphosphonate therapy.[43] This marker has been used to monitor disease with accelerated bone turnover. When used in cases with CNO, no clinically evident relapses occurred while uNTX/uCr was suppressed.

Concerns have been raised about using bisphosphonates in the pediatric population because long-term safety data are limited. The most common adverse events are minor flulike symptoms for a day after the infusion. Currently, osteonecrosis of the jaw is possible but is an unreported side effect of pamidronate use in children with CNO. This adverse event primarily occurs in elderly patients with myeloma. Because of this potential side effect, it is recommended to have pediatric patients have a dental screening and wisdom teeth extraction before pamidronate therapy whenever possible and postpone elective dental procedures for at least 6 months following therapy.[43]

No study has compared the efficacy of bisphosphonates with TNFα antagonists. There have been 2 larger observational studies that treated patients with either bisphosphonates or TNFα antagonists (3 and 2 in one cohort and 3 and 1 in the other cohort), but no data were included on the efficacy of these therapies (**Fig. 1**).[2,6]

Prognosis

In North America, CNO continues to be difficult to treat, with high rates of treatment nonresponders. In a study, only 43% of patients were in remission 22 months after diagnosis, and only 13% were in remission off therapy.[5] In general, European cohorts seem to have more favorable outcomes.[2,3] Functional and cosmetic consequences of hyperostosis are frequently seen.[2] Pathologic fractures are common and most frequently occur in the vertebrae.[2,3] Scoliosis, bony overgrowth, and generalized growth failure are possible long-term morbidities associated with CNO (**Box 1**).[2,5,6]

Summary

CNO is a diagnosis of exclusion that is established by the clinical presentation, imaging studies, and a culture-negative bone biopsy. Recently, there have been several advancements in understanding the cause and genetic links for CNO. Treatment

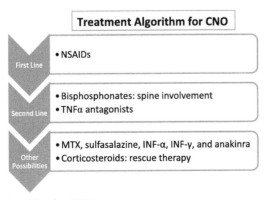

Treatment Algorithm for CNO

First Line
- NSAIDs

Second Line
- Bisphosphonates: spine involvement
- TNFα antagonists

Other Possibilities
- MTX, sulfasalazine, INF-α, INF-γ, and anakinra
- Corticosteroids: rescue therapy

Fig. 1. Treatment algorithm for CNO.

Box 1
Common morbidities associated with CNO

Pathologic fractures

Scoliosis

Bony overgrowth/hyperostosis

Generalized growth failure

---

remains challenging. TNFα antagonist and bisphosphonates seem to be possible second-line agents for CNO. There are high rates of pathologic fractures and morbidity when untreated.

DISTINCT GENETIC AUTOINFLAMMATORY BONE SYNDROMES
Majeed Syndrome

Majeed syndrome is a rare autosomal recessive disorder first described by Majeed and colleagues[45] in 1989 that is characterized by a clinical triad of features: CRMO, congenital dyserythropoietic anemia (CDA), and inflammatory dermatosis.[45,46] The disease course of Majeed syndrome differs from CNO in that it is more severe, has an earlier age of onset, and is associated with CDA and inflammatory dermatosis (**Fig. 2**).[45,46]

The disease onset of Majeed syndrome is in infancy. This disease is associated with recurrent fevers, severe pain, chronic anemia, and soft tissue swelling that typically affects large joints. Frequent exacerbations, as often as 3 to 4 per month, each lasting a few days with short remissions, characterize disease in Majeed syndrome.[46,47] The distribution of the CRMO is similar to CNO in that it also tends to affect the metaphyses of long bones.[46,48] The inflammatory neutrophilic dermatosis, Sweet syndrome, is the associated skin manifestation.[45–47] The CDA seen with Majeed syndrome is variable in its presentation and severity and different from other known forms of CDA. This microcytic anemia typically appears by 9 months of age. Children with Majeed

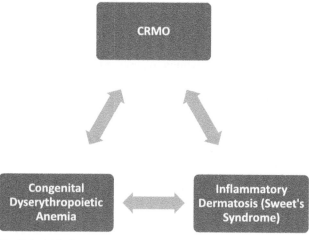

Fig. 2. Majeed's clinical triad.

syndrome often have multiple complications and poor outcomes that include growth retardation, failure to thrive, hepatomegaly, joint contractures, and muscle atrophy.[45–48] Neonatal cholestatic jaundice and mild neutropenia were seen in one patient.[48]

LPIN2 is the mutation responsible for Majeed syndrome and encodes LIPIN2.[17,48] LIPIN2 is part of the LIPIN family. This protein family plays a role in glycerolipid biosynthesis by acting as phosphatidate phosphatase (PAP).[49,50] Homozygous mutations in LPIN2 have been found in 4 families with 4 unique mutations: a missense mutation (S734L), a frame shift mutation (T180fs), a splice site mutation (R776Sfs), 2-base pair deletion in LIPIN2 (c.1312-1313delCT; p.Leu438fs+16X).[51] LPIN2 is expressed in multiple different organs: liver, lung, kidney, placenta, spleen, thymus, lymph node, prostate, testes, small intestine, and colon.[17] Mutations in LPIN1 in mice cause lipodystrophy, fatty liver, hypertriglyceridemia, glucose intolerance, peripheral neuropathy, and atherosclerosis. The LPIN2 mutation in humans does not seem to produce lipid abnormalities.[48] Recently, it has been suggested that the phenotypic picture seen with Majeed syndrome results from a loss of PAP activity in LIPIN2.[49] In an in vitro model, the mutation of serine to leucine at amino acid 734 (S734L) is required for appropriate PAP function. This mutation seems to impact the PAP activity without affecting the other lipid and metabolic functions of lipin2. It is still unclear how the dysfunction of LIPIN2 produces all of the phenotypic features of Majeed syndrome; however, Valdearcos and colleagues[52] recently demonstrated that LPIN2 dampens the proinflammatory signaling that is produced by macrophages when exposed to excessive saturated fatty acids.

Majeed syndrome can be difficult to treat. Typically, NSAIDs and oral corticosteroids have been used with variable success.[47] Recently, 2 brothers failed treatment with a TNF inhibitor, but treatment with IL-1 beta blockade resulted in clinical, laboratory, and radiologic improvement.[51] This finding supports the hypothesis that Majeed syndrome is an autoinflammatory syndrome.

DIRA

DIRA is a newly recognized autosomal recessive autoinflammatory disorder.[18,53–55] Prose and colleagues[56] described a child with what was likely DIRA in 1994, and it was recognized as a distinct syndrome in 2009.[18,19] DIRA is caused by a mutation in the ILIRN, is potentially life threatening, and can mimic neonatal sepsis.[18,55] A high index of suspicion is critical to prevent multisystem organ damage and death.

The characteristic clinical presentation includes generalized pustulosis, osteitis, periostitis, and systemic inflammation.[18,19,47,53–55] Within the first few weeks after birth, a pustular rash and systemic signs of inflammation develop.[18,19,53,55] Even though systemic inflammatory markers are markedly elevated, fever is usually absent.[18,19,53,55] Weeks after the rash presents, osteitis is detected.[18,53,55] The osteitis seen in DIRA is severe, with extensive bone involvement, a multifocal osteolytic pattern of disease, and marked periostitis.[18,19,53,55] These bony lesions typically affect long bones, vertebral bodies, and have a predilection for the proximal femur. The bone biopsy in DIRA is characterized by a purulent osteomyelitis that is culture negative with fibrosis and sclerosis.[18] Three radiographic characteristic findings are typically seen that include widening of the anterior rib ends, multifocal osteolytic lesions, and periosteal elevation of the long bones.[18,19,53,55] Other less common findings include heterotopic ossification of the proximal femurs, widening of the clavicles, metaphyseal osteolytic areas of long bones, and osteolytic skull lesions.[18] As with CNO, vertebral involvement and morbidities are common. Collapse of the vertebrae caused by osteolytic lesions can occur and cause cervical vertebral fusion (**Fig. 3**).[18,53]

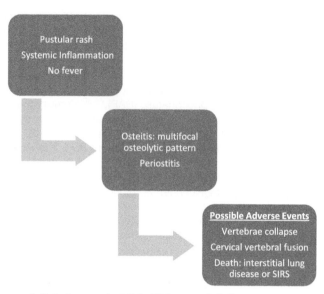

Fig. 3. Summary of clinical course in DIRA. SIRS, systemic inflammatory response syndrome.

DIRA is caused by a mutation in the *ILIRN*. There are presently 6 known mutations in the *ILIRN*.[18,19,53,55] The most common mutation is E77X. Other mutations seen are N52KfsX25, Q54X, D72-176del, T47Tfs, and 175-kb deletion on chromosome 2q13. All but 1 child had homozygous mutations in the gene.[18,19,53] One child was a compound heterozygote (E77X and T47TfsX4).[57] The 75 kb chromosomal deletion on chromosome 2q13 includes the *ILIRN* gene and 5 other IL-1 family members.[18,19] The genetic understanding of this disease has enabled improved outcomes because of the treatment of IL-1 blocking agents, such as anakinra.[47,54,58] Before the use of anakinra, there was a 33% mortality rate.[47] These children died of systemic inflammatory response syndrome (SIRS) early in life (n = 2) or pulmonary interstitial disease in childhood (n = 1). Long-term outcome data of children treated with anakinra are unknown.

Cherubism

Cherubism is an autosomal-dominant autoinflammatory bone disorder affecting the maxilla and mandible.[59–62] The bony changes of the jaw give these children's faces a chubby-cheeked appearance; hence, the disorder was named after their likeness to cherubs depicted in Renaissance art. Children present in childhood (2–7 years) with a large multilocular, cystic lesion of the mandible or less commonly the maxilla.[59–62] Similar multilocular cysts can be found in Noonan syndrome and is considered part of the Noonan spectrum.[63]

Cherubism is an autoinflammatory disorder that is driven by 2 mechanisms: macrophage activity leading to high levels of TNFα with subsequent inflammation and osteoclast activation causing excessive bone resorption.[63] In 2001, 3 heterozygous missense mutations in the SH3 binding protein 2 (*SH3BP2*) were identified, primarily affecting amino acid 415, 418, and 420.[63] Since that time, 3 additional mutations were identified: amino acid 420, 418, and 419.[63] SH3BP2 is an adapter protein involved in innate and adaptive immune system signaling through interacting and forming complexes with binding and scaffolding proteins.[63] In various immune cells, especially osteoclasts, SH3BP2 can cause phosphorylation and, therefore, affect signal pathways.[63] Mutations in this regulator cause uncontrolled bone resorption of the jaw. This genetic locus is commonly deleted in bladder cancer and contained within the locus for Wolf-Hirschhorn syndrome, which is a syndrome characterized by craniofacial malformations, intellectual disability, muscle hypotonia, and heart defects.[63]

Cherubism continues to be difficult to treat. Recently, 2 patients have been unsuccessfully treated with adalimumab.[64] There has been another recent case report of a patient receiving adalimumab and oral bisphosphonate with no clinical improvement. However, this child was only treated with these therapies for a short period of time.[65]

SAPHO Syndrome in Childhood

SAPHO syndrome is an autoinflammatory disease that affects both skin and bones, which has been diagnosed primarily in adults.[66,67] The bone manifestations seen in SAPHO are generally described as CRMO. Palmoplantar pustulosis, severe acne, or psoriasis are the typical skin manifestations and have a neutrophilic predominance.[11,66,67] Recently, SAPHO has also been described in childhood. It is unclear if it is a distinct entity or is a more severe form of CRMO.

The cause for SAPHO remains unknown. Recent studies suggest the polymorphonuclear cell dysfunction could be a possible cause of SAPHO. *LPIN2*, *PSTPIP2*, and *NOD2* mutations do not seem to be associated with SAPHO.[68] Recently, a child and mother were reported who both had a clinical presentation of SAPHO and had abnormal polymorphonuclear leukocytes (PMN) intracellular production of reactive oxygen species.[69] It has been proposed that *P acnes* might stimulate IL-8 and IL-18 release by PMNs leading to the pathogenesis of SAPHO.[70]

The first-line treatment of childhood SAPHO is typically NSAIDs.[11] Other agents that have been used are methotrexate, oral corticosteroids, colchicine, and sulfasalazine. Ben Abdelghani and colleagues[71] studied 6 adults treated with TNFα antagonist for SAPHO syndrome and 66.6% had a beneficial response. Bisphosphonates have also been used. In a recent case series, all 7 patients had a marked clinical improvement with pamidronate.[72] In this study, some children were classified as SAPHO without the classic skin manifestations and may have better been classified as CRMO.

Juvenile Mandibular Chronic Osteomyelitis

Diffuse sclerosing osteomyelitis is a sclerosing osteomyelitis of the jaw first described by Carl Garré in 1893.[73] Recently, the name *juvenile mandibular chronic osteomyelitis* (JMCO) has been used to describe this disease in children.[73] The mean age of presentation of JMCO is 13 years.[73] JMCO is characterized by a mixed osteolytic and sclerotic process that can cause mandibular nerve canal enlargement and adjacent soft tissue involvement.[73] Typically, unilateral mandible involvement is seen.[73] Similar findings can occur in patients with jaw involvement in typical CRMO. It is unclear if these are the same disease entity (ie, JMCO is CNO of the mandible) or they are distinct clinical entities.

SUMMARY

CNO is an autoinflammatory bone disease that is culture negative and has no demonstrable organism on histopathology. It is a systemic disease that affects many organ systems in addition to bones and has high rates of comorbid autoinflammatory/autoimmune diseases. This disease can also be part of a larger genetic syndrome such as seen with DIRA and Majeed syndrome. Recently, TNFα antagonists and pamidronate has shown great promise in treating CNO in NSAID-resistant disease. Early control is essential to decrease morbidities, such as pathologic fractures and scoliosis.

REFERENCES

1. Masters SL, Simon A, Aksentijevich I, et al. Horror autoinflammaticus: the molecular pathophysiology of autoinflammatory disease (*). Annu Rev Immunol 2009; 27:621–68.
2. Jansson A, Renner ED, Ramer J, et al. Classification of non-bacterial osteitis: retrospective study of clinical, immunological and genetic aspects in 89 patients. Rheumatology (Oxford) 2007;46:154–60.
3. Girschick HJ, Zimmer C, Klaus G, et al. Chronic recurrent multifocal osteomyelitis: what is it and how should it be treated? Nat Clin Pract Rheumatol 2007;3: 733–8.
4. Jansson AF, Müller TH, Gliere L, et al. Clinical score for nonbacterial osteitis in children and adults. Arthritis Rheum 2009;60:1152–9.
5. Borzutzky A, Stern S, Reiff A, et al. Pediatric chronic nonbacterial osteomyelitis. Pediatrics 2012;130:e1190–7.
6. Catalano-Pons C, Comte A, Wipff J, et al. Clinical outcome in children with chronic recurrent multifocal osteomyelitis. Rheumatology (Oxford) 2008;47:1397–9.
7. Giedion A, Holthusen W, Masel LF, et al. Subacute and chronic "symmetrical" osteomyelitis. Ann Radiol (Paris) 1972;15:329–42.
8. Probst FP, Bjorksten B, Gustavson KH. Radiological aspect of chronic recurrent multifocal osteomyelitis. Ann Radiol (Paris) 1978;21:115–25.
9. Girschick HJ, Raab P, Surbaum S, et al. Chronic non-bacterial osteomyelitis in children. Ann Rheum Dis 2005;64:279–85.
10. Gikas PD, Islam L, Aston W, et al. Nonbacterial osteitis: a clinical, histopathological, and imaging study with a proposal for protocol-based management of patients with this diagnosis. J Orthop Sci 2009;14:505–16.
11. Beretta-Piccoli BC, Sauvain MJ, Gal I, et al. Synovitis, acne, pustulosis, hyperostosis, osteitis (SAPHO) syndrome in childhood: a report of ten cases and review of the literature. Eur J Pediatr 2000;159:594–601.
12. Schilling F, Wagner AD. Azithromycin: an anti-inflammatory effect in chronic recurrent multifocal osteomyelitis? A preliminary report. Z Rheumatol 2000;59: 352–3.
13. Edlund E, Johnsson U, Lidgren L, et al. Palmoplantar pustulosis and sternocostoclavicular arthro-osteitis. Ann Rheum Dis 1988;47:809–15.
14. Hofmann SR, Schwarz T, Möller JC, et al. Chronic non-bacterial osteomyelitis is associated with impaired Sp1 signaling, reduced IL10 promoter phosphorylation, and reduced myeloid IL-10 expression. Clin Immunol 2011;141: 317–27.
15. Hofmann SR, Morbach H, Schwarz T, et al. Attenuated TLR4/MAPK signaling in monocytes from patients with CRMO results in impaired IL-10 expression. Clin Immunol 2012;145:69–76.
16. Hofmann SR, Roesen-Wolff A, Hahn G, et al. Update: cytokine dysregulation in chronic nonbacterial osteomyelitis (CNO). Int J Rheumatol 2012;2012: 310206.
17. Ferguson PJ, Chen S, Tayeh MK, et al. Homozygous mutations in LPIN2 are responsible for the syndrome of chronic recurrent multifocal osteomyelitis and congenital dyserythropoietic anaemia (Majeed syndrome). J Med Genet 2005; 42:551–7.

18. Aksentijevich I, Masters SL, Ferguson PJ, et al. An autoinflammatory disease with deficiency of the interleukin-1-receptor antagonist. N Engl J Med 2009; 360:2426–37.
19. Reddy S, Jia S, Geoffrey R, et al. An autoinflammatory disease due to homozygous deletion of the IL1RN locus. N Engl J Med 2009;360:2438–44.
20. Ferguson PJ, Bing X, Vasef MA, et al. A missense mutation in pstpip2 is associated with the murine autoinflammatory disorder chronic multifocal osteomyelitis. Bone 2006;38:41–7.
21. Grosse J, Chitu V, Marquardt A, et al. Mutation of mouse Mayp/Pstpip2 causes a macrophage autoinflammatory disease. Blood 2006;107:3350–8.
22. Yeung YG, Soldera S, Stanley ER. A novel macrophage actin-associated protein (MAYP) is tyrosine-phosphorylated following colony stimulating factor-1 stimulation. J Biol Chem 1998;273:30638–42.
23. Wu Y, Dowbenko D, Lasky LA. PSTPIP 2, a second tyrosine phosphorylated, cytoskeletal-associated protein that binds a PEST-type protein-tyrosine phosphatase. J Biol Chem 1998;273:30487–96.
24. Shoham NG, Centola M, Mansfield E, et al. Pyrin binds the PSTPIP1/CD2BP1 protein, defining familial Mediterranean fever and PAPA syndrome as disorders in the same pathway. Proc Natl Acad Sci U S A 2003;100:13501–6.
25. Golla A, Jansson A, Ramser J, et al. Chronic recurrent multifocal osteomyelitis (CRMO): evidence for a susceptibility gene located on chromosome 18q21.3-18q22. Eur J Hum Genet 2002;10:217–21.
26. Beck C, Morbach H, Beer M, et al. Chronic nonbacterial Osteomyelitis in childhood: prospective follow-up during the first year of anti-inflammatory treatment. Arthritis Res Ther 2010;12:R74.
27. Morbach H, Dick A, Beck C, et al. Association of chronic non-bacterial osteomyelitis with Crohn's disease but not with CARD15 gene variants. Rheumatol Int 2010;30:617–21.
28. Khanna G, Sato TS, Ferguson P. Imaging of chronic recurrent multifocal osteomyelitis. Radiographics 2009;29:1159–77.
29. Mandell GA, Contreras SJ, Conard K, et al. Bone scintigraphy in the detection of chronic recurrent multifocal osteomyelitis. J Nucl Med 1998;39:1778–83.
30. Wipff J, Adamsbaum C, Kahan A, et al. Chronic recurrent multifocal osteomyelitis. Joint Bone Spine 2011;78:555–60.
31. Fritz J, Tzaribatchev N, Claussen CD, et al. Chronic recurrent multifocal osteomyelitis: comparison of whole-body MR imaging with radiography and correlation with clinical and laboratory data. Radiology 2009;252:842–51.
32. Jurik AG, Egund N. MRI in chronic recurrent multifocal osteomyelitis. Skeletal Radiol 1997;26:230–8.
33. Guérin-Pfyffer S, Guillaume-Czitrom S, Tammam S, et al. Evaluation of chronic recurrent multifocal osteitis in children by whole-body magnetic resonance imaging. Joint Bone Spine 2012;79:616–20.
34. Sato TS, Ferguson PJ, Khanna G. Primary multifocal osseous lymphoma in a child. Pediatr Radiol 2008;38:1338–41.
35. Ferguson PJ, El-Shanti HI. Autoinflammatory bone disorders. Curr Opin Rheumatol 2007;19:492–8.
36. Abril JC, Ramirez A. Successful treatment of chronic recurrent multifocal osteomyelitis with indomethacin: a preliminary report of five cases. J Pediatr Orthop 2007;27:587–91.
37. Twilt M, Laxer RM. Clinical care of children with sterile bone inflammation. Curr Opin Rheumatol 2011;23:424–31.

38. Eleftheriou D, Gerschman T, Sebire N, et al. Biologic therapy in refractory chronic non-bacterial osteomyelitis in childhood. Rheumatology (Oxford) 2010;49:1505–12.

39. Deutschmann A, Mache CJ, Bodo K, et al. Successful treatment of chronic recurrent multifocal Osteomyelitis with tumor necrosis factor-alpha blockage. Pediatrics 2005;116:1231–3.

40. Marangoni RG, Halpern AS. Chronic recurrent multifocal osteomyelitis primarily affecting the spine treated with anti-TNF therapy. Spine (Phila Pa 1976) 2010;35: E253–6.

41. Simm PJ, Allen RC, Zacharin MR. Bisphosphonate treatment in chronic recurrent multifocal osteomyelitis. J Pediatr 2008;152:571–5.

42. Gleeson H, Wiltshire E, Briody J, et al. Childhood chronic recurrent multifocal osteomyelitis: pamidronate therapy decreases pain and improves vertebral shape. J Rheumatol 2008;35:707–12.

43. Miettunen PM, Wei X, Kaura D, et al. Dramatic pain relief and resolution of bone inflammation following pamidronate in 9 pediatric patients with persistent chronic recurrent multifocal osteomyelitis (CRMO). Pediatr Rheumatol Online J 2009;7:2.

44. Hospach T, Langendoerfer M, von Kalle T, et al. Spinal involvement in chronic recurrent multifocal osteomyelitis (CRMO) in childhood and effect of pamidronate. Eur J Pediatr 2010;169:1105–11.

45. Majeed HA, Kalaawi M, Mohanty D, et al. Congenital dyserythropoietic anemia and chronic recurrent multifocal osteomyelitis in three related children and the association with Sweet syndrome in two siblings. J Pediatr 1989;115:730–4.

46. Majeed HA, Al-Tarawna M, El-Shanti H, et al. The syndrome of chronic recurrent multifocal osteomyelitis and congenital dyserythropoietic anaemia. Report of a new family and a review. Eur J Pediatr 2001;160:705–10.

47. Ferguson PJ, Sandu M. Current understanding of the pathogenesis and management of chronic recurrent multifocal osteomyelitis. Curr Rheumatol Rep 2012;14:130–41.

48. Al-Mosawi ZS, Al-Saad KK, Ijadi-Maghsoodi R, et al. A splice site mutation confirms the role of LPIN2 in Majeed syndrome. Arthritis Rheum 2007;56:960–4.

49. Donkor J, Zhang P, Wong S, et al. A conserved serine residue is required for the phosphatidate phosphatase activity but not the transcriptional coactivator functions of lipin-1 and lipin-2. J Biol Chem 2009;284:29968–78.

50. Donkor J, Sariahmetoglu M, Dewald J, et al. Three mammalian lipins act as phosphatidate phosphatases with distinct tissue expression patterns. J Biol Chem 2007;282:3450–7.

51. Herlin T, Fiirgaard B, Bjerre M, et al. Efficacy of anti-IL-1 treatment in Majeed syndrome. Ann Rheum Dis 2013;72:410–3.

52. Valdearcos M, Esquinas E, Meana C, et al. Lipin-2 reduces proinflammatory signaling induced by saturated fatty acids in macrophages. J Biol Chem 2012;287:10894–904.

53. Jesus AA, Osman M, Silva CA, et al. A novel mutation of IL1RN in the deficiency of interleukin-1 receptor antagonist syndrome: description of two unrelated cases from Brazil. Arthritis Rheum 2011;63:4007–17.

54. Altiok E, Aksoy F, Perk Y, et al. A novel mutation in the interleukin-1 receptor antagonist associated with intrauterine disease onset. Clin Immunol 2012;145:77–81.

55. Schnellbacher C, Ciocca G, Menendez R, et al. Deficiency of interleukin-1 receptor antagonist responsive to anakinra. Pediatr Dermatol 2012. [Epub ahead of print].

56. Prose NS, Fahrner LJ, Miller CR, et al. Pustular psoriasis with chronic recurrent multifocal osteomyelitis and spontaneous fractures. J Am Acad Dermatol 1994; 31:376–9.

57. Stenerson M, Dufendach K, Aksentijevich I, et al. The first reported case of compound heterozygous IL1RN mutations causing deficiency of the interleukin-1 receptor antagonist. Arthritis Rheum 2011;63:4018–22.

58. Ter Haar N, Lachmann H, Ozen S, et al. Treatment of autoinflammatory diseases: results from the Eurofever Registry and a literature review. Ann Rheum Dis 2013; 72(5):678–85.

59. Ueki Y, Tiziani V, Santanna C, et al. Mutations in the gene encoding c-Abl-binding protein SH3BP2 cause cherubism. Nat Genet 2001;28:125–6.

60. Tiziani V, Reichenberger E, Buzzo CL, et al. The gene for cherubism maps to chromosome 4p16. Am J Hum Genet 1999;65:158–66.

61. Jones WA, Gerrie J, Pritchard J. Cherubism: familial fibrous dysplasia of the jaws. J Bone Joint Surg Br 1950;32-B:334–47.

62. Mangion J, Rahman N, Edkins S, et al. The gene for cherubism maps to chromosome 4p16.3. Am J Hum Genet 1999;65:151–7.

63. Reichenberger EJ, Levine MA, Olsen BR, et al. The role of SH3BP2 in the pathophysiology of cherubism. Orphanet J Rare Dis 2012;7:S5.

64. Hero M, Suomalainen A, Hagström J, et al. Anti-tumor necrosis factor treatment in cherubism–clinical, radiological and histological findings in two children. Bone 2013;52:347–53.

65. Pagnini I, Simonini G, Mortilla M, et al. Ineffectiveness of tumor necrosis factor-alpha inhibition in association with bisphosphonates for the treatment of cherubism. Clin Exp Rheumatol 2011;29:147.

66. Chamot AM, Benhamou CL, Kahn MF, et al. Acne-pustulosis-hyperostosis-osteitis syndrome: results of a national survey. 85 cases. Rev Rhum Mal Osteoartic 1987;54:187–96.

67. Benhamou CL, Chamot AM, Kahn MF. Synovitis-acne-pustulosis hyperostosis-osteomyelitis syndrome (SAPHO): a new syndrome among the spondyloarthropathies? Clin Exp Rheumatol 1988;6:109–12.

68. Hurtado-Nedelec M, Chollet-Martin S, Chapeton D, et al. Genetic susceptibility factors in a cohort of 38 patients with SAPHO syndrome: a study of PSTPIP2, NOD2, and LPIN2 genes. J Rheumatol 2010;37:401–9.

69. Ferguson PJ, Lokuta MA, El-Shanti HI, et al. Neutrophil dysfunction in a family with a SAPHO syndrome-like phenotype. Arthritis Rheum 2008;58:3264–9.

70. Hurtado-Nedelec M, Chollet-Martin S, Nicaise-Roland P, et al. Characterization of the immune response in the synovitis, acne, pustulosis, hyperostosis, osteitis (SAPHO) syndrome. Rheumatology (Oxford) 2008;47:1160–7.

71. Ben Abdelghani K, Dran DG, Gottenberg JE, et al. Tumor necrosis factor-alpha blockers in SAPHO syndrome. J Rheumatol 2010;37:1699–704.

72. Kerrison C, Davidson JE, Cleary AG, et al. Pamidronate in the treatment of childhood SAPHO syndrome. Rheumatology (Oxford) 2004;43:1246–51.

73. Kadom N, Egloff A, Obeid G, et al. Juvenile mandibular chronic osteomyelitis: multimodality imaging findings. Oral Surg Oral Med Oral Pathol Oral Radiol Endod 2011;111:e38–43.

Treatment of Juvenile Idiopathic Arthritis in the Biologic Age

Matthew L. Stoll, MD, PhD, MSCS*, Randy Q. Cron, MD, PhD

KEYWORDS

- Juvenile idiopathic arthritis • Treatment • Biologic therapy • Randomized trials

KEY POINTS

- Juvenile idiopathic arthritis (JIA) is a heterogeneous group of diseases, with potentially different treatment responses among the varying categories.
- Methotrexate continues to be widely used and effective in the management of JIA.
- Interleukin-1 and Interleukin-6 blockade are both highly effective in children with systemic JIA (sJIA).
- With the exception of sJIA, children with all categories of JIA generally respond well to tumor necrosis factor (TNF) inhibition; certain complications of JIA (uveitis and inflammatory bowel disease) respond better to anti-TNF monoclonal antibodies than to etanercept.
- Abatacept is safe and effective in children with polyarticular JIA, and may also have a role in the management of uveitis.
- Rituximab may be effective in JIA, although its precise role remains undefined.

SUBTYPES OF JUVENILE IDIOPATHIC ARTHRITIS

Juvenile idiopathic arthritis (JIA) is a heterogeneous group, currently parsed into 7 distinct subtypes.[1] Although a discussion of the clinical and pathophysiologic differences between the subtypes is beyond the scope of this review, a brief discussion of them is in order. It is likely that many of the JIA subtypes are genetically and pathophysiologically distinct, and may respond differently to the therapies currently available.

Oligoarticular

Oligoarticular JIA (oJIA) typically has onset in early childhood, with a peak age at onset of 2 to 3 years.[2] Most patients are female and antinuclear antibody (ANA)

Disclosures: None.
Department of Pediatrics, University of Alabama at Birmingham, CPP N210M, 1600 7th Avenue South, Birmingham, AL 35233, USA
* Corresponding author.
E-mail address: mstoll@peds.uab.edu

positive, with an increased risk of asymptomatic uveitis.[2] Some of these patients will never develop more than 5 involved joints and are thus said to have persistent oJIA; if 5 or more joints develop after at least 6 months of disease, the child is diagnosed with extended oJIA.

RF⁻ Polyarticular

Rheumatoid factor (RF)⁻ polyarticular JIA (pJIA) is diagnosed if a child has at least 5 involved joints within the first 6 months of disease, and if a test for RF is negative. This heterogeneous group includes children with similar demographic and clinical features as oJIA, as well as children with a symmetric course similar phenotypically to RF⁺ disease. About 50% of these children test positive for ANA, and it has been argued that this ANA-positive subgroup of children with RF⁻ pJIA, oJIA, and psoriatic JIA (psJIA; see later discussion) constitutes a homogeneous group.[2]

RF⁺ Polyarticular

Diagnosis of RF⁺ pJIA requires only 5 swollen joints, plus at least 2 positive tests for RF 3 months apart within the first 6 months of the disease. In practice, meeting the serologic requirements within the specified time frame is often the most challenging aspect of diagnosis, given delays in referral. Clinically, these patients typically have far more than 5 affected joints, as they resemble their adult counterparts diagnosed with rheumatoid arthritis (RA).[3] The similarities extend to shared genetics, additional laboratory studies, and extra-articular complications.[3]

Psoriatic JIA

Diagnosis of psJIA requires frank psoriasis in the context of a child with arthritis, or the presence of 2 or more psoriatic-like findings, namely nail pits, dactylitis, and positive family history in a first-degree relative (in the absence of exclusion criteria).[1] psJIA is a heterogeneous group, consisting of an early-onset cohort similar clinically to children with early-onset oJIA and pJIA; and a late-onset group that is more similar to adults with psoriatic arthritis (PsA) and to other children with spondyloarthritis (SpA).[4]

Enthesitis-Related Arthritis

Enthesitis-related arthritis (ERA) constitutes juvenile SpA and best corresponds to the undifferentiated SpA category used in adult classification systems. Although it is rare for children to have frank ankylosis, many of these children have SpA features, including male predominance, enthesitis, evidence of sacroiliitis on magnetic resonance imaging, and positive test for HLA-B27.[5]

Systemic JIA

Systemic JIA (sJIA) is defined by occurrence of systemic features, including high spiking fevers, rash, hepatosplenomegaly, lymphadenopathy, and serositis. Laboratory testing often reveals markedly elevated inflammatory markers, although some of the laboratory values can become spuriously normal in the setting of macrophage activation syndrome (MAS).[6] Although arthritis is required for diagnosis as per the International League of Associations for Rheumatology (ILAR) criteria,[1] it is not uncommon for the systemic features to predominate at first, before or simultaneously with the onset of arthritis.[7]

Undifferentiated Arthritis

Undifferentiated arthritis is not a single diagnosis, but rather reflects a catch-all category of children who do not meet any or who meet 2 or more of the other ILAR categories.[1] Examples include a child with clear features of sJIA, who has a parent with psoriasis; a child with RF+ pJIA who, owing to referral delays, did not have 2 separate positive tests for RF within 6 months of onset of disease; and a child with both HLA-B27–positive axial spondyloarthritis and psoriasis. Because of its evident heterogeneity, this category is not discussed further herein.

OVERVIEW OF TRIAL DESIGNS

Conventional randomized controlled trials (RCTs), including all of the studies in the prebiologic era, were designed such that children were randomized to receive study drug versus active or placebo comparator for a prespecified duration. At the end of the study period, the primary outcome is assessed (**Fig. 1**A). In most recent pediatric rheumatology studies, the primary outcome is a composite outcome of the pediatric American College of Rheumatology (pACR) core set of domains: physician global assessment of disease activity, parent/patient assessment of overall well-being, functional ability, number of joints with active arthritis, number of joints with limited range of motion, and an inflammatory marker.[8] Specifically, a typical primary outcome is a pACR-30 response, which by definition requires at least 30% improvement in at least 3 domains with at least 30% worsening in no more than 1 domain.

More recently, a study design was introduced to the field that maintains the randomization process in a controlled setting, but avoids exposure to placebo for prolonged periods of time (**Fig. 1**B). In these withdrawal trials, all subjects are initially treated with active therapy. Subsequently, those who respond to the therapy in the open-label portion of the study, typically with at least a pACR-30 response, are then carried forward into the randomized, blinded portion of the study, in which children are randomized to active drug versus placebo. Once a child flares, he or she is

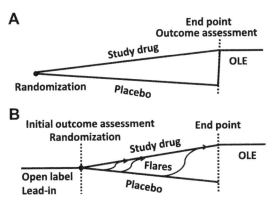

Fig. 1. Designs for randomized controlled trials in pediatric rheumatology. In the standard trial design (*A*), all subjects who meet inclusion criteria are randomized to receive placebo versus active drug. After a predetermined period of time (eg, 24 weeks), the subjects in the two arms are compared. The alternative design (*B*) starts with an open-label lead-in period, in which all enrollees receive active drug. After a predetermined period of time, subjects with at least an adequate response to the study drug are invited to participate in the double-blind portion of the study, in which subjects are randomized to either remain on the study drug or switch to placebo. The end point occurs at either the initial flare or after a predetermined period. Any subject on the placebo arm who achieves the end point, including a flare, is automatically switched to the active drug arm. Both study designs often have an open-label extension (OLE), from which additional safety information is obtained.

then removed from the controlled portion of the study and is offered the drug open-label. The outcome is either the percentage of subjects in both groups who flare over a specific period of time (eg, 24 weeks), or the time to flare. Although this study design avoids long-term exposure to placebo in subjects other than those who maintain a good response to the placebo agent, it is open to criticism on the grounds that the only children who are randomized are those who show an initial response; furthermore, interpretation of the safety data in the control arm is clouded by prior receipt of the study drug.[9]

TREATMENT OF JIA
Nonsteroidal Anti-Inflammatory Drugs

Once start of the art, current recommendations give scant emphasis to nonsteroidal anti-inflammatory drug (NSAID) therapy.[10] Specifically, NSAIDs were recommended for children with oJIA absent of any poor prognostic features for a limited trial period of 1 to 2 months, and were considered to be of uncertain benefit as monotherapy in any other context. Their role in SpA remains unclear, as they seem to be the only therapeutic class that can prevent progression of ankylosis among patients with established ankylosing spondylitis.[11] Whether these findings apply to pediatric patients, in whom frank ankylosing spondylitis is rare, is a matter of conjuncture.

Corticosteroids

Like NSAIDs, oral corticosteroids (CS) were once given a prominent place on the treatment paradigm, but current guidelines are silent on their use.[10] Adverse events associated with long-term oral CS use are well recognized, although no studies have demonstrated lasting benefit.

Unlike oral CS, intra-articular CS injections (IACI) play a prominent role in the management of children with JIA. IACI are recommended as initial therapy in children with oJIA,[10] as nearly 50% of such injections can result in remission lasting at least 1 year.[12] Among the IACI preparations, triamcinolone hexacetonide has been shown to result in longer-lasting remission compared with triamcinolone acetonide[13]; however, on a patient level, no consistent predictors identify patients who are likely to respond to local therapy alone.[12] IACI may also be of benefit in selected cases as adjunctive therapy, among patients who are currently receiving systemic immunosuppression. Even in the context of systemic immunosuppression, adjunctive IACI may be preferred by the patient because of the rapid onset of symptomatic relief. Furthermore, in some cases, particularly with the temporomandibular joint, active arthritis can persist even in otherwise quiescent disease and despite aggressive use of systemic therapy for arthritis.[14]

Conventional Disease-Modifying Antirheumatic Drugs
Methotrexate

Methotrexate (MTX) remains the most widely used conventional disease-modifying antirheumatic drug (DMARD) in the management of JIA.[15] It is standard concurrent therapy in most of the trials involving biological therapies in children with JIA. Current guidelines recommend its use in children with oJIA refractory to NSAIDs or IACI, as well as in children with pJIA and sJIA complicated by active arthritis; its role in ERA remains unclear.[10] MTX can be given both orally and subcutaneously, with the latter potentially of greater benefit.[16] MTX is typically well tolerated by children, with most of the adverse events affecting the gastrointestinal tract; monitoring of blood counts and liver tests is required.[10]

Sulfasalazine

Like MTX, sulfasalazine (SSZ) has been used for decades in the management of inflammatory arthritis.[16] SSZ has never been compared head-to-head with MTX in treating JIA. However, indirect comparisons show that MTX appears to be better tolerated and may be more effective in most patients without spondyloarthritis.[17] Current guidelines support its use in ERA but not in other types of JIA.[10] In particular, SSZ should probably be avoided in children with sJIA.[18]

Leflunomide

Leflunomide (LEF) appears to be infrequently used in JIA. There are no placebo-controlled trials; a head-to-head comparison with MTX showed them to have roughly equal efficacy and tolerability.[19] A significant safety concern with LEF is that it is teratogenic and undergoes enterohepatic circulation for up to 2 years,[20] a combination of factors that make it less desirable in many pediatric patients. Its current role in the management of JIA is uncertain.[10]

Biologics

Overview

To date, there have been 15 RCTs of biologics in the treatment of children with JIA **(Table 1)**. For the most part, the trials, along with data from large registries, have confirmed what is evident in practice. These therapies have revolutionized the management of JIA, and have given a generation of children a possibility unimaginable as recently as 20 years ago: the chance of a normal childhood.[21–39]

Biologics as a group are generally defined as large, complex molecules that require some type of living organism for their synthesis.[40] There are several different types of drug designs **(Fig. 2)**, one of which consists of soluble receptor antagonists; this category includes etanercept, rilonacept, and abatacept. All 3 of these medicines are fusion proteins consisting of a soluble receptor to a proinflammatory cytokine or cell-surface molecule, fused to the human immunoglobulin G (IgG) Fc portion to stabilize it in the circulation. Because these drugs bind effectively to the target protein but lack downstream signaling, they serve as decoy receptors, thus downregulating immunologic responses. A second major design type consists of monoclonal antibodies directed against either a specific cytokine (eg, interleukin [IL]-1β for canakinumab, TNF for adalimumab and infliximab) or a specific cell-surface protein (eg, IL-6 receptor for tocilizumab, CD20 for rituximab). In the case of rituximab, the result is depletion of cells bearing the target protein. Finally, the drug anakinra merits its own category, as it is virtually identical to an endogenously produced anti-inflammatory protein (see later discussion).

The monoclonal antibodies are either fully or partially humanized. If a bench scientist were to inject TNF into a laboratory animal and collect polyclonal antibodies from the serum or even monoclonal antibodies from the spleen, this preparation would have very limited therapeutic effectiveness and tolerability in humans. Such ineffectiveness and intolerability would be due to neutralizing antibodies in the human recipients, leading to limited half-life, serum sickness, and anaphylaxis. Thus all of the monoclonal antibodies consist of a human Fc region, fused to the therapeutic Fab segment. Furthermore, even chimeric molecules containing animal-derived Fab regions can be immunogenic, so several of the agents are fully humanized.

TNF inhibitors: etanercept and monoclonal antibodies

Three TNF inhibitors, namely adalimumab, etanercept, and infliximab, have been extensively used in children with JIA, although only adalimumab and etanercept have been approved by the Food and Drug Administration (FDA) for that purpose. Etanercept

Table 1
RCTs of biologics in JIA

Authors,[Ref.] Year	Study Drug	Study Population	Primary Outcome	Outcome Met?
Lovell et al,[25] 2000	Etanercept	Polyarticular-course JIA	Disease flare by 4 mo	Yes
Smith et al,[26] 2005	Etanercept	JIA with uveitis	Improved uveitis at 6 mo	No
Ruperto et al,[27] 2007	Infliximab	Polyarticular-course JIA	pACR-30 at 14 wk	No
Lovell et al,[29] 2008	Adalimumab	Polyarticular-course JIA	Disease flare by 32 wk	Yes
Ruperto et al,[28] 2008	Abatacept	Polyarticular-course JIA	Time to flare	Yes
Yokota et al,[30] 2008	Tocilizumab	sJIA	Maintenance of pACR-30 response and low CRP	Yes
Ilowite et al,[31] 2009	Anakinra	pJIA	Disease flare by 16 wk[a]	No
Quartier et al,[32] 2011	Anakinra	sJIA	pACR-30, absence of fever, 50% decrease (or normalization) of inflammatory markers	Yes
De Benedetti et al,[36] 2012	Tocilizumab	sJIA	pACR-30, absence of fever	Yes
Tynjala et al,[33] 2011	Infliximab[b]	pJIA	pACR-75 at 54 wk	Yes
Horneff et al,[34] 2012	Adalimumab	Juvenile AS	ASAS-40 at 12 wk	No
Ruperto et al,[37] 2012	Canakinumab	sJIA	pACR-30 at 15 d	Yes
Ruperto et al,[37] 2012	Canakinumab	sJIA	Time to flare	Yes
Wallace et al,[35] 2012	Etanercept[c]	pJIA	Clinically inactive disease at 6 mo	No
Brunner et al,[39] 2012	Tocilizumab	pJIA	Disease flare by 40 wk	Yes

Abbreviations: AS, ankylosing spondylitis; ASAS, Assessment of SpondyloArthritis international Society response criteria; CRP, C-reactive protein; JIA, juvenile idiopathic arthritis; pJIA, polyarticular JIA; pACR, pediatric American College of Rheumatology response; sJIA, systemic JIA.

[a] Owing to poor enrollment, the primary outcome was switched from efficacy to safety analysis; the safety outcome was met.

[b] Tynjala study: infliximab + methotrexate (MTX) is compared with MTX alone and with MTX + sulfasalazine + hydroxychloroquine.

[c] Wallace study: etanercept + prednisone + MTX is compared with placebo + MTX.

is a fusion protein consisting of the extracellular ligand-binding domain of the p75 TNF receptor, linked to the Fc portion of human IgG1.[41] By contrast, adalimumab and infliximab are monoclonal antibodies against TNF: the former is fully humanized, whereas the latter has murine components to the variable region.[41]

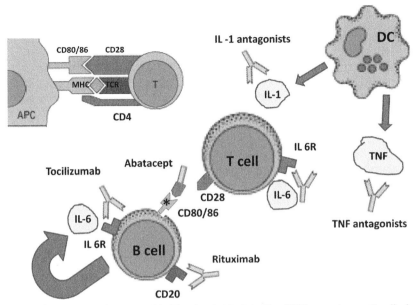

Fig. 2. Medications used to treat JIA. Rituximab binds to the CD20 receptor on B cells, leading to depletion. Tocilizumab blocks the interaction between interleukin (IL)-6 and its receptor, preventing downstream signaling. Abatacept blocks T-cell/B-cell costimulation. As a class, the tumor necrosis factor (TNF) and IL-1 antagonists block TNF and IL-1, respectively. For both TNF and IL-1 inhibition, the specific agents vary in their mechanisms of action. See the text for details.

Effectiveness Data from several large registries have shown TNF inhibitors to be safe and effective in the management of JIA; combined, these studies included 1669 children followed for 1 to 6 years (**Table 2**).[21–24,38,42,43] This efficacy has been borne out in several RCTs. Specifically, Lovell and colleagues[25] enrolled 69 subjects with a polyarticular-course JIA, of whom 51 obtained a pACR-30 response in the 12-week open-label portion of the study and were randomized to receive etanercept versus placebo for up to 4 months, thus constituting the first published withdrawal study in pediatric rheumatology. Over the 4-month study, withdrawals because of flare were observed in significantly fewer patients treated with etanercept compared with placebo. Similar results were obtained in a withdrawal study evaluating adalimumab in

Table 2			
Registries of TNF inhibitors in JIA			
Country of Origin	**Authors,[Ref.] Year**	**N**	**Duration of Follow-Up (y)**
France	Quartier et al,[43] 2003	61	1
Germany	Horneff et al,[38] 2004	322	4
Netherlands	Prince et al,[23] 2009	146	2.5
USA/Canada	Giannini et al,[24] 2009	397	3
Hungary	Sevcic et al,[22] 2011	72	1
Poland	Zuber et al,[21] 2011	188	2 (effectiveness); 6 (safety)
United Kingdom	Southwood et al,[42] 2011	483	941 patient-years

children with JIA.[29] Of note, the single placebo-controlled RCT of infliximab failed to meet its primary aim of a significantly higher American College of Rheumatology (ACR)-30 response at 14 weeks, although the infliximab-treated patients did have a significantly lower swollen joint count than the placebo-treated patients.[27] However, a more recent study comparing infliximab and MTX with either MTX alone or triple therapy (MTX, SSZ, hydroxychloroquine) showed that over a period of 54 weeks, using an ambitious end point of a pACR-75 response, infliximab plus MTX was superior to both other treatment arms; this end point was met by all 19 patients in the infliximab group, compared with 10 of 20 (50%) in the MTX arm and 13 of 20 (65%) of those on combination DMARD therapy (P<.0001).[33] Thus most practitioners consider all 3 agents to be viable options, with the choice of first therapy dictated by factors such as insurance coverage, patient convenience, and safety. In addition, the monoclonal antibodies appear to be more effective in the management of particular granulomatous complications of JIA, such as uveitis[44] and inflammatory bowel disease,[45] and are thus preferred in such contexts.

As reflected in the study design of most of the RCTs involving TNF inhibitors in children with pJIA, most practitioners combine TNF inhibitors with MTX or other nonbiological DMARDs, when tolerated. Data from the German etanercept registry supports this practice, as children taking etanercept plus MTX demonstrated improved treatment responses in comparison with those taking etanercept alone, without an increase in adverse events.[46] The RCT of adalimumab in children with JIA compared adalimumab-treated subjects who were on baseline MTX with adalimumab-treated subjects not on baseline MTX, finding a slightly but not statistically significant improved treatment response among those patients on baseline MTX.[29] There are no randomized studies in children comparing TNF inhibitors as monotherapy versus combination treatment consisting of TNF inhibitors and conventional DMARDs, nor are there any data supporting combinations of TNF inhibitors with additional biologics.

The usefulness of dose escalation in children who have had an incomplete response to standard doses is a matter of debate. There are no reports of dose escalation of etanercept in JIA. However, a study of Greek children with pJIA reported 7 children who had improved responses to weekly compared with biweekly dosing of adalimumab.[47] Infliximab doses as high as 20 mg/kg have been reported in children with JIA-associated uveitis.[48] In addition, Tambralli and colleagues[49] recently reported on 58 children with JIA who were treated with doses ranging from 10 to 20 mg/kg of infliximab, at intervals as close together as every 2 weeks. These high doses of infliximab were well tolerated and, at least in some cases, were more effective than standard doses. To the authors' knowledge, there are no published reports on the use of the relatively newer TNF inhibitors golimumab and certolizumab to treat the arthritis associated with JIA, although there is also no obvious theoretical reason that they should not work.

Mirroring the data in adults, TNF inhibitors have been shown to be effective in multiple different subtypes of JIA.[25,29,33] Most of the RCTs were in children with a polyarticular course, which can include oligoarticular and even systemic onset (see **Table 1**); children with psJIA, ERA, and sJIA with active systemic features have typically been excluded. However, several open-label studies have shown TNF inhibitors to be effective in pediatric SpA,[50] and a recent RCT showed promise, albeit the primary aim was not met.[34] There are no studies of TNF inhibitors in psJIA, although the improved outcomes of children in recent case series on comparison with older series may be attributable to the use of aggressive therapy, including TNF inhibitors.[51] The one category of JIA in which TNF inhibitors have been disappointing is sJIA; observational and controlled studies have shown that such patients respond less well to TNF inhibitors than those with pJIA (see **Fig. 2**).[25,38,43]

Safety Registry and trial data have shown TNF inhibitors to be safe in children with JIA.[21–35] In 2008, the FDA released a report of 48 children with a variety of underlying disorders who developed a malignancy while under treatment with a TNF inhibitor over a 10-year period.[52] This study has been criticized on methodological grounds, including failure to take into account background risk of underlying diseases plus concomitant therapies in some of the patients.[53] More recently, highly reassuring data have emerged from large database studies, comparing malignancy and infection rates in JIA patients treated with TNF inhibitors compared with those treated with conventional DMARDs or no therapy at all. In these studies, despite the inability to adjust for disease severity, no increased risk of infections or malignancy was detected among the patients treated with TNF inhibitors.[54,55]

Despite the overall reassuring safety profile, there have been case reports of serious infections and other adverse events in children taking TNF inhibitors, including septic arthritis, septic abscess, sepsis, tuberculosis, Hodgkin disease, onset of lupus, optic neuritis, and psoriasis.[41] Patients on such therapies therefore require close monitoring for potential complications.

Interleukin-1 inhibitors
IL-1 is a highly proinflammatory cytokine that appears to play a role in a variety of inflammatory conditions, following signaling through the IL-1 receptor.[56] The IL-1 receptor antagonist (IL-1Ra) is a naturally produced cytokine that bears substantial structural similarity to IL-1 but which, rather than activating through the receptor, serves as a competitive antagonist.[56] There are 3 commercially available IL-1 antagonists, all of which operate through different mechanisms. The first to be studied was anakinra, which save for a single amino acid substitution is structurally identical to the human IL-1Ra.[56] Rilonacept is a fusion protein containing the extracellular domain of the IL-1 receptor and the IL-1 receptor accessory protein attached to human IgG Fc. Because of its structure, rilonacept may also block the IL-1Ra, partially counteracting its anti-inflammatory properties. Canakinumab is a fully humanized monoclonal antibody directed against IL-1β,[56] and is now FDA-approved for sJIA.

Effectiveness A study of anakinra in children with polyarticular JIA did not reveal significant improvement.[31] However, anakinra has clearly found a place in the management of sJIA; a large case series has shown anakinra to be highly effective, often within days, in the management of the systemic features associated with sJIA, and also of benefit, although perhaps somewhat less so, in the articular features.[57] The efficacy of anakinra in sJIA was also borne out in a placebo-controlled trial in which 24 patients were randomized to anakinra versus placebo for a period of 1 month. In this study, outcome criteria included not only the pACR-30 response but also improvement in the C-reactive protein (CRP) and resolution of the systemic symptoms, and was met by 8 of 12 anakinra-treated patients versus 1 of 12 control subjects ($P = .003$).[32] Anakinra may be of particular benefit early in the disease course, when the systemic features are most prominent and the articular features less so; such was the observation of Nigrovic and colleagues,[57] who reported dramatic success in a cohort of 46 children treated with anakinra within the first few months of disease; in 15 cases, corticosteroids were avoided altogether. Dose escalation up to 10 mg/kg/d may be required in some cases.[58] Two separate but interrelated trials of canakinumab, one with a conventional design and the other with a withdrawal design, were recently published together.[37] In the first, subjects were randomized to receive canakinumab or placebo, with the primary outcome being an ACR-30 response plus absence of fever; this was met by 36 of 43 (84%) subjects treated with canakinumab, compared with 4 of

41 (10%) control subjects ($P<.001$). In the withdrawal study, which all of the subjects enrolled in the initial study were permitted to enter, the median time to flare was 236 days in the placebo group and was unmeasurable in the canakinumab group, owing to less than 50% of the subjects actually flaring ($P = .003$).[37] A trial of rilonacept in children with sJIA has yet to be published.

An emerging role for IL-1 inhibition is in the management of MAS, a potentially lethal complication of multiple rheumatic diseases, especially sJIA.[6] There is substantial clinical and laboratory overlap between features of MAS and of active sJIA,[6] so reported effectiveness of anakinra in the management of MAS secondary to sJIA comes as little surprise.[59]

Safety The overall safety data of IL-1 inhibition has been reassuring. Large RCTs of anakinra in adults with RA as well as smaller studies of anakinra and canakinumab in children with polyarticular or systemic JIA did not identify significantly increased risks of any type of serious adverse events.[31,32,37,57,60] Despite its overall reassuring safety profile, there have been scattered case reports of unusual or opportunistic infections in patients taking anakinra, including visceral leishmaniasis, multiple-organism sepsis, and tuberculosis reactivation.[41] Thus caution should be exercised, particularly because the underlying diseases for which anakinra is typically used share clinical features with serious infections, such as fever and lymphadenopathy.

Abatacept

Abatacept is a soluble fusion protein consisting of the cytotoxic T cell lymphocyte antigen 4 (CTLA-4) fused with the Fc region of human IgG.[61] The concept behind this molecule is that T cell activation generally requires 2 separate events: presentation of a peptide antigen by the major histocompatibility complex to the T cell receptor; and some form of costimulation involving binding of a ligand on an antigen-presenting cell (APC) to its cognate receptor on a T cell.[61] An important costimulatory molecule on APCs is the CD80/86 complex, which binds to CD28 as well as to CTLA-4 on T cells. Soluble CTLA-4-Ig (abatacept) binds to the CD80/86 complex, blocking costimulation via CD28.[61] It is approved for pJIA.

Effectiveness An RCT of abatacept in children with polyarticular-course JIA refractory to biological or nonbiological DMARDs was published in 2008.[28] In this study, 122 of 190 subjects completed the 4-month open-label period with a pACR-30 response, and were enrolled in the double-blind portion. For these, the median time to flare was 6 months for the placebo-treated patients and was unable to be assessed in the abatacept arm, owing to an insufficient number of events ($P = .0002$). The trial showed abatacept to be effective, meeting the primary aim of increased time to flare in comparison with placebo.[28] An additional important finding in the open-label arm was that patients who had received prior therapy with a TNF inhibitor were less likely to have attained pACR-30, -50, -70, and -90 responses, although statistical testing was not reported. Abatacept may also be of benefit in the management of uveitis associated with JIA,[62] albeit there are no prospective or controlled studies. Finally, there is a single report of effective combination therapy of anakinra with abatacept in the management of 4 children with refractory sJIA.[58]

Safety Trials in children with JIA[28] and adults with RA have shown abatacept to be well tolerated, with a meta-analysis of RCTs of adult studies that included both the double-blind and the open-label portions of the trials concluding that the overall risk of serious infections requiring hospitalizations among abatacept-treated RA patients is commensurate with that of RA patients taking nonbiological DMARDs.[63] A separate study indicated that abatacept appears to be associated with a lower risk of serious adverse events compared with other biologics.[64]

Tocilizumab

Like IL-1, IL-6 is a highly proinflammatory cytokine that helps mediate several features associated with chronic inflammation, including fever, anemia of chronic disease, elevated levels of acute-phase reactants, and fatigue.[65] A partially humanized antibody against the IL-6 receptor was first reported in 1993,[41] and now has indications for sJIA and pJIA.

Effectiveness The only published pediatric trials of tocilizumab are in children with sJIA. Two phase III placebo-controlled withdrawal trials demonstrated its efficacy.[30,36] In the study by Yokota and colleagues,[30] 56 children refractory to conventional DMARDs were recruited for the open-label lead-in portion of the study, of whom 51 achieved an pACR-30 response and 43 were recruited into the double-blind portion; of those, only 4 of 17 (23%) of the placebo-treated patients maintained a pACR-30 and a low CRP, compared with 16 of 20 (80%) in the tocilizumab group (P<.0001).[30] In the study by De Benedetti and colleagues,[36] 112 subjects were randomized to tocilizumab versus placebo for 12 weeks, with the primary aim of a pACR-30 response and absence of fever being met in 64 of 75 (85%) tocilizumab-treated patients, compared with 9 of 37 (24%) control patients (P<.0001). In addition, the 12-month open-label extension data published in the same report demonstrated substantial improvement in the arthritis as well as in the systemic symptoms. Radiographic improvement has also been reported with tocilizumab therapy.[66] A completed trial of tocilizumab in children with pJIA was presented at the 2012 American College of Rheumatology conference which, at the time of writing, has not yet been published.[39] In this withdrawal study, tocilizumab was administered open-label for 16 weeks to 188 subjects, of whom 166 entered the double-blind portion of the trial. Of these, over the 40-week double-blind portion of the trial, flares were reported in significantly more placebo-treated than tocilizumab-treated (48% vs 26%) subjects.

Safety Although tocilizumab has not overall been associated with an increased risk of infections in comparison with placebo,[64] there does appear to be an increased risk of both serious respiratory infections and gastrointestinal perforations, at least in adults.[67] Additional safety concerns in adult studies include lipid abnormalities and elevated liver function tests.[67] The latter has also been observed in the pediatric studies, as have lymphopenia, neutropenia, and gastrointestinal hemorrhage.[30,68] In addition, the study by De Benedetti and colleagues[36] did demonstrate an increased risk of total and serious infections in the children who received the study drug, including a case of fatal pneumococcal sepsis.

Rituximab

Rituximab is a chimeric monoclonal antibody directed against the human CD20 receptor, consisting of a human IgG1 heavy chain bound to a murine anti-CD20 antibody.[69] The mechanism of action is unclear; the simplistic explanation that it works by preventing pathogenic autoantibody production is belied by the variety of additional functions of B cells, including cytokine production and antigen presentation.

Effectiveness There are very few data regarding the use of rituximab to treat children with JIA. The largest study was a prospective uncontrolled study of 55 children with JIA, who were treated every 6 months as needed for disease flares and followed for up to 96 weeks, with remission occurring in 50% of cases at 1 year and in nearly 100% of the 25 children followed for the entire period.[70] Interestingly this study included a large number of subjects with sJIA, indicating that the mechanism of action may not be through prevention of autoantibody formation. Uveitis associated with JIA may also respond well to rituximab.[71]

Safety The most frequent adverse events are infusion reactions which, while typically minor, can result in anaphylaxis.[72] The risk of infections appears to be low in subjects with rheumatic diseases[64]; however, cases of progressive multifocal leukoencephalopathy, a nearly always fatal infection, have been reported following therapy with rituximab, albeit the overall risk appears to be low.[73] An additional noninfectious risk is interstitial lung disease, with a recent review reporting 121 such cases potentially attributable to rituximab.[74] The pediatric data are less extensive, but the safety profile also appears to be reassuring.[70]

SUMMARY

The last 15 years have witnessed an explosion of new therapeutic options for children with rheumatic diseases. Multiple studies have demonstrated that TNF inhibitors and abatacept are excellent options for children with pJIA and refractory oJIA, with the role of tocilizumab and rituximab unclear. TNF inhibitors clearly have an important role in the management of children with ERA; the potential utility of other classes of biologics in ERA is uncertain, owing to the absence of studies in children and the so far unimpressive data in adults. Although there are no trials limited to children with psJIA, and most other studies have excluded this subtype, there is every reason to be optimistic that TNF inhibitors will be effective; the roles of other classes of biologics also remain unclear.

Finally, physicians have excellent options for sJIA, the category that historically has resulted in the most severe morbidity and mortality,[75] with therapeutic targeting of both IL-1 and IL-6 signaling pathways demonstrating substantial promise. Thanks to novel biological therapies, children with JIA are no longer relegated to wheelchairs but rather are found running on soccer fields and basketball courts.

REFERENCES

1. Petty RE, Southwood TR, Manners P, et al. International League of Associations for Rheumatology classification of juvenile idiopathic arthritis: second revision, Edmonton, 2001. J Rheumatol 2004;31:390–2.
2. Ravelli A, Felici E, Magni-Manzoni S, et al. Patients with antinuclear antibody-positive juvenile idiopathic arthritis constitute a homogeneous subgroup irrespective of the course of joint disease. Arthritis Rheum 2005;52:826–32.
3. Tebo AE, Jaskowski T, Davis KW, et al. Profiling anti-cyclic citrullinated peptide antibodies in patients with juvenile idiopathic arthritis. Pediatr Rheumatol Online J 2012;10:29.
4. Stoll ML, Zurakowski D, Nigrovic LE, et al. Patients with juvenile psoriatic arthritis comprise two distinct populations. Arthritis Rheum 2006;54:3564–72.
5. Stoll ML, Bhore R, Dempsey-Robertson M, et al. Spondyloarthritis in a pediatric population: risk factors for sacroiliitis. J Rheumatol 2010;37:2402–8.
6. Ravelli A, Grom AA, Behrens EM, et al. Macrophage activation syndrome as part of systemic juvenile idiopathic arthritis: diagnosis, genetics, pathophysiology and treatment. Genes Immun 2012;13:289–98.
7. Behrens EM, Beukelman T, Gallo L, et al. Evaluation of the presentation of systemic onset juvenile rheumatoid arthritis: data from the Pennsylvania

Systemic Onset Juvenile Arthritis Registry (PASOJAR). J Rheumatol 2008;35: 343–8.

8. Giannini EH, Ruperto N, Ravelli A, et al. Preliminary definition of improvement in juvenile arthritis. Arthritis Rheum 1997;40:1202–9.

9. Lehman TJ. Are withdrawal trials in paediatric rheumatic disease helpful? Lancet 2008;372:348–50.

10. Beukelman T, Patkar NM, Saag KG, et al. 2011 American College of Rheumatology recommendations for the treatment of juvenile idiopathic arthritis: initiation and safety monitoring of therapeutic agents for the treatment of arthritis and systemic features. Arthritis Care Res (Hoboken) 2011;63:465–82.

11. Haroon N, Kim TH, Inman RD. NSAIDs and radiographic progression in ankylosing spondylitis. Bagging big game with small arms? Ann Rheum Dis 2012; 71:1593–5.

12. Gotte AC. Intra-articular corticosteroids in the treatment of juvenile idiopathic arthritis: safety, efficacy, and features affecting outcome. A comprehensive review of the literature. Open Access Rheumatol Res Rev 2009;1:37–49.

13. Zulian F, Martini G, Gobber D, et al. Triamcinolone acetonide and hexacetonide intra-articular treatment of symmetrical joints in juvenile idiopathic arthritis: a double-blind trial. Rheumatology (Oxford) 2004;43:1288–91.

14. Stoll ML, Sharpe T, Beukelman T, et al. Risk factors for temporomandibular joint arthritis in children with juvenile idiopathic arthritis. J Rheumatol 2012;39: 1880–7.

15. Beukelman T, Ringold S, Davis TE, et al. Disease-modifying antirheumatic drug use in the treatment of juvenile idiopathic arthritis: a cross-sectional analysis of the CARRA Registry. J Rheumatol 2012;39:1867–74.

16. Kemper AR, Van Mater HA, Coeytaux RR, et al. Systematic review of disease-modifying antirheumatic drugs for juvenile idiopathic arthritis. BMC Pediatr 2012;12:29.

17. Prieur AM, Quartier P. Comparative tolerability of treatments for juvenile idiopathic arthritis. BioDrugs 2000;14:159–83.

18. Brooks CD. Sulfasalazine for the management of juvenile rheumatoid arthritis. J Rheumatol 2001;28:845–53.

19. Silverman E, Mouy R, Spiegel L, et al. Leflunomide or methotrexate for juvenile rheumatoid arthritis. N Engl J Med 2005;352:1655–66.

20. Prakash A, Jarvis B. Leflunomide: a review of its use in active rheumatoid arthritis. Drugs 1999;58:1137–64.

21. Zuber Z, Rutkowska-Sak L, Postepski J, et al. Etanercept treatment in juvenile idiopathic arthritis: the Polish registry. Med Sci Monit 2011;17:SR35–42.

22. Sevcic K, Orban I, Brodszky V, et al. Experiences with tumour necrosis factor-{alpha} inhibitors in patients with juvenile idiopathic arthritis: Hungarian data from the National Institute of Rheumatology and Physiotherapy Registry. Rheumatology (Oxford) 2011;50:1337–40.

23. Prince FH, Twilt M, ten Cate R, et al. Long-term follow-up on effectiveness and safety of etanercept in juvenile idiopathic arthritis: the Dutch national register. Ann Rheum Dis 2009;68:635–41.

24. Giannini EH, Ilowite NT, Lovell DJ, et al. Long-term safety and effectiveness of etanercept in children with selected categories of juvenile idiopathic arthritis. Arthritis Rheum 2009;60:2794–804.

25. Lovell DJ, Giannini EH, Reiff A, et al. Etanercept in children with polyarticular juvenile rheumatoid arthritis. Pediatric Rheumatology Collaborative Study Group. N Engl J Med 2000;342:763–9.

26. Smith JA, Thompson DJ, Whitcup SM, et al. A randomized, placebo-controlled, double-masked clinical trial of etanercept for the treatment of uveitis associated with juvenile idiopathic arthritis. Arthritis Rheum 2005;53:18–23.

27. Ruperto N, Lovell DJ, Cuttica R, et al. A randomized, placebo-controlled trial of infliximab plus methotrexate for the treatment of polyarticular-course juvenile rheumatoid arthritis. Arthritis Rheum 2007;56:3096–106.

28. Ruperto N, Lovell DJ, Quartier P, et al. Abatacept in children with juvenile idiopathic arthritis: a randomised, double-blind, placebo-controlled withdrawal trial. Lancet 2008;372:383–91.

29. Lovell DJ, Ruperto N, Goodman S, et al. Adalimumab with or without methotrexate in juvenile rheumatoid arthritis. N Engl J Med 2008;359:810–20.

30. Yokota S, Imagawa T, Mori M, et al. Efficacy and safety of tocilizumab in patients with systemic-onset juvenile idiopathic arthritis: a randomised, double-blind, placebo-controlled, withdrawal phase III trial. Lancet 2008;371:998–1006.

31. Ilowite N, Porras O, Reiff A, et al. Anakinra in the treatment of polyarticular-course juvenile rheumatoid arthritis: safety and preliminary efficacy results of a randomized multicenter study. Clin Rheumatol 2009;28:129–37.

32. Quartier P, Allantaz F, Cimaz R, et al. A multicentre, randomised, double-blind, placebo-controlled trial with the interleukin-1 receptor antagonist anakinra in patients with systemic-onset juvenile idiopathic arthritis (ANAJIS trial). Ann Rheum Dis 2011;70:747–54.

33. Tynjala P, Vahasalo P, Tarkiainen M, et al. Aggressive combination drug therapy in very early polyarticular juvenile idiopathic arthritis (ACUTE-JIA): a multicentre randomised open-label clinical trial. Ann Rheum Dis 2011;70:1605–12.

34. Horneff G, Fitter S, Foeldvari I, et al. Double blind, placebo-controlled randomized trial with adalimumab for treatment of juvenile onset ankylosing spondylitis (JoAS): significant short term improvement. Arthritis Res Ther 2012;14:R230.

35. Wallace CA, Giannini EH, Spalding SJ, et al. Trial of early aggressive therapy in polyarticular juvenile idiopathic arthritis. Arthritis Rheum 2012;64:2012–21.

36. De Benedetti F, Brunner HI, Ruperto N, et al. Randomized trial of tocilizumab in systemic juvenile idiopathic arthritis. N Engl J Med 2012;367:2385–95.

37. Ruperto N, Brunner HI, Quartier P, et al. Two randomized trials of canakinumab in systemic juvenile idiopathic arthritis. N Engl J Med 2012;367:2396–406.

38. Horneff G, Schmeling H, Biedermann T, et al. The German etanercept registry for treatment of juvenile idiopathic arthritis. Ann Rheum Dis 2004;63:1638–44.

39. Brunner H, Ruperto N, Zuber Z, et al. Efficacy of safety of tocilizumab in patients with polyarticular juvenile idiopathic arthritis: data from a phase 3 trial [abstract]. Arthritis Rheum 2012;64:S682.

40. Fox DA. Biological therapies: a novel approach to the treatment of autoimmune disease. Am J Med 1995;99:82–8.

41. Stoll ML, Gotte AC. Biological therapies for the treatment of juvenile idiopathic arthritis: lessons from the adult and pediatric experiences. Biologics 2008;2:229–52.

42. Southwood TR, Foster HE, Davidson JE, et al. Duration of etanercept treatment and reasons for discontinuation in a cohort of juvenile idiopathic arthritis patients. Rheumatology (Oxford) 2011;50:189–95.

43. Quartier P, Taupin P, Bourdeaut F, et al. Efficacy of etanercept for the treatment of juvenile idiopathic arthritis according to the onset type. Arthritis Rheum 2003;48:1093–101.

44. Foeldvari I, Nielsen S, Kummerle-Deschner J, et al. Tumor necrosis factor-alpha blocker in treatment of juvenile idiopathic arthritis-associated uveitis refractory

to second-line agents: results of a multinational survey. J Rheumatol 2007;34: 1146–50.

45. Assasi N, Blackhouse G, Xie F, et al. Patient outcomes after anti TNF-alpha drugs for Crohn's disease. Expert Rev Pharmacoecon Outcomes Res 2010;10:163–75.

46. Horneff G, De Bock F, Foeldvari I, et al. Safety and efficacy of combination of etanercept and methotrexate compared to treatment with etanercept only in patients with juvenile idiopathic arthritis (JIA): preliminary data from the German JIA Registry. Ann Rheum Dis 2009;68:519–25.

47. Trachana M, Pratsidou-Gertsi P, Pardalos G, et al. Safety and efficacy of adalimu-mab treatment in Greek children with juvenile idiopathic arthritis. Scand J Rheu-matol 2011;40:101–7.

48. Sukumaran S, Marzan K, Shaham B, et al. High dose infliximab in the treatment of refractory uveitis: does dose matter? ISRN Rheumatol 2012;2012:765380.

49. Tambralli A, Beukelman T, Weiser P, et al. High doses of infliximab in the man-agement of juvenile idiopathic arthritis. J Rheumatol, in press.

50. Tse SM, Burgos-Vargas R, Laxer RM. Anti-tumor necrosis factor alpha blockade in the treatment of juvenile spondylarthropathy. Arthritis Rheum 2005;52: 2103–8.

51. Stoll ML, Punaro M. Psoriatic juvenile idiopathic arthritis: a tale of two sub-groups. Curr Opin Rheumatol 2011;23:437–43.

52. Diak P, Siegel J, La Grenade L, et al. Tumor necrosis factor alpha blockers and malignancy in children: forty-eight cases reported to the Food and Drug Admin-istration. Arthritis Rheum 2010;62:2517–24.

53. Cron RQ, Beukelman T. Guilt by association—what is the true risk of malig-nancy in children treated with etanercept for JIA? Pediatr Rheumatol Online J 2010;8:23.

54. Beukelman T, Haynes K, Curtis JR, et al. Rates of malignancy associated with juvenile idiopathic arthritis and its treatment. Arthritis Rheum 2012;64:1263–71.

55. Beukelman T, Xie F, Chen L, et al. Rates of hospitalized bacterial infection asso-ciated with juvenile idiopathic arthritis and its treatment. Arthritis Rheum 2012; 64:2773–80.

56. Dinarello CA, Simon A, van der Meer JW. Treating inflammation by blocking interleukin-1 in a broad spectrum of diseases. Nat Rev Drug Discov 2012;11: 633–52.

57. Nigrovic PA, Mannion M, Prince FH, et al. Anakinra as first-line disease-modi-fying therapy in systemic juvenile idiopathic arthritis: report of forty-six patients from an international multicenter series. Arthritis Rheum 2011;63:545–55.

58. Record JL, Beukelman T, Cron RQ. Combination therapy of abatacept and ana-kinra in children with refractory systemic juvenile idiopathic arthritis: a retrospec-tive case series. J Rheumatol 2011;38:180–1.

59. Miettunen PM, Narendran A, Jayanthan A, et al. Successful treatment of severe paediatric rheumatic disease-associated macrophage activation syndrome with interleukin-1 inhibition following conventional immunosuppressive therapy: case series with 12 patients. Rheumatology (Oxford) 2011;50:417–9.

60. Mertens M, Singh JA. Anakinra for rheumatoid arthritis. Cochrane Database Syst Rev 2009;(1):CD005121.

61. Cron RQ. A signal achievement in the treatment of arthritis. Arthritis Rheum 2005;52:2229–32.

62. Kenawy N, Cleary G, Mewar D, et al. Abatacept: a potential therapy in refractory cases of juvenile idiopathic arthritis-associated uveitis. Graefes Arch Clin Exp Ophthalmol 2011;249:297–300.

63. Simon TA, Askling J, Lacaille D, et al. Infections requiring hospitalization in the abatacept clinical development program: an epidemiological assessment. Arthritis Res Ther 2010;12:R67.

64. Singh JA, Wells GA, Christensen R, et al. Adverse effects of biologics: a network meta-analysis and Cochrane overview. Cochrane Database Syst Rev 2011;(2):CD008794.

65. Ohsugi Y. Recent advances in immunopathophysiology of interleukin-6: an innovative therapeutic drug, tocilizumab (recombinant humanized anti-human interleukin-6 receptor antibody), unveils the mysterious etiology of immune-mediated inflammatory diseases. Biol Pharm Bull 2007;30:2001–6.

66. Inaba Y, Ozawa R, Imagawa T, et al. Radiographic improvement of damaged large joints in children with systemic juvenile idiopathic arthritis following tocilizumab treatment. Ann Rheum Dis 2011;70:1693–5.

67. Ruderman EM. Overview of safety of non-biologic and biologic DMARDs. Rheumatology (Oxford) 2012;51(Suppl 6):vi37–43.

68. Woo P, Wilkinson N, Prieur AM, et al. Open label phase II trial of single, ascending doses of MRA in Caucasian children with severe systemic juvenile idiopathic arthritis: proof of principle of the efficacy of IL-6 receptor blockade in this type of arthritis and demonstration of prolonged clinical improvement. Arthritis Res Ther 2005;7:R1281–8.

69. Grillo-Lopez AJ, White CA, Varns C, et al. Overview of the clinical development of rituximab: first monoclonal antibody approved for the treatment of lymphoma. Semin Oncol 1999;26:66–73.

70. Alexeeva EI, Valieva SI, Bzarova TM, et al. Efficacy and safety of repeat courses of rituximab treatment in patients with severe refractory juvenile idiopathic arthritis. Clin Rheumatol 2011;30:1163–72.

71. Heiligenhaus A, Miserocchi E, Heinz C, et al. Treatment of severe uveitis associated with juvenile idiopathic arthritis with anti-CD20 monoclonal antibody (rituximab). Rheumatology (Oxford) 2011;50:1390–4.

72. Kimby E. Tolerability and safety of rituximab (MabThera). Cancer Treat Rev 2005;31:456–73.

73. Molloy ES, Calabrese LH. Progressive multifocal leukoencephalopathy associated with immunosuppressive therapy in rheumatic diseases: evolving role of biologic therapies. Arthritis Rheum 2012;64:3043–51.

74. Hadjinicolaou AV, Nisar MK, Parfrey H, et al. Non-infectious pulmonary toxicity of rituximab: a systematic review. Rheumatology (Oxford) 2012;51:653–62.

75. Schneider R, Laxer RM. Systemic onset juvenile rheumatoid arthritis. Baillieres Clin Rheumatol 1998;12:245–71.

Update on Juvenile Spondyloarthritis

Anusha Ramanathan, MD[a], Hemalatha Srinivasalu, MD[b],
Robert A. Colbert, MD, PhD[c],*

KEYWORDS

- Juvenile spondyloarthritis • Enthesitis-related arthritis • Juvenile psoriatic arthritis
- HLA-B27 • Axial spondyloarthritis

KEY POINTS

- Juvenile spondyloarthritis can be viewed on a continuum with adult-onset disease.
- Spondyloarthritis in children presents with peripheral arthritis and enthesitis more frequently than inflammatory back pain.
- Sacroiliitis may be more common in children with juvenile spondyloarthritis than expected based on symptoms.
- Validated measures of clinical disease activity, imaging, and biomarkers are needed to identify children with axial spondyloarthritis.
- New therapeutic targets in the IL-23/IL-17 axis hold great promise for improving treatment options and outcomes in spondyloarthritis.

INTRODUCTION

Spondyloarthritis (SpA) encompasses a group of disorders linked by overlapping clinical manifestations and genetic predisposition. SpA typically includes ankylosing spondylitis (AS), psoriatic arthritis (PsA), reactive arthritis (ReA), arthritis associated with inflammatory bowel disease (IBD), and undifferentiated spondyloarthritis (USpA). Newer classification systems developed for adults with SpA focus on identifying individuals with axial or predominantly peripheral involvement. All forms of SpA can begin during childhood, and can be considered on a continuum with adult

R.A. Colbert was supported by the NIAMS Intramural Research Program, Z01 AR041184.
[a] Division of Rheumatology, Keck School of Medicine of USC, Children's Hospital of Los Angeles, 4650 Sunset Boulevard, MS#60, Los Angeles, CA 90027, USA; [b] Division of Rheumatology, Children's National Medical Center, George Washington University, 111 Michigan Avenue, North West, Washington, DC 20010, USA; [c] Pediatric Translational Research Branch, National Institute of Arthritis, Musculoskeletal and Skin Diseases (NIAMS), National Institutes of Health, Building 10 / CRC / Rm 1-5142, 10 Center Drive, Bethesda, MD 20892, USA
* Corresponding author.
E-mail address: colbertr@mail.nih.gov

Rheum Dis Clin N Am 39 (2013) 767–788
http://dx.doi.org/10.1016/j.rdc.2013.06.002
0889-857X/13/$ – see front matter Published by Elsevier Inc.

rheumatic.theclinics.com

disease. Nevertheless, there are important differences in presentation and outcome that depend on age at onset. This article highlights these differences, what has been learned about the genetics and pathogenesis of SpA, and important unmet needs for future studies.

CLASSIFICATION

Rosenberg and Petty[1] emphasized the importance of enthesitis and peripheral arthritis in the absence of back pain when they described seronegative enthesopathy and arthropathy (SEA) syndrome as a form of juvenile SpA (JSpA) distinct from other forms of chronic childhood arthritis. When the International League of Associations for Rheumatology (ILAR) formulated new classification criteria for chronic childhood arthritis, the term juvenile idiopathic arthritis (JIA) was adopted and divided into 7 subtypes (**Box 1**).[2] Using the ILAR system, most forms of JSpA are encompassed by enthesitis-related arthritis (ERA), juvenile PsA, and undifferentiated arthritis (**Box 2**). Exclusion criteria render ERA and PsA nonoverlapping, whereas children with chronic arthritis who do not fit into any category, or meet criteria for more than one category, are considered to have undifferentiated arthritis.

The ILAR classification is generally accepted for systemic, oligoarticular, and polyarticular forms of JIA, whereas it can be confusing for the concept of SpA as a group of overlapping disorders. The pros and cons of the ILAR classification system for JSpA have been the subject of much discussion.[3] For the purposes of this article, we use ERA, PsA, and undifferentiated arthritis as defined by ILAR when discussing specific studies in which patients were classified using this system. In other places we refer to JSpA as a term that broadly encompasses SpA in childhood. Juvenile AS is used to describe children who fulfill the modified New York criteria (**Box 3**) before age 16, and juvenile-*onset* AS for the 10% to 20% who have symptoms before age 16 but do not meet criteria for AS until later.

Box 1
International League of Associations for Rheumatology (ILAR) classification of juvenile idiopathic arthritis (JIA)

1. Systemic
2. Oligoarthritis
   a. Persistent
   b. Extended
3. Polyarthritis (rheumatoid factor [RF] negative)
4. Polyarthritis (RF positive)
5. Psoriatic arthritis
6. Enthesitis-related arthritis
7. Undifferentiated arthritis
   a. Fits no other category
   b. Fits more than 1 category

Data from Petty RE, Southwood TR, Manners P, et al. International League of Associations for Rheumatology classification of juvenile idiopathic arthritis: second revision, Edmonton, 2001. J Rheum 2004;31:390–2.

Box 2
ILAR categories encompassing juvenile spondyloarthritis (JSpA)

Enthesitis-related arthritis (ERA)

Arthritis and enthesitis

or

Arthritis or enthesitis with at least 2 of the following:

- Sacroiliac joint tenderness and/or inflammatory spinal pain
- Presence of HLA-B27
- Onset of arthritis in a male older than 6 years
- Family history in at least one first-degree relative of ankylosing spondylitis (AS), ERA, sacroiliitis with inflammatory bowel disease (IBD), reactive arthritis, or acute anterior uveitis
- Acute (symptomatic) anterior uveitis

Exclusions

1. Psoriasis or a history of psoriasis in the patient or a first-degree relative
2. Presence of immunoglobulin M (IgM) RF on at least 2 occasions at least 3 months apart
3. Systemic JIA in the patient

Psoriatic arthritis

Arthritis and psoriasis

or

Arthritis plus at least 2 of the following:

- Dactylitis
- Nail pitting or onycholysis
- Psoriasis in a first-degree relative

Exclusions

1. Arthritis in an HLA-B27–positive male beginning after the sixth birthday
2. AS, ERA, sacroiliitis with IBD, reactive arthritis or acute anterior uveitis, or a history of 1 of these disorders in a first-degree relative
3. Presence of IgM RF on at least 2 occasions at least 3 months apart
4. Systemic JIA in the patient

Undifferentiated arthritis

Arthritis that fulfills none of the ILAR categories, or fulfills criteria in 2 or more categories

Adapted from Petty RE, Southwood TR, Manners P, et al. International League of Associations for Rheumatology classification of juvenile idiopathic arthritis: second revision, Edmonton, 2001. J Rheum 2004;31:390–2.

The recent development of criteria by the Assessment of Spondyloarthritis International Society (ASAS) classifying adults with SpA based on primarily axial (**Box 4**) or peripheral (**Box 5**) involvement has reinforced the concept of SpA as a disease continuum.[4,5] Before the emergence of the ASAS criteria, "undifferentiated SpA" was most often classified based on the European Spondyloarthropathy Study Group (ESSG)[6] or Amor and colleagues'[7] criteria. Using the ASAS criteria, "axial SpA" identifies individuals who have radiographic sacroiliitis but lack clinical criteria for AS, those who have

> **Box 3**
> **Modified New York criteria for AS**
>
> *Clinical criteria*
>
> 1. Low back pain for at least 3 months improved by exercise and not relieved by rest
> 2. Limitation of lumbar spine motion in sagittal and frontal planes
> 3. Chest expansion decreased relative to normal values for age and sex
>
> *Radiological criterion*
>
> Unilateral sacroiliitis grade 3–4, or
>
> Bilateral sacroiliitis grade 2–4
>
> *Definite AS*
>
> Radiological criterion and at least 1 clinical criterion
>
> *Radiographic grading of sacroiliac changes:*
>
> Grade 0 = Normal
>
> Grade 1 = Suspicious
>
> Grade 2 = Sclerosis, some erosions
>
> Grade 3 = Severe erosions, widening of the joint space, some ankylosis
>
> Grade 4 = Complete ankylosis
>
> *Adapted from* Van der Linden S, Valkenburg HA, Cats A. Evaluation of diagnostic criteria for ankylosing spondylitis. A proposal, for modification of the New York criteria. Arthritis Rheum 1984;27:361–8.

magnetic resonance imaging (MRI) evidence of sacroiliitis (bone marrow edema adjacent to the sacroiliac joint), and subjects with no imaging evidence of sacroiliitis, but have HLA-B27 and SpA features that are highly predictive of eventual axial disease. It remains unknown what percentage of individuals with axial SpA will eventually meet full criteria for AS. Nevertheless, considering the 7-year to 8-year lag between the onset of symptoms and a diagnosis of AS,[8] the identification of patients with axial SpA affords an opportunity to ask whether early aggressive treatment can change the course and outcome of disease. Whether this can be achieved with tumor necrosis factor (TNF) inhibitors is an important unresolved question.

Many pediatric rheumatologists perceive the need to reclassify JSpA in a way that harmonizes with the adult classification system, including criteria that identify children with axial involvement.[9] This group is at greatest risk for progression to AS, and may benefit the most from early intervention. Although the ASAS criteria for axial SpA (see **Box 4**) are both sensitive (83%) and specific (84%) when applied to adults, they require at least 3 months of back pain as a starting point, and thus have limited sensitivity in children with SpA.

CLINICAL FEATURES
Enthesitis

Inflammation at entheses, where ligaments, tendons, fascia, and joint capsules attach to bones, is a defining characteristic of SpA, and can cause pain, swelling, and tenderness (**Fig. 1**). Enthesitis can be evaluated clinically by placing pressure on the enthesis with the dominant thumb until the nail bed blanches. If a dolorimeter is used, typically up to 40 lb/in^2 is applied to determine whether the patient is tender. In our experience,

---

Box 4
Assessment of Spondyloarthritis International Society (ASAS) classification criteria for axial SpA

Sacroiliitis on imaging[a] + $\geq$1 SpA feature[b]

HLA-B27 plus $\geq$2 other SpA features[b]

[a] Active (acute) inflammation on MRI highly suggestive of sacroiliitis associated with SpA or definite radiographic sacroiliitis according to modified New York criteria.

[b] SpA features:

- Inflammatory back pain
- Arthritis
- Enthesitis (heel)
- Uveitis
- Dactylitis
- Psoriasis
- Crohn disease/ulcerative colitis
- Good inflammatory response to nonsteroidal anti-inflammatory drugs
- Family history for SpA
- HLA-B27
- Elevated C-reactive protein

From Rudwaleit M, van der Heijde D, Landewe R, et al. The development of Assessment of SpondyloArthritis international Society classification criteria for axial spondyloarthritis (part II): validation and final selection. Ann Rheum Dis 2009;68:777–83; with permission.

---

it is not uncommon to exert greater than 40 lb/in^2 with thumb pressure; however, this varies between examiners. Therefore, the use of a dolorimeter can improve both inter-rater and even intra-rater reliability.

Entheseal pain and tenderness can occur in other JIA subtypes, and is sometimes seen in otherwise healthy children.[10] Pain and tenderness at or near entheses is also common in children with overuse or traction injuries, such as apophysitis (eg, Sever and Osgood-Schlatter syndrome), and can be confused with tender points in fibromyalgia.[11] As a presenting symptom, enthesitis is more common in juvenile than adult SpA. A cross-sectional study using the Childhood Arthritis and Rheumatology Research Alliance (CARRA) registry revealed that patients with ERA had higher pain intensity and poorer health status compared with other subtypes of JIA, with enthesitis, sacroiliac tenderness, and use of nonsteroidal anti-inflammatory drugs (NSAIDs) independently associated with increased pain intensity.[12] In addition, enthesitis early in disease was predictive of ongoing disease activity at 1 year and beyond.[13]

Several indices have been developed to assess enthesitis in adult SpA (**Table 1**). Sites that are common to 3 or more indices are shaded in **Table 1**. There are currently no universally accepted enthesitis indices for JSpA, although involvement of the patellae and heel insertion sites is common. Clinical evaluation alone tends to overestimate enthesitis, and thus ultrasound and whole-body (WB) MRI are being explored as research tools to study the specificity of clinical examination, and better understand the pathophysiology of this important clinical feature. Imaging studies to validate clinical findings may be beneficial when testing the efficacy of new biologics.

> **Box 5**
> **ASAS classification criteria for Peripheral SpA**
>
> Arthritis[a] or enthesitis or dactylitis, PLUS either
>
> One or more of the following:
>
> - Uveitis (anterior)
> - Psoriasis
> - Crohn disease or ulcerative colitis
> - Preceding infection (within 1 month)
> - HLA-B27
> - Sacroiliitis on imaging
>
> Two or more of the following:
>
> - Arthritis
> - Enthesitis
> - Dactylitis
> - Inflammatory back pain (ever)
> - Family history of SpA
>
>   [a] Peripheral arthritis; predominantly lower limb and/or asymmetric.
>   *Adapted from* Rudwaleit M, van der Heijde D, Landewe R, et al. The Assessment of Spondy-
> loArthritis International Society classification criteria for peripheral spondyloarthritis and for
> spondyloarthritis in general. Ann Rheum Dis 2011;70:25–31.

Ultrasound is noninvasive, relatively inexpensive, and can be performed in the clinic. Its use in rheumatology has become more widespread in recent years. Although heavily operator-dependent, it is emerging as a valid diagnostic tool in SpA,[14–16] and can be used to visualize synovitis, tendonitis, and enthesis. Features of enthesitis that are captured by ultrasonography include thickening, calcification, bony erosions, and tendon hypoechogenicity.[17] Although there is increasing evidence to support the

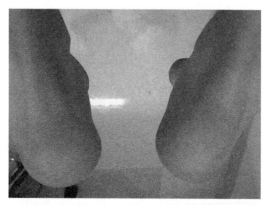

Fig. 1. Achilles tendon enthesitis. Heels of a 19-year-old HLA-B27–positive male with enthesitis and peripheral arthritis. Area of right Achilles tendon insertion on calcaneus is swollen, slightly erythematous, and tender to palpation, despite ongoing treatment with a TNF inhibitor. (Image provided by Dr. Carlos Rose, AI DuPont Hospital for Children, Wilmington, DE.)

Table 1
Entheseal sites in enthesitis indices

Site	Leeds[a]	Gladman[b]	MASES[c]	Mander[d]	Major[e]	SPARCC[f]
Nuchal crests				X		
Manubriosternal				X		
Costochondral			X[g]	X		
Rotator cuff insertion at shoulder		X				
Greater tuberosity of humerus				X		X
Medial humeral epicondyle				X	X	X
Lateral humeral epicondyle	X			X	X	X
Iliac crest			X	X	X	
Anterior superior iliac spine			X	X		
Greater trochanter of femur				X	X	X
Medial femoral condyle	X			X		
Lateral femoral condyle				X		
Superior pole of patella						X
Inferior pole of patella						X[h]
Tibial tuberosity		X				
Insertion of Achilles tendon	X	X	X	X	X	X
Plantar fascia to calcaneus		X		X	X	X
Cervical spinous process				X		
Thoracic spinous process				X		
Lumbar spinous process			X[i]	X		
Ischial tuberosity				X		
Posterior superior iliac spine			X	X		
Total number of entheseal sites	6	8	13	66	12	16

Shading indicates where a particular anatomic site is listed in 3 or more indices.
[a] Leeds Enthesitis Index.[98]
[b] Enthesitis index developed by Gladman et al for PsA.[99]
[c] Maastricht Ankylosing Spondylitis Enthesitis Score.[100]
[d] Enthesitis index developed by Mander et al for ankylosing spondylitis.[100,101]
[e] Major Enthesitis Index developed for ankylosing spondylitis.[102]
[f] Spondyloarthritis Research Consortium of Canada (SPARCC) Enthesitis Index.[103]
[g] Includes first and seventh costochondral junctions.
[h] Patellar ligament insertion into inferior pole of patella or tibial tubercle.
[i] Fifth lumbar spinous process.

use of ultrasound in detecting and monitoring enthesitis in SpA, better consensus on abnormal findings that define enthesitis lesions and standardization of methods is needed.[14] In the pediatric population, studies comparing enthesitis in SpA to apophysitis, overuse injury, and even fibromyalgia might be useful to help discriminate inflammatory enthesitis where tendon hypoechogenicity, vascularization on power Doppler, and erosions have been documented.[18]

WB MRI is frequently used to determine the presence and extent of bone marrow edema in suspected AS (**Figs. 2** and **3**),[19] to assess enthesitis in various forms of SpA,[20] and to evaluate active inflammatory lesions and structural damage in patients with nonradiographic axial SpA.[21] Few studies to date have explored the utility of WB MRI in the pediatric population. Preliminary data suggest that arthritis may be underestimated by clinical examination compared with WB MRI, whereas enthesitis is

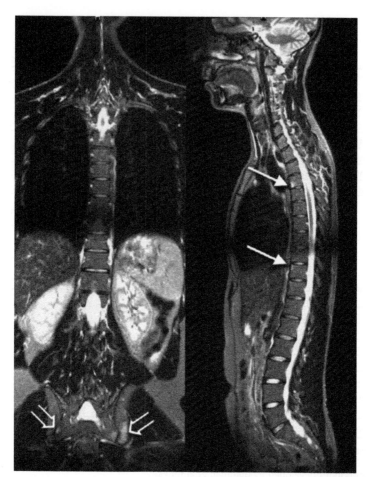

Fig. 2. WB MRI in suspected early AS. A 28-year-old HLA-B27–positive man with inflammatory back pain for 7 months was evaluated. STIR images show (*left*) bone marrow edema
adjacent to the lower portions of sacroiliac joints (*open arrows*), and (*right*) in anterior cor-
ners (*closed arrows*) of thoracic vertebral bodies. (*Reproduced from* Weber U, Pfirrmann CW,
Kissling RO, et al. Whole body MR imaging in ankylosing spondylitis: a descriptive pilot
study in patients with suspected early and active confirmed ankylosing spondylitis. BMC
Musculoskelet Disord 2007;8:20; with permission.)

overestimated.[22] We have made a similar observation, noting poor agreement
between enthesitis by clinical examination and WB MRI.[23]

Enthesitis is a key clinical and pathologic feature of JSpA, including ILAR-classified
ERA and PsA. A clinical enthesitis index supported by objective imaging evidence of
abnormalities is needed. This is critical for development of therapeutic trials and would
likely be a key component of any disease activity measure developed for JSpA.

Peripheral Arthritis

Peripheral arthritis in JSpA typically involves large joints of the lower extremities and
tends to be asymmetric. Hip involvement is more frequent in JSpA than in adult-
onset disease, and in long-term outcome studies is associated with more frequent

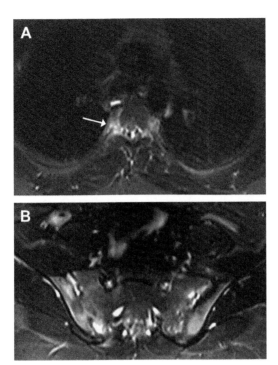

Fig. 3. WB MRI of a 16-year-old HLA-B27–positive boy with a 1-year history of knee and hip pain, and 6 months of inflammatory back pain. Patient was on indomethacin at the time of imaging. STIR images of (*A*) thoracic region showing enhanced signal at costovertebral junction (*arrow*), and (*B*) pelvis showing bone marrow edema on both the iliac and sacral sides of the sacroiliac joints bilaterally.

hip arthroplasty.[24,25] Hip arthritis is also a significant risk factor for sacroiliitis.[26] Tarsitis is also more common in JSpA than other forms of JIA or adult SpA. In a recent study from Spain, it was present in nearly one-third of children with JSpA and was often misdiagnosed as soft tissue infection.[27]

Axial Arthritis

Inflammatory back pain (IBP) has various definitions. ASAS has defined it as beginning before 40 years of age, insidious in onset, occurring at night, and improving with exercise but not with rest.[28] It often awakens patients at night, is typically associated with morning stiffness, and improves initially with NSAIDs. It sometimes results in buttock pain, which can alternate from side to side. Persistent IBP for at least 3 months is common in adults with axial arthritis, and thus is a major criterion required to classify an individual with axial SpA (see **Box 4**). In contrast, IBP is not a common clinical feature of JSpA. Although this has generally been interpreted to indicate lack of axial and in particular sacroiliac involvement in JSpA, this may not always be the case. Stoll and colleagues[26] demonstrated that although sacroiliitis was present in 37% of their patients with JSpA, 21% had "silent" sacroiliitis detected only by imaging and were lacking suggestive symptoms or physical examination findings. In this study, hip arthritis was a major risk factor for sacroiliitis, whereas dactylitis was negatively associated. In another study by Pagnini and colleagues,[29] 30% of children with ERA developed sacroiliitis documented clinically or by imaging, which was detectable by MRI as early as 1 year after disease onset. The main predictors of sacroiliitis in this cohort were active joint and enthesitis counts at onset.

Detecting sacroiliitis

Spinal involvement in AS is first detected in the sacroiliac joints in the vast majority of patients (**Fig. 4**). Given the insensitivity of plain radiography for early sacroiliitis, criteria for defining active sacroiliitis by MRI have been developed[30] and are used in the ASAS

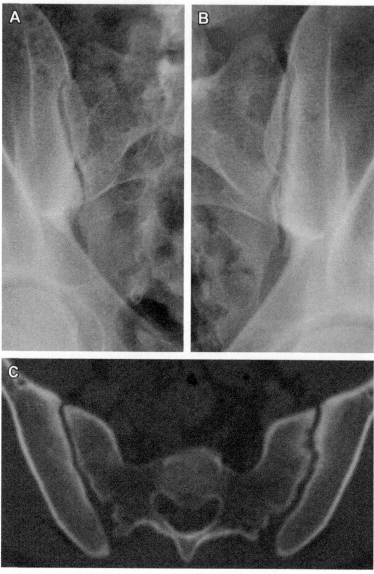

Fig. 4. Radiographic images of sacroiliac joints of a 19-year-old HLA-B27–positive male with 2-year history of intermittent lower back pain and 1 episode of acute anterior uveitis. Plain radiographs (*A, B*) and computed tomography scan (*C*) of sacroiliac joints. *A* and *B* reveal minimal sclerosis bilaterally with joint space widening (grade II). (*C*) Erosions and sclerosis.

classification scheme for axial SpA. The presence of either subchondral or periarticular bone marrow edema (BME) on STIR (short τ inversion recovery) imaging, or osteitis on T1 postgadolinium images, are considered highly suggestive of active sacroiliitis (**Fig. 5**). Importantly, the presence of enthesitis, synovitis, or capsulitis on MRI without concomitant bone marrow edema, although consistent with sacroiliitis, is not considered evidence of *active* sacroiliitis.[30] Although gadolinium is helpful to detect active synovitis, STIR sequences are sufficient to detect active BME.[31] Therefore, it is frequently preferable to obtain STIR MRI alone when evaluating children for sacroiliitis, considering the risks associated with gadolinium administration and the discomfort associated with placement of an intravenous catheter.

In the absence of IBP or stiffness, alternating buttock pain, or hip pain, it can be difficult to judge when to pursue further sacroiliac imaging in children with SpA. This is an important question, as the presence of sacroiliitis may have implications for treatment and long-term prognosis. The sensitivity of tenderness along the sacroiliac joint margin, reduced lumbosacral flexion (Schober test), or a positive Patrick test (or FABER test, for pain elicited by flexion, abduction, and external rotation of the leg) for predicting sacroiliac joint inflammation is not known, but in our experience is low. If sacroiliitis is suspected, radiographs are often obtained. Although they are low yield in early disease, as previously discussed, they provide an important baseline and can be helpful for future comparison considering the subtle changes that can sometimes indicate ongoing sacroiliitis (see **Box 3**). STIR MRI of the pelvis can be obtained without the need for sedation in most school-age children suspected of having axial SpA. In rare cases in which imaging is necessary in younger children, it may be necessary to provide sedation to obtain high-quality images.

Extra-articular Manifestations

Uveitis
Acute anterior uveitis (AAU) is the most common extra-articular manifestation of JSpA, and is also more frequent in HLA-B27–positive individuals even in the absence of arthritis or other features of SpA. AAU generally presents as unilateral, acute-onset ocular inflammation resulting in redness, pain, and photophobia. Up to one-third of patients with AS will develop AAU sometime during the course of their disease, with

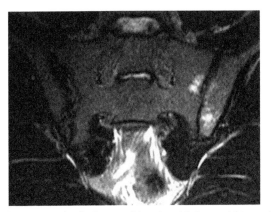

Fig. 5. STIR image from WB MRI of 19-year-old male with 2-year history of intermittent hip and alternating buttock pain, but lacking IBP. Bone marrow edema is apparent on sacral and iliac sides of left sacroiliac joint. Patient had previous MRI showing bone marrow edema adjacent to the right sacroiliac joint correlating with right-sided symptoms.

the highest risk being associated with HLA-B27, and about 50% experience at least one recurrence.[32] Although HLA-B27–positive AAU is frequently considered in the SpA category even in the absence of articular features, a new diagnosis of AAU can also lead to the recognition of preexisting nonspecific symptoms that are in fact due to other SpA features.[33] More than 50% of patients with HLA-B27–positive AAU will eventually be diagnosed with another form of SpA, including AS.[33]

AAU should be contrasted with the chronic uveitis associated with other forms of JIA (including early-onset PsA) that is most often asymptomatic. The risk of chronic uveitis is increased in patients positive for antinuclear antibodies, and ophthalmologic screening with a slit-lamp examination can detect early asymptomatic disease, enabling prompt treatment and reducing the risk of vision loss. Guidelines for screening children classified with juvenile rheumatoid arthritis (before the adoption of JIA criteria) have been published,[34] but do not address JSpA or ERA. For children with JSpA who are antinuclear antibody (ANA) negative but at risk for AAU, we provide education and counseling about obtaining prompt evaluation for ocular symptoms, and recommend yearly ophthalmologic examination. Children with early-onset PsA should be tested for ANA and screened according to current guidelines for oligoartic-ular or polyarticular arthritis.[34]

Gastrointestinal Inflammation

There is a strong link between gut inflammation and arthritis, particularly in SpA. Peripheral and axial arthritis occurs in up to 30% of patients with IBD. Conversely, 6.5% of patients with AS eventually develop IBD, but nearly 60% have subclinical gastrointestinal inflammation.[35,36] The prevalence of gut inflammation in JSpA is not known. IBD-associated arthritis is not specifically addressed by the ILAR classification system, except as an exclusion for PsA, and, consequently, children would mostly be classified as having ERA or undifferentiated arthritis. Interestingly, elevated levels of fecal calprotectin, a marker of intestinal inflammation, were seen in a small series of patients with ERA compared with healthy, other JIA, and other connective tissue dis-ease controls.[37] In a follow-up study, MR enterography performed on 5 patients with JIA and elevated fecal calprotectin, including 4 with JSpA, showed evidence of intes-tinal inflammation.[38]

Other Extra-articular Manifestations

Long-standing AS is associated with atherosclerotic and nonatherosclerotic cardiac manifestations.[17] Atherosclerotic consequences include an increased risk for myocar-dial infarction, with a twofold increased risk for ischemic heart disease noted in a Swedish population.[39] Nonatherosclerotic complications, including aortitis, aortic regurgitation, and aortic and mitral valve thickening without regurgitation, have been reported, even in relatively early AS.[40] Although cardiac manifestations of JSpA are relatively mild,[41] they can occur, making cardiac risk factors and functional assess-ment important for long-term care.

PSORIATIC ARTHRITIS (PsA)

Juvenile PsA appears to be composed of 2 distinct clinical subgroups.[42] One is char-acterized by early onset (peak age of 1–2 years) with features similar to oligoarticular and polyarticular JIA, including a predilection for females with a positive ANA, chronic uveitis, and an HLA-DR5 association. The second subgroup reflects later onset (peak age between 8 and 12 years), association with HLA-B27 but not ANA, equal sex ratio, and more frequent dactylitis, enthesitis, nail pitting, and axial involvement.[42,43] Clinical and genetic characteristics of the latter group are more representative of the SpA continuum. Reclassification of JSpA in a manner that recognizes these subgroups may be helpful for future studies and in communicating the different implications for outcome. Recent studies suggest that nail involvement in PsA may have an anatomic basis reflecting the presence of a bone-enthesis-nail complex.[44–47] In this context, distal interphalangeal joint involvement along with onycholysis and nail pitting in PsA are considered components of extensor tendon enthesopathy rather than synovitis.

GENETIC SUSCEPTIBILITY AND PATHOGENESIS

Significant advances in understanding genetic susceptibility to SpA have been made in the past several years.[48] Most of these discoveries pertain to AS and PsA, as well as the underlying conditions of psoriasis and IBD. Several concepts have begun to emerge from this work. First, there are significant overlaps between genes that predispose to AS and risk genes for psoriasis and PsA, and between AS and IBD, including both Crohn disease and ulcerative colitis. Some degree of shared genetic predisposition might be expected because of the clinical features common to various forms of SpA. In contrast, there is currently no overlap between AS and autoimmune diseases, such as rheumatoid arthritis and systemic lupus erythematosus. Second, genes in pathways relevant to the interleukin (IL)-23/IL-17 axis[49] are involved in susceptibility to AS, most notably the IL-23 receptor (*IL23R*) and the p40 subunit of IL-12 (*IL12B*) (which combines with IL-23p19 to produce the active IL-23 cytokine). These genes are also implicated in susceptibility to IBD and psoriasis. *STAT3*, another gene involved in transmitting cellular cytokine signals, including the response to IL-23, is also implicated in susceptibility to AS and IBD. A third important lesson from genome-wide association studies (GWAS) in AS that is also true for other complex genetic diseases, is that most heritability remains to be explained. For example, in AS only about 25% of overall heritability has been accounted for[48] despite large-scale studies involving several thousand affected individuals and even greater numbers of controls in the several GWAS performed to date. HLA-B27 accounts for the vast majority (23.3% of the 25.4%) of the known heritability, with newly discovered genes or gene regions accounting for the remaining 2.1%. The unidentified heritability may be related to rare variants and/or copy number differences not detected by commonly used high throughput methods of single nucleotide polymorphism (SNP) detection, and/or gene-gene interactions that remain to be thoroughly assessed. Although there have been no GWAS performed in ERA or juvenile PsA, it is interesting that a small pediatric study confirmed associations between *IL23R* variants and PsA in 93 individuals, and *ERAP1* SNPs and ERA in 74 subjects.[50] Although HLA-B27 is clearly associated with JSpA, its true prevalence in ERA and juvenile PsA cannot be determined because it is used for classification in the ILAR criteria.

Considerable evidence implicating the IL-23/IL-17 axis in SpA pathogenesis has accumulated over the past several years. Studies have documented IL-23 and IL-17 overexpression and expansion of Th17 T cells in both IBD and arthritis in HLA-B27 transgenic rats,[51,52] as well as in synovial fluid and peripheral blood from patients with SpA.[53,54] In rats, IL-23 overproduction has been linked to HLA-B27 misfolding and endoplasmic reticulum (ER) stress through activation of the unfolded protein response,[51] whereas loss of tolerizing dendritic cells may be important as well.[55] Human macrophages from subjects with HLA-B27–positive SpA produce more IL-23 without evidence of ongoing ER stress through a mechanism that remains to be defined.[56] Interestingly, dimers of HLA-B27 heavy chains expressed on the cell surface of antigen-processing–deficient cells can trigger leukocyte immunoglobulin-like receptors in the killer immunoglobulin receptor (KIR) family, particularly KIR3DL2.[57] When present on CD4+ Th17 T cells, KIR3DL2 activation can promote survival and increase IL-17 production, providing another possible link between HLA-B27 and Th17 cytokines in pathogenesis. The discovery of *ERAP1* (formerly *ARTS1*) as a risk gene,[58] and subsequently a gene-gene interaction with HLA-B27 in AS,[59] suggests that qualitative and/or quantitative differences in peptides that affect HLA-B27 folding and assembly, peptide presentation, and/or cell surface dimerization are important in disease susceptibility and pathogenesis.

Further support for the important role of IL-23 in SpA comes from a recent article showing that systemic delivery of this cytokine in mice can result in peripheral and axial enthesitis (without synovitis), aortic root inflammation, and osteoproliferation.[60] The location of IL-23–driven inflammation in this model was found to be a consequence of a newly discovered population of entheseal-resident T cells expressing the IL-23 receptor. These cells also express other transcription factors that direct the production of Th17 cytokines, including IL-17A, TNF-α, and IL-22, but differ from classical Th17 T cells in that they are CD4 negative. IL-22 was particularly important for induction of bone remodeling.

TREATMENT

The approach to managing JSpA is guided in large part by evidence from studies in adults with SpA and children with other forms of JIA. NSAIDs are often the first line of therapy recommended in both axial and peripheral SpA,[61] as they improve symptoms and can reduce inflammation.[62] Traditional disease-modifying antirheumatic drugs (DMARDs), such as methotrexate and sulfasalazine, are of limited utility for axial disease, despite their efficacy in other forms of inflammatory arthritis, such as polyarticular JIA and rheumatoid arthritis. There is some evidence supporting the use of sulfasalazine in juvenile AS and SEA syndrome, but improvement was limited to patient and physician global assessment of disease activity and not in primary outcome measures.[63] Other open-label studies of sulfasalazine in juvenile AS, ERA, and PsA have shown improvement in clinical symptoms, inflammatory markers, and remission rates.[64,65] These DMARDs have not been effective for axial disease or enthesopathy, although they are still used for peripheral arthritis and some extra-articular manifestations.[66] TNF inhibitors (TNFi) consistently reduce inflammation and signs and symptoms of AS/SpA in adults, and not surprisingly have also shown benefit for JSpA. Infliximab improved arthritis, enthesitis, inflammatory markers, pain, and physical function in a 3-month double-blind placebo-controlled trial in JSpA.[67] Open-label trials in juvenile AS and ERA have shown improvement in all clinical outcomes with the use of both infliximab[68,69] and etanercept,[70–73] and more recently a double-blind placebo-controlled trial of adalimumab demonstrated efficacy in juvenile-onset AS.[74]

Specific recommendations for the treatment of JIA were recently published.[75] Treatment groups for nonsystemic JIA were established based on the cumulative number of peripheral joints involved (≤4 or ≥5 joints), and whether or not active sacroiliitis was present. Following these recommendations, active sacroiliitis lowers the threshold for the initiation of a TNFi. Active sacroiliitis was not defined, although the need for both clinical and imaging evidence was noted. Because active disease cannot be determined by plain radiography, a positive sacroiliac MRI as defined by the ASAS criteria would seem appropriate. Parameters used to determine how quickly one should advance from NSAIDs, methotrexate, or sulfasalazine to a TNFi include clinical presentation, prognosis and disease activity measures. Poor prognosis is defined as radiographic damage (erosions or joint space narrowing) of any joint. However, in someone with JSpA who may have little peripheral or only sacroiliac arthritis, erosions may be a late finding and joint space widening may occur rather than narrowing.[76] Given the lack of efficacy of methotrexate and sulfasalazine for axial disease in adult trials, it may be prudent to move more rapidly from NSAIDs to a TNFi when active sacroiliitis is present. Treatment recommendations for adults with axial SpA include the initiation of a TNFi when disease activity persists despite at least two 4-week courses of NSAIDs at optimal doses, with no requirement for DMARD failure.[77] Peripheral disease is considered refractory when it remains active despite current or past intake of sulfasalazine or local corticosteroids.[77] Predictors of a positive response to TNFi therapy in adults include short disease duration, younger age, better functional status, elevated inflammatory markers, HLA-B27 positivity, and higher spinal MRI scores.[78–81] Many of these predictors suggest that early active disease in younger patients will be more responsive to TNFi. Exercise and physical therapy for JSpA are also important adjuncts to therapy that should not be ignored.

The question of whether TNFi can slow syndesmophyte growth and axial progression in AS remains a subject of great debate.[82] Although continuous use of NSAIDs has been shown to slow radiographic progression, the effect is small.[83] This is measured with the Modified Stoke AS Spine Score (mSASSS), with increases of 1 unit or more per year considered progression. Initial studies comparing patients on TNFi in large clinical trials to historical controls in the Outcome in AS International Study (OASIS) cohort suggested that despite having a marked effect on controlling disease activity and inflammation, TNFi were unable to slow the growth of syndesmophytes measured with the mSASSS.[84–86] However, newer data are emerging that may challenge this concept. Haroon and colleagues[87] analyzed 334 patients with AS from several centers in North America who had been followed prospectively. Patients receiving TNFi at least 50% of the time with axial symptoms had a significantly lower rate of mSASSS progression than those not receiving TNFi. Predictors of progression included baseline inflammatory markers, smoking status, and the mSASSS. These results are encouraging and suggest that TNFi can modify axial progression. It will be important to confirm these results in additional studies. TNFi currently approved for use in AS are etanercept, infliximab, and adalimumab. Golimumab is approved for active AS and PsA in adults and several adult trials with certolizumab pegol are under way with preliminary efficacy and similar safety profiles as other TNFi.[88,89]

We are not aware of any studies on the efficacy of other biologic therapies in juvenile SpA. In adults with SpA, rituximab, anakinra, and abatacept have been evaluated primarily in small open-label pilot studies. Rituximab and anakinra have shown modest benefit in TNFi-naïve patients.[90,91] Multiple studies have failed to find any major improvement with abatacept in AS or SpA,[92,93] and the IL-6 inhibitor tocilizumab was not efficacious in axial SpA.[94] Newer and more promising therapies include the anti–IL-17A antibody, secukinumab, which provided favorable results in a proof-of-concept trial in AS, including the open-label extension phase up to 24 months.[95,96] The oral phosphodiesterase-4 inhibitor, apremilast, has also shown evidence of efficacy in AS.[97] The recently elucidated role of IL-23 in SpA with its relationship to HLA-B27 and as a driver of enthesitis[60] (see the Summary) may provide another therapeutic target for juvenile SpA in the coming years.

SUMMARY

Juvenile SpA occurs on a continuum with adult disease, although there are differences in presentation and outcome that pediatric and adult rheumatologists need to be familiar with. Major unmet needs include criteria to readily identify children with early axial involvement, and validated measures of disease activity. Significant advances in our understanding of genetic susceptibility and pathogenesis have identified new target genes for entheseal inflammation in SpA and may explain unique aspects of the phenotype previously thought to be a consequence of autoreactive CD8+ T cells. TNF blockade continues to be a key treatment strategy, suppressing inflammation and providing symptom relief for a large number of patients suffering from SpA. New research suggests that IL-23, IL-17, and IL-22 could be equally important disease mediators. The ongoing development and clinical testing of antibodies that target these cytokines and/or their receptors hold considerable promise for improving the outcome for patients including children with SpA.

REFERENCES

1. Rosenberg AM, Petty RE. A syndrome of seronegative enthesopathy and arthropathy in children. Arthritis Rheum 1982;25:1041–7.
2. Petty RE, Southwood TR, Manners P, et al. International League of Associations for Rheumatology classification of juvenile idiopathic arthritis: second revision, Edmonton, 2001. J Rheumatol 2004;31:390–2.
3. Colbert RA. Classification of juvenile spondyloarthritis: enthesitis-related arthritis and beyond. Nat Rev Rheumatol 2010;6:477–85.
4. Rudwaleit M, van der Heijde D, Landewe R, et al. The development of Assessment of SpondyloArthritis International Society classification criteria for axial spondyloarthritis (part II): validation and final selection. Ann Rheum Dis 2009; 68:777–83.
5. Rudwaleit M, van der Heijde D, Landewe R, et al. The Assessment of SpondyloArthritis International Society classification criteria for peripheral spondyloarthritis and for spondyloarthritis in general. Ann Rheum Dis 2011;70:25–31.
6. Dougados M, van der Linden S, Juhlin R, et al. The European Spondyloarthropathy Study Group preliminary criteria for the classification of spondyloarthropathy. Arthritis Rheum 1991;34:1218–27.
7. Amor B, Dougados M, Mijiyawa M. Criteres de classification des spondyloarthropathies. Rev Rhum Mal Osteoartic 1990;57:85–9.
8. Feldtkeller E, Khan MA, van der Heijde D, et al. Age at disease onset and diagnosis delay in HLA-B27 negative vs. positive patients with ankylosing spondylitis. Rheumatol Int 2003;23:61–6.
9. Burgos-Vargas R. The assessment of the spondyloarthritis international society concept and criteria for the classification of axial spondyloarthritis and peripheral spondyloarthritis: a critical appraisal for the pediatric rheumatologist. Pediatr Rheumatol Online J 2012;10:14.
10. Sherry DD, Sapp LR. Enthesalgia in childhood: site-specific tenderness in healthy subjects and in patients with seronegative enthesopathic arthropathy. J Rheumatol 2003;30:1335–40.
11. Weiss PF. Diagnosis and treatment of enthesitis-related arthritis. Adolesc Health Med Ther 2012;2012:67–74.
12. Weiss PF, Beukelman T, Schanberg LE, et al. Enthesitis-related arthritis is associated with higher pain intensity and poorer health status in comparison with other categories of juvenile idiopathic arthritis: the Childhood Arthritis and Rheumatology Research Alliance Registry. J Rheumatol 2012;39:2341–51.
13. Weiss PF, Klink AJ, Behrens EM, et al. Enthesitis in an inception cohort of enthesitis-related arthritis. Arthritis Care Res (Hoboken) 2011;63:1307–12.

14. Gandjbakhch F, Terslev L, Joshua F, et al. Ultrasound in the evaluation of enthesitis: status and perspectives. Arthritis Res Ther 2011;13:R188.
15. Jousse-Joulin S, Breton S, Cangemi C, et al. Ultrasonography for detecting enthesitis in juvenile idiopathic arthritis. Arthritis Care Res (Hoboken) 2011;63: 849–55.
16. Bandinelli F, Milla M, Genise S, et al. Ultrasound discloses entheseal involvement in inactive and low active inflammatory bowel disease without clinical signs and symptoms of spondyloarthropathy. Rheumatology 2011;50:1275–9.
17. Eder L, Barzilai M, Peled N, et al. The use of ultrasound for the assessment of enthesitis in patients with spondyloarthritis. Clin Radiol 2013;68:219–23.
18. Marchesoni A, De Lucia O, Rotunno L, et al. Entheseal power Doppler ultrasonography: a comparison of psoriatic arthritis and fibromyalgia. J Rheumatol Suppl 2012;89:29–31.
19. Weber U, Pfirrmann CW, Kissling RO, et al. Whole body MR imaging in ankylosing spondylitis: a descriptive pilot study in patients with suspected early and active confirmed ankylosing spondylitis. BMC Musculoskelet Disord 2007;8:20.
20. Coates LC, Hodgson R, Conaghan PG, et al. MRI and ultrasonography for diagnosis and monitoring of psoriatic arthritis. Best Pract Res Clin Rheumatol 2012; 26:805–22.
21. Althoff CE, Sieper J, Song IH, et al. Active inflammation and structural change in early active axial spondyloarthritis as detected by whole-body MRI. Ann Rheum Dis 2013;72(6):967–73.
22. Rachlis AC, Babyn PS, Lobo-Mueller E, et al. Whole body magnetic resonance imaging in juvenile spondyloarthritis: will it provide vital information compared to clinical exam alone? Arthritis Rheum 2011;63(Suppl 10):749.
23. Srinivasalu H, Hill SC, Montealegre Sanchez G, et al. Whole body magnetic resonance imaging in evaluation of enthesitis in spondyloarthropathy. Arthritis Rheum 2012;64(Suppl 10):S848.
24. Gensler LS, Ward MM, Reveille JD, et al. Clinical, radiographic and functional differences between juvenile-onset and adult-onset ankylosing spondylitis: results from the PSOAS cohort. Ann Rheum Dis 2008;67:233–7.
25. Lin YC, Liang TH, Chen WS, et al. Differences between juvenile-onset ankylosing spondylitis and adult-onset ankylosing spondylitis. J Chin Med Assoc 2009;72:573–80.
26. Stoll ML, Bhore R, Dempsey-Robertson M, et al. Spondyloarthritis in a pediatric population: risk factors for sacroiliitis. J Rheumatol 2010;37:2402–8.
27. Alvarez-Madrid C, Merino R, De Inocencio J, et al. Tarsitis as an initial manifestation of juvenile spondyloarthropathy. Clin Exp Rheumatol 2009;27:691–4.
28. Sieper J, van der Heijde D, Landewe R, et al. New criteria for inflammatory back pain in patients with chronic back pain: a real patient exercise by experts from the Assessment of SpondyloArthritis international Society (ASAS). Ann Rheum Dis 2009;68:784–8.
29. Pagnini I, Savelli S, Matucci-Cerinic M, et al. Early predictors of juvenile sacroiliitis in enthesitis-related arthritis. J Rheumatol 2010;37:2395–401.
30. Rudwaleit M, Jurik AG, Hermann KG, et al. Defining active sacroiliitis on magnetic resonance imaging (MRI) for classification of axial spondyloarthritis: a consensual approach by the ASAS/OMERACT MRI group. Ann Rheum Dis 2009;68:1520–7.
31. Sieper J, Rudwaleit M, Baraliakos X, et al. The Assessment of SpondyloArthritis international Society (ASAS) handbook: a guide to assess spondyloarthritis. Ann Rheum Dis 2009;68(Suppl 2):ii1–44.

32. Wendling D. Uveitis in seronegative arthritis. Curr Rheumatol Rep 2012;14: 402–8.
33. Chang JH, McCluskey PJ, Wakefield D. Acute anterior uveitis and HLA-B27. Surv Ophthalmol 2005;50:364–88.
34. Cassidy J, Kivlin J, Lindsley C, et al. Ophthalmologic examinations in children with juvenile rheumatoid arthritis. Pediatrics 2006;117:1843–5.
35. Jacques P, Van Praet L, Carron P, et al. Pathophysiology and role of the gastro-intestinal system in spondyloarthritides. Rheum Dis Clin North Am 2012;38: 569–82.
36. Deepthi RV, Bhat SP, Shetty SM, et al. Juvenile spondyloarthritis with micro-scopic colitis. Indian Pediatr 2012;49:579–80.
37. Stoll ML, Punaro M, Patel AS. Fecal calprotectin in children with the enthesitis-related arthritis subtype of juvenile idiopathic arthritis. J Rheumatol 2011;38: 2274–5.
38. Stoll ML, Patel AS, Punaro M, et al. MR enterography to evaluate sub-clinical in-testinal inflammation in children with spondyloarthritis. Pediatr Rheumatol Online J 2012;10:6.
39. Bremander A, Petersson IF, Bergman S, et al. Population-based estimates of common comorbidities and cardiovascular disease in ankylosing spondylitis. Arthritis Care Res (Hoboken) 2011;63:550–6.
40. Park SH, Sohn IS, Joe BH, et al. Early cardiac valvular changes in ankylosing spondylitis: a transesophageal echocardiography study. J Cardiovasc Ultra-sound 2012;20:30–6.
41. Stamato T, Laxer RM, de Freitas C, et al. Prevalence of cardiac manifestations of juvenile ankylosing spondylitis. Am J Cardiol 1995;75:744–6.
42. Stoll ML, Zurakowski D, Nigrovic LE, et al. Patients with juvenile psoriatic arthritis comprise two distinct populations. Arthritis Rheum 2006;54:3564–72.
43. Stoll ML, Punaro M. Psoriatic juvenile idiopathic arthritis: a tale of two sub-groups. Curr Opin Rheumatol 2011;23:437–43.
44. Aydin SZ, Castillo-Gallego C, Ash ZR, et al. Ultrasonographic assessment of nail in psoriatic disease shows a link between onychopathy and distal interphalan-geal joint extensor tendon enthesopathy. Dermatology 2012;225:231–5.
45. Tan AL, Tanner SF, Waller ML, et al. High-resolution [18F]fluoride positron emis-sion tomography of the distal interphalangeal joint in psoriatic arthritis—a bone-enthesis-nail complex. Rheumatology (Oxford) 2013;52:898–904.
46. McGonagle DG, Helliwell P, Veale D. Enthesitis in psoriatic disease. Derma-tology 2012;225:100–9.
47. Tan AL, Benjamin M, Toumi H, et al. The relationship between the extensor tendon enthesis and the nail in distal interphalangeal joint disease in psoriatic arthritis—a high-resolution MRI and histological study. Rheumatology 2007;46:253–6.
48. Reveille JD. Genetics of spondyloarthritis—beyond the MHC. Nat Rev Rheuma-tol 2012;8:296–304.
49. Layh-Schmitt G, Colbert RA. The interleukin-23/interleukin-17 axis in spondyloar-thritis. Curr Opin Rheumatol 2008;20:392–7.
50. Hinks A, Martin P, Flynn E, et al. Subtype specific genetic associations for juve-nile idiopathic arthritis: ERAP1 with the enthesitis related arthritis subtype and IL23R with juvenile psoriatic arthritis. Arthritis Res Ther 2011;13:R12.
51. Delay ML, Turner MJ, Klenk EI, et al. HLA-B27 misfolding and the unfolded pro-tein response augment interleukin-23 production and are associated with Th17 activation in transgenic rats. Arthritis Rheum 2009;60:2633–43.

52. Glatigny S, Fert I, Blaton MA, et al. Proinflammatory Th17 cells are expanded and induced by dendritic cells in spondylarthritis-prone HLA-B27-transgenic rats. Arthritis Rheum 2012;64:110–20.
53. Wendling D, Cedoz JP, Racadot E, et al. Serum IL-17, BMP-7, and bone turnover markers in patients with ankylosing spondylitis. Joint Bone Spine 2007; 74:304–5.
54. Singh R, Aggarwal A, Misra R. Th1/Th17 cytokine profiles in patients with reactive arthritis/undifferentiated spondyloarthropathy. J Rheumatol 2007;34: 2285–90.
55. Utriainen L, Firmin D, Wright P, et al. Expression of HLA-B27 causes loss of migratory dendritic cells in a rat model of spondylarthritis. Arthritis Rheum 2012;64:3199–209.
56. Zeng L, Lindstrom MJ, Smith JA. Ankylosing spondylitis macrophage production of higher levels of interleukin-23 in response to lipopolysaccharide without induction of a significant unfolded protein response. Arthritis Rheum 2011;63: 3807–17.
57. Bowness P, Ridley A, Shaw J, et al. Th17 cells expressing KIR3DL2+ and responsive to HLA-B27 homodimers are increased in ankylosing spondylitis. J Immunol 2011;186:2672–80.
58. Burton PR, Clayton DG, Cardon LR, et al. Association scan of 14,500 nonsynonymous SNPs in four diseases identifies autoimmunity variants. Nat Genet 2007; 39:1329–37.
59. Evans DM, Spencer CC, Pointon JJ, et al. Interaction between ERAP1 and HLA-B27 in ankylosing spondylitis implicates peptide handling in the mechanism for HLA-B27 in disease susceptibility. Nat Genet 2011;43:761–7.
60. Sherlock JP, Joyce-Shaikh B, Turner SP, et al. IL-23 induces spondyloarthropathy by acting on ROR-gammat+ CD3+CD4-CD8- entheseal resident T cells. Nat Med 2012;18:1069–76.
61. Zochling J, van der Heijde D, Burgos-Vargas R, et al. ASAS/EULAR recommendations for the management of ankylosing spondylitis. Ann Rheum Dis 2006;65: 442–52.
62. Jarrett SJ, Sivera F, Cawkwell LS, et al. MRI and clinical findings in patients with ankylosing spondylitis eligible for anti-tumour necrosis factor therapy after a short course of etoricoxib. Ann Rheum Dis 2009;68:1466–9.
63. Burgos-Vargas R, Vazquez-Mellado J, Pacheco-Tena C, et al. A 26 week randomised, double blind, placebo controlled exploratory study of sulfasalazine in juvenile onset spondyloarthropathies. Ann Rheum Dis 2002;61:941–2.
64. Huang JL, Chen LC. Sulphasalazine in the treatment of children with chronic arthritis. Clin Rheumatol 1998;17:359–63.
65. van Rossum MA, Fiselier TJ, Franssen MJ, et al. Sulfasalazine in the treatment of juvenile chronic arthritis: a randomized, double-blind, placebo-controlled, multicenter study. Dutch Juvenile Chronic Arthritis Study Group. Arthritis Rheum 1998;41:808–16.
66. Dougados M, Baeten D. Spondyloarthritis. Lancet 2011;377:2127–37.
67. Burgos-Vargas R, Casasola-Vargas J, Gutierrez-Suarez R, et al. Efficacy, safety, and tolerability of infliximab in juvenile-onset spondyloarthropathies (JO-SpA): results of a three-month, randomized, double-blind, placebo-controlled trial phase. Arthritis Rheum 2007;56:S319.
68. Schmeling H, Horneff G. Infliximab in two patients with juvenile ankylosing spondylitis. Rheumatol Int 2004;24:173–6.

69. Tse SM, Burgos-Vargas R, Laxer RM. Anti-tumor necrosis factor alpha blockade in the treatment of juvenile spondylarthropathy. Arthritis Rheum 2005;52:2103–8.
70. Henrickson M, Reiff A. Prolonged efficacy of etanercept in refractory enthesitis-related arthritis. J Rheumatol 2004;31:2055–61.
71. Horneff G, De Bock F, Foeldvari I, et al. Safety and efficacy of combination of etanercept and methotrexate compared to treatment with etanercept only in patients with juvenile idiopathic arthritis (JIA): preliminary data from the German JIA Registry. Ann Rheum Dis 2009;68:519–25.
72. Otten MH, Prince FH, Armbrust W, et al. Factors associated with treatment response to etanercept in juvenile idiopathic arthritis. JAMA 2011;306:2340–7.
73. Otten MH, Prince FH, Twilt M, et al. Tumor necrosis factor-blocking agents for children with enthesitis-related arthritis—data from the Dutch arthritis and biologicals in children register, 1999-2010. J Rheumatol 2011;38:2258–63.
74. Horneff G, Fitter S, Foeldvari I, et al. Double-blind, placebo-controlled randomized trial with adalimumab for treatment of juvenile onset ankylosing spondylitis (JoAS): significant short term improvement. Arthritis Res Ther 2012;14:R230.
75. Beukelman T, Patkar NM, Saag KG, et al. 2011 American College of Rheumatology recommendations for the treatment of juvenile idiopathic arthritis: initiation and safety monitoring of therapeutic agents for the treatment of arthritis and systemic features. Arthritis Care Res (Hoboken) 2011;63:465–82.
76. Guglielmi G, Cascavilla A, Scalzo G, et al. Imaging findings of sacroiliac joints in spondyloarthropathies and other rheumatic conditions. Radiol Med 2011;116:292–301.
77. Braun J, van den Berg R, Baraliakos X, et al. 2010 update of the ASAS/EULAR recommendations for the management of ankylosing spondylitis. Ann Rheum Dis 2011;70:896–904.
78. Rudwaleit M, Listing J, Brandt J, et al. Prediction of a major clinical response (BASDAI 50) to tumour necrosis factor alpha blockers in ankylosing spondylitis. Ann Rheum Dis 2004;63:665–70.
79. Davis JC Jr, Van der Heijde DM, Dougados M, et al. Baseline factors that influence ASAS 20 response in patients with ankylosing spondylitis treated with etanercept. J Rheumatol 2005;32:1751–4.
80. Rudwaleit M, Claudepierre P, Wordsworth P, et al. Effectiveness, safety, and predictors of good clinical response in 1250 patients treated with adalimumab for active ankylosing spondylitis. J Rheumatol 2009;36:801–8.
81. Rudwaleit M, Schwarzlose S, Hilgert ES, et al. MRI in predicting a major clinical response to anti-tumour necrosis factor treatment in ankylosing spondylitis. Ann Rheum Dis 2008;67:1276–81.
82. Maksymowych WP, Elewaut D, Schett G. Motion for debate: the development of ankylosis in ankylosing spondylitis is largely dependent on inflammation. Arthritis Rheum 2012;64:1713–9.
83. Wanders A, Heijde D, Landewe R, et al. Nonsteroidal antiinflammatory drugs reduce radiographic progression in patients with ankylosing spondylitis: a randomized clinical trial. Arthritis Rheum 2005;52:1756–65.
84. van der Heijde D, Landewe R, Baraliakos X, et al. Radiographic findings following two years of infliximab therapy in patients with ankylosing spondylitis. Arthritis Rheum 2008;58:3063–70.
85. van der Heijde D, Landewe R, Einstein S, et al. Radiographic progression of ankylosing spondylitis after up to two years of treatment with etanercept. Arthritis Rheum 2008;58:1324–31.

86. van der Heijde D, Salonen D, Weissman BN, et al. Assessment of radiographic progression in the spines of patients with ankylosing spondylitis treated with adalimumab for up to 2 years. Arthritis Res Ther 2009;11:R127.
87. Haroon N, Inman RD, Learch TJ, et al. The impact of TNF-inhibitors on radiographic progression in ankylosing spondylitis. Arthritis Rheum 2013;64. [Epub ahead of print].
88. Sieper J, Kivitz AJ, Van Tubergen AM, et al. Rapid improvements in patient reported outcomes with certolizumab pegol in patients with axial spondyloarthritis, including ankylosing spondylitis and non-radiographic axial spondyloarthritis: 24 week results of a phase 3 double blind randomized placebo-controlled study. Arthritis Rheum 2012;64(Suppl 10):S558.
89. Landewe R, Rudwaleit M, van der Heijde D, et al. Effect of certolizumab pegol on signs and symptoms of ankylosing spondylitis and non-radiographic axial spondyloarthritis: 24 week results of a double-blind randomized placebo-controlled phase 3 axial spondyloarthritis study. Arthritis Rheum 2012;64(Suppl 10):S777.
90. Song IH, Heldmann F, Rudwaleit M, et al. Different response to rituximab in tumor necrosis factor blocker-naive patients with active ankylosing spondylitis and in patients in whom tumor necrosis factor blockers have failed: a twenty-four-week clinical trial. Arthritis Rheum 2010;62:1290–7.
91. Bennett AN, Tan AL, Coates LC, et al. Sustained response to anakinra in ankylosing spondylitis. Rheumatology 2008;47:223–4.
92. Song IH, Heldmann F, Rudwaleit M, et al. Treatment of active ankylosing spondylitis with abatacept: an open-label, 24-week pilot study. Ann Rheum Dis 2011; 70:1108–10.
93. Lekpa FK, Farrenq V, Canoui-Poitrine F, et al. Lack of efficacy of abatacept in axial spondylarthropathies refractory to tumor-necrosis-factor inhibition. Joint Bone Spine 2012;79:47–50.
94. Sieper J, Porter-Brown B, Thompson L, et al. Assessment of short-term symptomatic efficacy of tocilizumab in anklyosing spondylitis: results of randomized, placebo-controlled trials. Ann Rheum Dis 2013. [Epub ahead of print].
95. Baeten D, et al. The anti-IL-17A monoclonal antibody secukinumab (AIN457) showed good safety and efficacy in the treatment of active ankylosing spondylitis. Ann Rheum Dis 2011;70(Suppl 3):127.
96. Baraliakos X, Braun J, Laurent DD, et al. Long term inhibition of interleukin (IL)-17A with secukinumab improves clinical symptoms and reduces spinal inflammation as assessed by magnetic resonance imaging in patients with ankylosing spondylitis. Arthritis Rheum 2012;64(Suppl 10):S574.
97. Pathen E, Abraham S, Van Rossen E, et al. Efficacy and safety of apremilast, an oral phosphodiesterase 4 inhibitor, in ankylosing spondylitis. Ann Rheum Dis 2012. [Epub ahead of print].
98. Gladman DD, Inman RD, Cook RJ, et al. International spondyloarthritis interobserver reliability exercise—the INSPIRE study: II. Assessment of peripheral joints, enthesitis, and dactylitis. J Rheumatol 2007;34:1740–5.
99. Gladman DD, Cook RJ, Schentag C, et al. The clinical assessment of patients with psoriatic arthritis: results of a reliability study of the spondyloarthritis research consortium of Canada. J Rheumatol 2004;31:1126–31.
100. Heuft-Dorenbosch L, Spoorenberg A, van Tubergen A, et al. Assessment of enthesitis in ankylosing spondylitis. Ann Rheum Dis 2003;62:127–32.
101. Mander M, Simpson JM, McLellan A, et al. Studies with an enthesis index as a method of clinical assessment in ankylosing spondylitis. Ann Rheum Dis 1987; 46:197–202.

102. Braun J, Brandt J, Listing J, et al. Treatment of active ankylosing spondylitis with Infliximab—a double-blind placebo controlled multicenter trial. Lancet 2002; 359:1187–93.

103. Maksymowych WP, Mallon C, Morrow S, et al. Development and validation of the Spondyloarthritis Research Consortium of Canada (SPARCC) Enthesitis Index. Ann Rheum Dis 2009;68:948–53.

Update in Pediatric Inflammatory Bowel Disease

Shervin Rabizadeh, MD, MBA*, Marla Dubinsky, MD

KEYWORDS

- Inflammatory bowel disease • Pediatrics • Crohn disease • Ulcerative colitis

KEY POINTS

- The number of children with inflammatory bowel disease (IBD) is on the increase.
- Crohn disease and ulcerative colitis, the main subtypes of this intestinal inflammatory disease, affect both children and adults.
- Children are developing physically, emotionally, and immunologically. The interface between this development and IBD affects presentation, diagnosis, and management.
- This review focuses on the special aspects of pediatric IBD and how these influence management of children with IBD.

INTRODUCTION

Inflammatory bowel disease (IBD) impairs the quality of life of many children and adults. The disorder of intestinal inflammation results from chronic conditions such as Crohn disease and ulcerative colitis. Twenty percent of patients diagnosed with IBD are in the pediatric age range, although they are mostly more than 6 years of age.[1] The incidence of this chronic inflammatory condition is on the increase in children. Studies in Sweden, Norway and the United States have shown this dramatic increase, with an estimated incidence of 7 to 10 children of 100,000 developing IBD in any given year.[2–4] There are an estimated 50,000 to 100,000 children who currently have IBD in the United States.[5] The incidence of Crohn disease in children seems to be twice that of ulcerative colitis.[2,4] Although most cases of IBD in children are diagnosed in the second to third decades of life, very young children (<6 years of age) can also present with IBD. In this group, ulcerative colitis seems to be as common as Crohn disease.[6] This review focuses on the special aspects of pediatric IBD and the implications for the diagnosis and management of this disease, which has significant morbidity.

Funded by: NIH, Grant number(s): 5K08DK089076; R21DK084554.

Department of Pediatrics, Pediatric Inflammatory Bowel Disease Center, Cedars-Sinai Medical Center, 8635 West 3rd Street, Suite 1165W, Los Angeles, CA 90048, USA

* Corresponding author.

E-mail address: Shervin.Rabizadeh@cshs.org

PATHOGENESIS

Although the cause is unclear, IBD is believed to result from an interaction of genetics, host immunity, and environmental factors. One of the most important risk factors for developing IBD is a positive family history of the disorder.[7] Other possible factors include a child's living conditions,[8,9] maternal smoking, and older maternal age during pregnancy.[10] Controversial factors include the protective role of breast-feeding and whether certain vaccines, in particular measles vaccines, are risk factors for developing IBD.[11] The most recent evidence does not suggest this latter association.[12]

Despite extensive effort, a gene defect responsible for pediatric onset IBD has not been identified. However, genetics seem to play a significant role in patients who present earlier in life. Monozygotic twins have a 50% concordance risk for Crohn disease and children of parents with Crohn disease have a 33% risk of developing the disease.[13,14] A single gene for IBD has yet to be identified but the number of susceptibility loci associated with IBD has grown exponentially. The gene for NOD2/CARD15 (caspase activation recruitment domain), an important protein in innate immunity, was 1 of the first associated risk alleles for Crohn disease, with a 20-fold to 40-fold increased risk of developing disease if a person has 2 risk alleles.[15] More recently, genome-wide association studies (GWAS) have identified more than 100 independent gene loci associated with the disease.[16] GWAS in children and young adults have reproduced loci implicated in the GWAS of adult-onset Crohn disease.[17] There is extensive crossover of genes between Crohn disease and ulcerative colitis, demonstrating the common link between these chronic inflammatory conditions and the spectrum of the disease.[16–18] The genetic loci identified in patients with Crohn disease and ulcerative colitis implicate many biologically relevant immune pathways, such as interleukin (IL)-23 and IL-10. For the most part, although overlap exists, Crohn disease gene variations seem to be in pathways involved in microbe recognition and immune system responses such as autophagy, whereas ulcerative colitis genes seem to be involved in intestinal barrier integrity and function.[16] In infants, 1 genetic mutation of significant interest is found in the IL-10 pathway.[19] This rare autosomal recessive mutation leads to an infantile form of severe IBD, which sometimes requires bone marrow transplantation.

DIAGNOSIS

Similar to adults, pediatric patients with IBD present most commonly with diarrhea and abdominal pain (**Table 1**). Rectal bleeding occurs more often in patients with ulcerative colitis, whereas patients with Crohn disease are more likely to have perianal disease. Weight loss is seen in most children with Crohn disease at the time of presentation. This malnutrition in these patients results from suboptimal dietary intake, increased gastrointestinal losses, malabsorption, and possibly increased requirements associated with chronic inflammatory activity. Patients may be mistakenly diagnosed with anorexia nervosa given the severity of their presentation and the fear that eating leads to worsening of symptoms.

Growth Failure

The issues related to growth are a unique aspect of pediatric IBD. Forty percent of children with Crohn disease have growth failure compared with less than 10% of patients with ulcerative colitis.[20] Evidence of impaired linear growth may be the only presenting sign of IBD and can precede gastrointestinal symptoms (**Fig. 1**). Growth failure is likely secondary to chronic malnutrition caused by inadequate intake, excessive losses, and increased energy requirement, as well as the effects of inflammation on growth.[21,22]

Table 1 Presenting symptoms of new onset Crohn disease and ulcerative colitis in children (most common to least common)	
Crohn Disease	**Ulcerative Colitis**
Abdominal pain	Rectal bleeding
Weight loss	Diarrhea
Growth failure	Urgency/tenesmus
Anemia	Abdominal pain
Diarrhea	Anemia
Perianal disease	Weight loss
Fevers	Fevers
Arthritis	Arthritis
Skin lesions	Skin lesions

Patients seem to have normal growth hormone levels, but insulinlike growth factor 1 is reduced, suggesting hormone insensitivity possibly secondary to inflammation instead of deficiency.[23] Medication can play a role in growth failure as well. Recurrent and chronic administration of high-dose corticosteroids may lead to decreased collagen production and hence decrease in linear growth.[24] The medical and self-esteem problems associated with growth failure in pediatric patients with IBD must be considered especially when contemplating usage of prolonged corticosteroid therapy.

Joint Involvement

Joint inflammation is a common extraintestinal manifestation of IBD. Up to a quarter of children with IBD have arthritis[25] and like other extraintestinal manifestations of IBD, joint symptoms can occur before or after intestinal symptoms. Axial joint manifestations in patients with IBD include ankylosing spondylitis (AS) and sacroiliitis. AS is more common in patients with ulcerative colitis although the overall incidence in patients with IBD is low. Most of these patients have the HLA-B27 haplotype[26] unlike patients with IBD with sacroiliitis who are often asymptomatic.[27] Recent GWASs have identified similar single nucleotide polymorphisms within T helper 17 (Th-17) cells in patients with spondyloarthritis such as AS, IBD, and psoriasis.[28] Treatment of IBD-related symptomatic axial disorders usually focuses on exercise and physical therapy.

Peripheral joint disease, involving the larger joints, is seen more with Crohn disease and is often associated with bowel inflammation, especially disease within the colon.[27] Treatment of the bowel inflammation with immunomodulatory medication such as methotrexate and biologic medications such as infliximab often lead to resolution of the peripheral joint inflammation.[27] Treatment with nonsteroidal inflammatory agents should be avoided, if possible, secondary to the risk for gastrointestinal mucosal injury.

Laboratory Testing

Similar to adults with IBD, standard diagnostic laboratory testing is used for pediatric patients. Patients are evaluated for anemia, iron deficiency, increase in markers of inflammation (ie, erythrocyte sedimentation rate [ESR], C-reactive protein, fecal calprotectin), and hypoalbuminemia as a marker of poor nutrition; stool studies are used to exclude infections as a cause of symptoms. Unique to pediatric patients with IBD is the fact that some, especially those with milder disease, may present with no laboratory abnormality. In 1 study, 21% of pediatric patients with mild Crohn

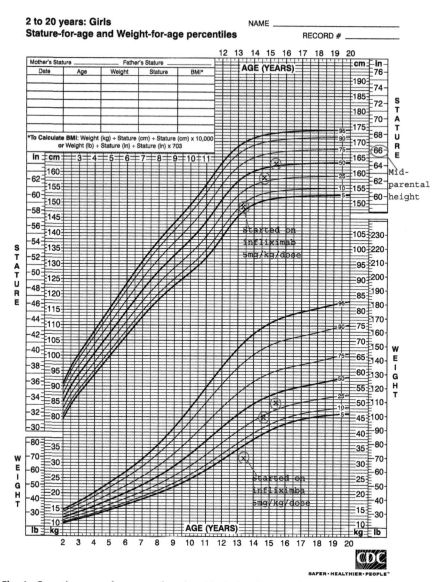

Fig. 1. Growth curve of a young female with Crohn disease who was started on infliximab. Height is well below the midparental height before initiation of infliximab. On anti-tumor necrosis factor therapy, the growth velocity dramatically improves to on par with the mid-parental height.

disease and 54% with mild ulcerative colitis had normal ESR, hemoglobin, platelet count, and albumin levels. In contrast, approximately 4% of those with moderate/severe disease had normal parameters.[29] Fecal calprotectin, a protein derived from neutrophils, is a marker that can be obtained noninvasively and is a good marker for diagnosing IBD and detecting flares.[30]

There is a growing knowledge regarding immunologic markers for categorizing patients with IBD. Antineutrophil cytoplasmic antibody (ANCA), anti-*Saccharomyces cerevisiae* antibody (ASCA), an antibody to the *Escherichia coli*–related outer membrane porin C and anti-Cbir1 antibody (antibody against flagellin) have been used to try to differentiate Crohn disease from ulcerative colitis as well to provide insight into prognosis. Perinuclear ANCA (pANCA) is detected in the serum of 60% to 70% of patients with ulcerative colitis and in only 15% to 25% of patients with Crohn disease.[31,32] This latter group presents an ulcerative colitis like picture of Crohn disease with predominant colonic disease. Anti-Cbir1 antibody has been shown to be present in approximately 50% of patients with Crohn disease who are pANCA positive as opposed to less than 5% of those with ulcerative colitis. This marker seems to help differentiate ulcerative colitis from those with Crohn disease who have ulcerative colitis–type symptoms.[33] On the other hand, ASCA (IgG or IgA) is highly predictive of Crohn disease,[32,34] especially in the absence of ANCA. Patients less than 7 years of age seem to express a different antibody profile because they are more likely to have antibody to Cbir1 compared with older children who have higher rates of ASCA.[35] Antibodies also serve a prognostic role. In children with Crohn, the sum of positive antibodies predicts more complicated disease. As the number and magnitude of these antibodies increases so does the incidence of internal penetrating and stricturing disease, leading to high surgery rates.[36]

Endoscopic Evaluation

Endoscopic evaluation remains the gold standard for the diagnosis of IBD. Children should undergo both an upper endoscopy and colonoscopy during the initial evaluation for IBD. The upper gastrointestinal tract may be involved in more than 50% of patients with IBD.[37] Although findings in the upper tract may be nonspecific, it can provide additional information in patients with indeterminate disease. Inflammation is most commonly noted in the stomach and although nonspecific gastritis is common in Crohn disease, it can also be present in patients with ulcerative colitis and hence it does not reliably differentiate between the 2 diseases.[38] Children with upper gastrointestinal disease can have symptoms such as nausea, vomiting, and weight loss, but a proportion can be asymptomatic. To maximize yield, biopsies of macroscopically involved and noninvolved tissue are performed in both the upper and lower gastrointestinal tract.

Small Bowel Imaging

Small bowel imaging is strongly recommended in all children suspected to have IBD, especially in patients who had unsuccessful ileal intubation or when the diagnosis is indeterminate. Historically, the small bowel follow through (SBFT) examination has been the radiologic technique of choice but with advancements in technology, other approaches such as such as ultrasonography, computer tomography (CT), magnetic resonance imaging (MRI), and video wireless capsule endoscopy have increased the options available for disease characterization. Ultrasonography provides a noninvasive radiation-free method to evaluate for bowel wall thickening with sensitivity of 75% to 95% and specificity of 67% to 100% for the diagnosis of Crohn disease.[39] Limitations of ultrasonography include operator dependency, technical difficulties depending on body habitus, and inability to evaluate superficial lesions. CT, especially with negative luminal contrast in CT enterography or CT enteroclysis studies, allows visualization of bowel wall inflammation as well as fistulas and abscesses[40,41] but exposes children to significant radiation. MRI has the advantage of limiting radiation but it is more costly and requires a child to lie still for an extended period. Oral enterography with intraluminal contrast and intravenous gadolinium has made MRI as diagnostically effective as or even superior to CT enterography and SBFT for detection of small bowel abnormalities and extraenteric complications.[42]

TREATMENT

The therapeutic goal in treating patients with IBD is mucosal healing and long-lasting remission. Treatment of pediatric patients with IBD should focus on the individual patient and requires a commonsense approach, with consideration of symptoms and quality of life, including growth, and minimizing side effects. There is a paucity of therapies approved specifically for children with IBD, therefore most of the treatment regimens are extrapolated from adult studies. Similar to adults with IBD, children with IBD have been treated in a stepwise approach with less powerful medication tried first. However, as experience with biologic therapies and immunomodulators has increased, this approach has been challenged with consideration toward changing the natural history of the disease in patients presenting so early in their lives.

Steroid-sparing strategies are preferable in the treatment of pediatric patients. Corticosteroids have multiple side effects, including impairment of growth and aesthetic complications (acne, cushingoid facies, and so forth). Hence minimizing or avoiding use of corticosteroids is always preferable in children with IBD.

Nutritional therapy is usually unique to pediatric patients. Although compliance can be an obstacle, a study of pediatric Crohn disease has shown that a short course of polymeric diet was more effective than corticosteroids in inducing healing.[43] This contradicts a Cochrane review meta-analysis that showed corticosteroids to be more efficacious than enteral therapy for inducing remission in Crohn disease.[44]

The benefits of early usage of immunomodulators in IBD were demonstrated in a pediatric trial for patients with Crohn disease. Children with Crohn disease were put on steroids alone or corticosteroids with 6-mercaptopurine (6-MP).[45] The latter group was significantly more likely to be off steroids and in remission after 600 days of therapy than the group treated with corticosteroid monotherapy. There was no difference in linear growth velocity between the groups.

The emergence of tumor necrosis factor α inhibitors (anti-TNFα) has added a powerful weapon to the arsenal in the fight against IBD. Most providers use biologics when they are unable to wean patients off steroids after 4 to 6 months of immunomodulatory therapy or if there is significant growth failure secondary to disease. The REACH trial (a randomized, multicenter, open-label study to evaluate the safety and efficacy of anti-TNF alpha chimeric monoclonal antibody [infliximab] in pediatric subjects with moderate-to-severe Crohn's disease) was the first of its kind in pediatric gastroenterology using a multicenter approach to study the efficacy and safety of infliximab in more than 110 children with Crohn disease. Close to 90% of patients had clinical response at 10 weeks and more than 50% were in remission at 54 weeks after starting of the medication.[46] This study demonstrated an increase in height velocity in patients treated with infliximab with dramatic catch-up growth (see **Fig. 1**). Infliximab has also been shown to be effective in pediatric ulcerative colitis, although the response is not as robust as in Crohn disease.[47] It is important to consider infliximab, surgery, or cyclosporine in pediatric patients who are hospitalized with severe ulcerative colitis and are not responsive to corticosteroids after 3 days.[47] In addition to infliximab, newer biologics already approved for treatment of adult patients with IBD are currently in trials for pediatric IBD. Adalimumab and certolizumab are anti-TNF medication not yet approved in pediatrics but are used in patients with significant adverse reactions and/or high antibody formation to infliximab. Similarly, natalizumab, an anti-integrin $\alpha4$, has been used in patients with refractory Crohn disease but special precautions need to be taken with patients who are JC virus positive because of the risk of progressive multifocal leukoencephalopathy. Newer treatments on the horizon include ustekinumab (anti-IL-12/IL-23 p40), which has been successful in the treatment of patients with psoriasis, psoriatic arthritis, and spondyloarthritis.[28]

Two areas of great interest in pediatric IBD treated with biologic therapies involve predicting which patients will respond to the treatment regimen and the debate on monotherapy (ie, biologic therapy only) versus concomitant therapy (ie, biologic plus immunomodulator). Research is ongoing to identify the phenotypic and genotypic features of pediatric patients who would be most predictive of primary nonresponse to biologic therapy.[48] This research would allow for creation of a predictive model that could be used to discuss a patient's potential for response to biologic therapy. In the ongoing argument regarding monotherapy versus concomitant therapy, the jury is still out for pediatric patients, balancing potential increased efficacy with reduction in antibody formation versus risk of malignancy, specifically hepatosplenic T-cell lymphoma (HSTCL). The recent SONIC trial has shown improved response rates in adults naive to immunomodulators on concomitant therapy versus monotherapy with no increased risk of malignancy.[49] However, HSTCL, a rare but unfortunately usually fatal lymphoma, has been reported in a handful of patients with IBD (primarily males and less than 21 years of age) treated with 6-MP/azathioprine alone, or these medications combined with infliximab or adalimumab.[50,51] HSTCL has not been reported in patients on concomitant biologic and methotrexate. Registry studies have tried to compute the risk of malignancy, including HSTCL, in patients with and without IBD on biologic therapy. Specific to IBD, compared with the colon cancer risk in untreated or poorly controlled patients, this risk of treatment-associated malignancy, although mildly increased, is substantially lower than the intrinsic risk from the disease. Providers need to have discussions with families to review the risks, benefits, and alternatives when considering monotherapy or concomitant therapy in pediatric patients with IBD.

Bone Health

Children with IBD may develop osteopenia as a result of inflammatory cytokine production, malnutrition, malabsorption or inadequate intake of calcium and vitamin D, prolonged inactivity, and/or corticosteroid therapy.[52] Compared with controls, children with IBD, especially those on prolonged courses of corticosteroids, may be at increased risk for fractures.[53] Bone mineral density (BMD) as determined by dual energy X-ray absorptiometry (DEXA) is an appropriate method for bone mass assessment. However, z scores instead of the standard t scores should be used to compare a child's BMD with a control of the same age and sex.[54] Quantitative CT is an alternative method for measuring BMD because it allows a true volumetric BMD but can involve higher radiation doses than DEXA.[55]

Psychosocial Issues

IBD not only causes physical issues but is also a psychosocial burden on children. Compared with healthy children, pediatric patients with IBD can have issues with behavioral/emotional functioning, particularly depression and anxiety, social functioning, and self-esteem. Depression and anxiety are common in children with IBD. Symptoms of depression and/or anxiety have been noted in 25% to 30% of children with IBD, and 10% to 30% meet the criteria for clinical depression or an anxiety disorder.[56] These rates are similar to those in children with other chronic illnesses.[56] Most studies have shown that disease activity can improve with treatment of psychological issues.[57,58] Programs such as summer camps for children with IBD, peer

Table 2	
Recommendations for avoidance of live agent vaccines in patients with IBD	
Condition or Treatments	**Avoid Live Agent Vaccines**
Active disease	Significant protein-calorie malnutrition
Corticosteroids	Prednisone 20 mg/d equivalent, or 2 mg/kg per day if less than 10 kg, for 2 wk or more, and within 3 mo of stopping
6-MP/azathipurine	While on medication or within 3 mo of stopping
Methotrexate	While on medication or within 3 mo of stopping
Biologics (ie, anti-TNF therapy)	While on medication or within 3 mo of stopping

groups, and counseling may be productive especially to improve self-esteem. Medical management of depression and anxiety can be helpful when indicated.

Immunizations

Protection against vaccine-preventable illnesses is critical in pediatric patients with IBD given the immune-compromised state of active disease and immunosuppression induced by most treatments such as immunomodulators and biologics. However, safety and efficacy of immunizations must be considered before they can be recommended for these patients. With the exception of live vaccines (measles, mumps, rubella; varicella; influenza intranasal spray), immunizations can be safely administered in patients with IBD even those on immunosuppressants and hence immunization in pediatric and adult patients with IBD should not deviate from recommended schedules in the general population.[59] Recommendations for live agent vaccines are listed in **Table 2**. For patients who do receive vaccines while immune suppressed, adequate immune response should be assessed and repeat dosing should be considered if the response is insufficient.

SUMMARY

The incidence of IBD in children is on the increase and approximately one-quarter of patients with IBD present in childhood. Pediatric patients with IBD can suffer both physically and psychosocially. An individualized therapeutic strategy in a child with IBD is necessary in terms of both medical and psychosocial management. Special attention should be paid to growth, immunizations, and mental health. IBD is a disorder with potential morbidities and lifelong challenges, therefore understanding the different entities that affect children with the disorder can improve overall care.

REFERENCES

1. Dubinsky M. Special issues in pediatric inflammatory bowel disease. World J Gastroenterol 2008;14:413–20.
2. Hildebrand H, Finkel Y, Grahnquist L, et al. Changing pattern of paediatric inflammatory bowel disease in northern Stockholm 1990–2001. Gut 2003;52:1432–4.
3. Perminow G, Brackmann S, Lyckander LG, et al. A characterization in childhood inflammatory bowel disease, a new population-based inception cohort from South-Eastern Norway, 2005-07, showing increased incidence in Crohn's disease. Scand J Gastroenterol 2009;44:446–56.

4. Kugathasan S, Judd RH, Hoffmann RG, et al. Epidemiologic and clinical characteristics of children with newly diagnosed inflammatory bowel disease in Wisconsin: a statewide population-based study. J Pediatr 2003;143:525–31.
5. Baldassano RN, Piccoli DA. Inflammatory bowel disease in pediatric and adolescent patients. Gastroenterol Clin North Am 1999;2:445–58.
6. Heyman MB, Kirschner BS, Gold BD, et al. Children with early-onset inflammatory bowel disease (IBD): analysis of a pediatric IBD consortium registry. J Pediatr 2005;6:35–40.
7. Ahmad T, Satsangi J, McGovern D, et al. The genetics of inflammatory bowel disease. Aliment Pharmacol Ther 2001;15:731–48.
8. Feeney MA, Murphy F, Clegg AJ, et al. A case-control study of childhood environmental risk factors for the development of inflammatory bowel disease. Eur J Gastroenterol Hepatol 2002;14:529–34.
9. Blanchard JF, Bernstein CN, Wajda A, et al. Small-area variations and sociodemographic correlates for the incidence of Crohn's disease and ulcerative colitis. Am J Epidemiol 2001;154:328–35.
10. Montgomery SM, Wakefield AJ, Ekbom A. Sex-specific risks for pediatric onset among patients with Crohn's disease. Clin Gastroenterol Hepatol 2003;1: 303–9.
11. Corrao G, Tragnone A, Caprilli R, et al. Risk of inflammatory bowel disease attributable to smoking, oral contraception and breastfeeding in Italy: a nationwide case-control study. Cooperative Investigators of the Italian Group for the Study of the Colon and the Rectum (GISC). Int J Epidemiol 1998;27:397–404.
12. Robertson DJ, Sandler RS. Measles virus and Crohn's disease: a critical appraisal of the current literature. Inflamm Bowel Dis 2001;7:51–7.
13. Laharie D, Debeugny S, Peeters M, et al. Inflammatory bowel disease in spouses and their offspring. Gastroenterology 2001;120:816–9.
14. Halfvarson J, Bodin L, Tysk C, et al. Inflammatory bowel disease in a Swedish twin cohort: a long-term follow-up of concordance and clinical characteristics. Gastroenterology 2003;124:1767–73.
15. Bonen DK, Cho JH. The genetics of inflammatory bowel disease. Gastroenterology 2003;124:521–36.
16. McCauley JL, Abreu MT. Genetics in diagnosing and managing inflammatory bowel disease. Gastroenterol Clin North Am 2012;31:513–22.
17. Imielinski M, Baldassano RN, Griffiths A, et al. Common variants at five new loci associated with early-onset inflammatory bowel disease. Nat Genet 2009;41: 1335–40.
18. Cho JH. The genetics and immunopathogenesis of inflammatory bowel disease. Nat Rev Immunol 2008;8:458–66.
19. Glocker EO, Kotlarz D, Boztug K, et al. Inflammatory bowel disease and mutations affecting the interleukin-10 receptor. N Engl J Med 2009;21:2033–45.
20. Kanof ME, Lake AM, Bayless TM. Decreased height velocity in children and adolescents before the diagnosis of Crohn's disease. Gastroenterology 1988;95: 1523–7.
21. Savage MO, Beattie RM, Camacho-Hubner C, et al. Growth in Crohn's disease. Acta Paediatr Suppl 1999;88:89–92.
22. Ballinger A. Fundamental mechanisms of growth failure in inflammatory bowel disease. Horm Res 2002;58(Suppl 1):7–10.
23. Ballinger AB, Azooz O, El-Haj T, et al. Growth failure occurs through a decrease in insulin-like growth factor 1 which is independent of undernutrition in a rat model of colitis. Gut 2000;46:694–700.

24. Hyams JS, Moore RE, Leichtner AM, et al. Relationship of type I procollagen to corticosteroid therapy in children with inflammatory bowel disease. J Pediatr 1988;112:893–8.

25. Passo MH, Fitzgerald JF, Brandt KD. Arthritis associated with inflammatory bowel disease in children: relationship of joint disease to activity and severity of bowel lesion. Dig Dis Sci 1986;31:492.

26. Rothfuss KS, Stange EF, Herrlinger KR. Extraintestinal manifestations and complications in inflammatory bowel disease. World J Gastroenterol 2006;12:4819.

27. Danese S, Semeraro S, Papa A, et al. Extraintestinal manifestations in inflammatory bowel disease. World J Gastroenterol 2005;11:7227.

28. Reveille JD. Genetics of spondyloarthritis - beyond the MHC. Nat Rev Rheumatol 2012;8:296–304.

29. Mack DR, Lanton C, Markowitz J, et al. Laboratory values for children with newly diagnosed inflammatory bowel disease. Pediatrics 2007;119:1113–9.

30. Kostakis ID, Cholidou KG, Vaiopoulos AG, et al. Fecal calprotectin in pediatric inflammatory bowel disease: a systematic review. Dig Dis Sci 2013;58:309–19.

31. Targan SR. The utility of ANCA and ASCA in inflammatory bowel disease. Inflamm Bowel Dis 1999;5:61–3 [discussion: 66–7].

32. Ruemmele FM, Targan SR, Levy G, et al. Diagnostic accuracy of serological assays in pediatric inflammatory bowel disease. Gastroenterology 1998;115:822–9.

33. Targan SR, Landers CJ, Yang H, et al. Antibodies to CBir1 flagellin define a unique response that is associated independently with complicated Crohn's disease. Gastroenterology 2005;128:2020–8.

34. Dubinsky MC, Ofman JJ, Urman M, et al. Clinical utility of serodiagnostic testing in suspected pediatric inflammatory bowel disease. Am J Gastroenterol 2001;96:758–65.

35. Markowitz J, Kugathasan S, Dubinsky MC, et al. Age of diagnosis influences serologic responses in children with Crohn's disease: a possible clue to etiology. Inflamm Bowel Dis 2009;15:714–9.

36. Dubinsky MC, Kugathasan S, Mei L, et al. Increased immune reactivity predict aggressive complicating Crohn's disease in children. Clin Gastroenterol Hepatol 2008;6:1105–11.

37. Castellaneta SP, Afzal NA, Greenberg M, et al. Diagnostic role of upper gastrointestinal endoscopy in pediatric inflammatory bowel disease. J Pediatr Gastroenterol Nutr 2004;39:257–61.

38. Sharif F, McDermott M, Dillon M, et al. Focally enhanced gastritis in children with Crohn's disease and ulcerative colitis. Am J Gastroenterol 2002;97:1415–20.

39. Fraquelli M, Colli A, Casazza G, et al. Role of US in detection of Crohn disease: meta-analysis. Radiology 2005;236:95–101.

40. Salbeni S, Rondonotti E, Iozzelli A, et al. Imaging of the small bowel in Crohn's disease: a review of old and new techniques. World J Gastroenterol 2007;13: 3279–87.

41. Bodily KD, Fletcher JG, Solem CA, et al. Crohn disease: mural attenuation and thickness at contrast-enhanced CT enterography: correlation with endoscopic and histologic findings of inflammation. Radiology 2006;238:505–16.

42. Lee SS, Kim AY, Yang SK, et al. Crohn's disease of the small bowel: comparison of CT enterography, MR enterography, and small-bowel follow-through as diagnostic techniques. Radiology 2009;251:751–61.

43. Borrelli O, Cordischi L, Cirulli M, et al. Polymeric diet alone versus corticosteroids in the treatment of active pediatric Crohn's disease: a randomized controlled open-label trial. Clin Gastroenterol Hepatol 2006;4:744–53.

44. Zachos M, Tondeur M, Griffiths AM. Enteral nutritional therapy for induction of remission in Crohn's disease. Cochrane Database Syst Rev 2007;(1):CD000542.
45. Markowitz J, Grancher K, Kohn N, et al. A multicenter trial of 6-mercaptopurine and prednisone in children with newly diagnosed Crohn's disease. Gastroenterology 2000;119:895–902.
46. Hyams J, Crandall W, Kugathasan S, et al. Induction and maintenance infliximab therapy for the treatment of moderate-to-severe Crohn's disease in children. Gastroenterology 2007;132:863–73.
47. Turner D, Mack D, Leleiko N, et al. Severe pediatric ulcerative colitis: a prospective multicenter study of outcomes and predictors of response. Gastroenterology 2010;138:2282–91.
48. Dubinsky MC, Mei L, Friedman M, et al. Genome wide association (GWA) predictors of anti-TNFalpha therapeutic responsiveness in pediatric inflammatory bowel disease. Inflamm Bowel Dis 2010;16:1357–66.
49. Sandborn WJ, Rutgeerts PJ, Reinisch W, et al. One year data from the Sonic Study: a randomized, double-blind trial comparing infliximab and infliximab plus azathioprine to azathioprine in patients with Crohn's disease naive to immunomodulators and biologic therapy. Gastroenterology 2009;136:A-116.
50. Rosh JR, Gross T, Mamula P, et al. Hepatosplenic T-cell lymphoma in adolescents and young adults with Crohn's disease: a cautionary tale? Inflamm Bowel Dis 2007;13:1024–30.
51. Cucciara S, Escher JC, Hildebrand H. Pediatric inflammatory bowel diseases and the risk of lymphoma: should we revise our treatment strategies. J Pediatr Gastroenterol Nutr 2009;48:257–67.
52. Sentongo TA, Semaeo EJ, Stettler N, et al. Vitamin D status in children, adolescents, and young adults with Crohn disease. Am J Clin Nutr 2002;76:1077–81.
53. Van Staa TP, Cooper C, Brusse LS, et al. Inflammatory bowel disease and the risk of fracture. Gastroenterology 2003;125:1591–7.
54. Sylvester FA. IBD and skeletal health: children are not small adults! Inflamm Bowel Dis 2005;11:1020–3.
55. Bachrach LK. Osteoporosis and measurement of bone mass in children and adolescents. Endocrinol Metab Clin North Am 2005;34:521–35.
56. Mackner L, Crandall W, Szigethy E. Psychosocial functioning in pediatric inflammatory bowel disease. Inflamm Bowel Dis 2006;12(3):239–44.
57. Mawdsley JE, Rampton DS. Psychological stress in IBD: new insights into pathogenic and therapeutic implications. Gut 2005;54:1481–91.
58. Deter HC, Keller W, von Wietersheim J, et al. Psychological treatment may reduce the need for healthcare in patients with Crohn's disease. Inflamm Bowel Dis 2007;13:745–52.
59. Sands BE, Cuffari C, Katz J, et al. Guidelines for immunizations in patients with inflammatory bowel disease. Inflamm Bowel Dis 2004;10:677–92.

Rheumatic Inflammatory Eye Diseases of Childhood

Andreas Reiff, MD[a],*, Sibel Kadayifcilar, MD[b], Seza Özen, MD[c]

KEYWORDS

- Inflammatory eye diseases • Uveitis • Blood eye/brain barrier
- Ocular coherence tomography

KEY POINTS

- Vision-threatening complications of pediatric uveitis are significant.
- The clinical presentation of inflammatory eye diseases in children is often asymptomatic, leading to a delay in diagnosis and causing a distinct challenge for treatment.
- A close collaboration with ophthalmologists and pediatric rheumatologists remains essential to improve the long-term outcome of these patients.

INTRODUCTION

Chronic inflammatory eye diseases (IEDs) are a common manifestation of pediatric rheumatologic diseases, potentially leading to lifelong vision impairment and disability. The mechanisms leading to the breach of the blood eye/brain barrier and the subsequent immune attack against a variety of intraocular mostly unidentified antigens remains poorly understood.

Pediatric rheumatologists need to be familiar with the various IEDs because they are often responsible for selecting and supervising treatment in close collaboration with the ophthalmologist. This article provides an update of recent developments in the pathogenesis and treatment of the most relevant ocular diseases encountered in rheumatologic practice.

Chronic inflammatory and degenerative eye diseases in children consist of a wide array of infectious, traumatic, malignant, or autoimmune conditions including conjunctivitis, keratitis, scleritis, and uveitis. Noninfectious uveitis remains one of the leading causes of preventable, irreversible vision loss, particularly in the Western world.[1,2] Most chronic, vision-threatening inflammatory eye conditions are autoimmune in nature.[3-5] Because initial symptoms are often subtle, patients are frequently unaware of a disease process and do not consult an ophthalmologist until they experience

[a] Division of Rheumatology, Children's Hospital Los Angeles, Los Angeles, CA, USA; [b] Department of Ophthalmology, School of Medicine, Hacettepe University, Ankara 06100, Turkey; [c] Department of Pediatrics, School of Medicine, Hacettepe University, Ankara 06100, Turkey
* Corresponding author.
E-mail address: areiff@chla.usc.edu

Rheum Dis Clin N Am 39 (2013) 801–832
http://dx.doi.org/10.1016/j.rdc.2013.05.005   **rheumatic.theclinics.com**
0889-857X/13/$ – see front matter © 2013 Elsevier Inc. All rights reserved.

visual impairment. This aspect is of particular importance in children since children have a higher rate of posterior uveitis which is associated with a higher risk for visison loss.[6,7] Complications from chronic eye disease or its treatment such as band keratopathy, synechiae, cataracts, glaucoma, and retinal edema can further compromise visual acuity and severely affect quality of life. **Table 1** summarizes the more common ocular manifestations in rheumatologic diseases.

UVEITIS

Uveitis remains the most common ocular manifestation in children with rheumatic diseases.[5,6] The term uveitis describes inflammation of individual or entire sections of the uveal tract, consisting of the iris, ciliary body, and choroid. The intraocular inflammation generally originates from the uvea, but may involve the overlying retina (retinitis) or the optic nerve (optic neuritis).[2]

Uveitis should not be used as a diagnostic designation, as it is an umbrella term for more than 50 different disease entities of infectious, malignant, or autoimmune background.[3] A potential underlying systemic autoimmune always has to be considered when patients present with signs and symptoms of IED, and disease management has to be adjusted accordingly.

Uveitis may be differentiated by its location within the eye to include anterior uveitis (iridocyclitis), intermediate uveitis (pars planitis), and posterior uveitis. Another way of differentiation is to use primary (idiopathic) uveitis to refer to intraocular inflammation of unknown cause, and secondary uveitis for ocular conditions that either are associated with a systemic disease (arthritis, sarcoidosis, vasculitis, and so forth), are of infectious or malignant origin, or represent independent ocular syndromes (eg, Vogt-Koyanagi-Harada [VKH] syndrome, Fuchs uveitis syndrome, birdshot retinitis).[8,9]

Primary uveitis is idiopathic in up to 60% of children, with anterior uveitis being the most common presentation, and accounts for roughly 40% of cases seen in tertiary referral centers.[10,11] Masquerade syndromes caused by intraocular cancers such as retinoblastoma or lymphoma can mimic IED.[1,2]

EPIDEMIOLOGY

In general, the incidence and prevalence of uveitis is lowest in the pediatric age group, increases with age, and is highest in patients 65 years and older.[12] Therefore pediatric cases account for less than 10% of all uveitis patients in larger series. In a study conducted in the United Kingdom, the incidence of pediatric uveitis increased with age from 3.15 per 100,000 children aged 0 to 5 years, to 6.06 per 100,000 of those between 11 and 15 years of age.[13] Similar to uveitis in adults, there are also ethnic and geographic differences in the prevalence and incidence, with highest observed rates in Scandinavia, followed by the United States and Asia, and lowest rates in India.[14–16] In a population-based study from Finland, the yearly incidence of uveitis was 4.3 per 100,000 in children and 27.2 per 100,000 in adults; prevalence rates were 27.9 and 93.1 per 100,000 respectively.[16]

Juvenile idiopathic arthritis (JIA) is the leading cause of anterior uveitis in Northern Europe and the United States, but is less common in the Mediterranean, the Middle East, and Asia.[7] Analysis of pooled data from 26 JIA series suggest a cumulative uveitis incidence of 8.3% (95% confidence interval [CI] 7.5%–9.1%). Over the last decade the incidence of uveitis appears to be on the increase, and is estimated to affect approximately 52.4 per 100,000 person-years with a period prevalence of 115.3 in 100,000 patients.[10,17,18] It is estimated that uveitis afflicts between 420,000 and 2 million Americans annually.[18]

Table 1
Clinically relevant inflammatory eye diseases of childhood and their disease associations

Disease and Frequency of Ocular Involvement	Uveitis Type	Ocular Clinical Presentation	Genetic Association	Other
JIA (oligoarticular) ~30% JIA (polyarticular) ~15%	Chronic nongranulomatous anterior uveitis Episcleritis in polyarticular JIA	Frequently asymptomatic Bilateral in ~70%	HLA-DRB1, -DQA1, -DQB1	ANA positivity increases risk RF positivity decreases risk
JIA (ERA) ~20% JIA (PsA) ~10%	Acute nongranulomatous anterior uveitis	Acute recurrent attacks of unilateral anterior uveitis, scleritis, episcleritis Bilateral conjunctivitis	HLA-B27	HLA-B27 positivity increases risk
Vogt-Koyanagi-Harada syndrome	Chronic granulomatous anterior or panuveitis	Bilateral Mutton-fat keratic precipitates in chronically ill and undertreated patients Choroiditis, exudative retinal changes, papillitis, glaucoma, and vitreitis can be seen	HLA-DR4 HLA-DQ4 HLA-DR53 HLA-DRB1*0405	Sensorineural hearing loss, vitiligo, poliosis
Pars planitis	Chronic nongranulomatous intermediate uveitis/vitreitis	Asymmetrical onset but frequent bilateral involvement Snowbanking or snowball formation	HLA-DR2 HLA-DR15	High risk for optic disc edema, CME, vitreous hemorrhage
Behçet syndrome (70%, initial in 20%)	Anterior iridocyclitis, posterior	Bilateral in 75%	HLA-B51, HLA-B5, R92Q TNFRSF1A mutation	High risk for retinal vasculitis, retinal and optic nerve atrophy
Tubulointerstitial nephritis and uveitis syndrome	Chronic nongranulomatous anterior uveitis	Unilateral or bilateral interstitial keratitis, episcleritis photophobia, lacrimation, eye pain	HLA-DQA1*01, HLA-DQB1*05, HLA-DRB1*01	Nephritis, fever, arthralgias, weight loss, abdominal and flank pain
Cogan syndrome	Chronic nongranulomatous anterior uveitis		HLA-A9 (Aw24), Bw35, and Cw4	Vestibuloauditory dysfunction, sensorineural hearing loss

Abbreviations: ANA, antinuclear antibody; CME, cystoid macular edema; ERA, enthesitis-related arthritis; HLA, human leukocyte antigen; JIA, juvenile idiopathic arthritis; PsA, psoriatic arthritis; RF, rheumatoid factor.

PATHOGENESIS

The etiology and pathogenesis of uveitis is not fully understood, and varies among the different forms. A variety of susceptibility genes related to uveitis and age-related macular degeneration have recently been described.[19] The most striking human leukocyte antigen (HLA) class I and II associations for uveitis are HLA-DR4 for sympathetic ophthalmia and VKH disease, and the linkage of HLA-A29 with birdshot retinopathy.[20]

Based on studies in various animal models of experimental autoimmune uveitis (ie, EAU mouse model) and studies in human autoimmune uveitis, an aberrant immune response against mostly unknown retinal antigens driven by autoreactive CD4+ T cells, including Th1 and Th17 cells, seems to play a central role in intraocular inflammation.[21–26] Of interest, peripheral CD4+CD25+FOXP3+ T cells normalized in patients with active uveitis after they had received treatment for their uveitis, suggesting that these cells are involved in the uveitic disease process and contribute to the patients' clinical improvement.[27]

Moreover, significantly elevated ocular and systemic cytokine levels, especially those of interleukin (IL)-1β and tumor necrosis factor (TNF), suggest that the intraocular disease is driven by a systemic inflammatory response.[28] In fact, it has been hypothesized that these 2 cytokines, in conjunction with vascular endothelial growth factor (VEGF), are the main factors leading to the breakdown of the blood-retinal barrier (BRB) by opening tight junctions between retinal vascular endothelial cells, resulting in an increase in transendothelial vesicular transport activity and a subsequent exposure of the inner eye to autoreactive cells.[29] It has been postulated that during the inflammatory response, disease-specific antigens are expressed on retinal vessels recruiting more inflammatory cells into the eye.[30,31] Within days, the retina acquires structural damage[32] through an early interferon (IFN)-γ and IL-2 driven Th1-type attack, followed by a more predominant Th2-type presence in the resolution phase.[24] The ensuing infiltration of T lymphocytes and leukocytes from the systemic vasculature into the eye is a complex multistep process mediated by CXCR4, a chemokine receptor mainly expressed on T cells, neutrophils, and monocytes.[33]

Once the BRB has been breached, IL-1 and IL-6 may act as intraocular amplification signals, disrupting the delicate local immunologic homeostasis within the eye and maintaining local inflammation.[34]

In addition, other proinflammatory cytokines such as IL-2, IL-4, IL-8, IL-12, IL-15, and IL-17, chemokines, and matrix metalloproteinases play an important role in maintaining the chronic inflammation in the eye.[35–37] Of note, the cytokine dominance may vary among the various types of autoimmune uveitis, in that IL-1 and TNF appear to be the predominant cytokines in anterior uveitis, whereas IL-6 may be more predominant in VKH syndrome, and IL-6 and IL-12 more dominant in Behçet syndrome.[38–41]

DIAGNOSIS AND CLINICAL PRESENTATION

Children who present with acute anterior uveitis are usually photophobic and complain about eye pain and headaches, whereas children with chronic uveitis are frequently asymptomatic or minimally symptomatic. Consequently, chronic uveitis can result in profound and irreversible vision loss, especially when ocular complications are unrecognized and improperly treated. Some of the more frequent complications include cataract formation, synechiae, band keratopathy, glaucoma, retinal detachment, cystoid macular edema, and neovascularization of the retina, optic nerve, and iris.[1,5,42]

A comprehensive evaluation of the patient's history and a thorough physical examination are imperative to assess the underlying etiology of the IED. In addition, a meticulous slit-lamp examination by an experienced ophthalmologist will clarify the type and extent of the intraocular disease process.

Key parameters for an ocular examination include:

- The number of cells in the anterior chamber
- Flare (vitreal protein concentration measured by photometry)
- Intraocular pressure (10–20 mm Hg)
- Visual acuity

Recently, the use of ocular coherence tomography (OCT) has been recommended as a noninvasive tool to obtain quantitative and qualitative data of associated changes in the macula and the retinal nerve fiber layers of children and adults with acute anterior uveitis. The benefit of using OCT may be in the detection of posterior segment manifestations that may not be discoverable by slit-lamp examination.[43–45] In addition, a recent study reported that anterior uveitis seems to be associated with impaired biomechanical strength of the cornea, although no correlations with disease duration or attack frequency were determined.[46]

In a retrospective Italian study including 257 patients younger than 16 years (mean age at onset of uveitis was 8.54 ± 3.98 years, 54.5% girls), children with anterior uveitis comprised the largest group (47.8%), whereas children with posterior uveitis (24.9%) were reported less frequently when compared with series decades ago. On the other hand, intermediate uveitis was seen in 19.4% and panuveitis in 7.8% of the patients. Ocular involvement was bilateral in 67.8%. Infectious uveitis represented 31% of all cases. Causes of severe visual loss were cataract, macular scars, macular edema/maculopathy, and secondary glaucoma. At follow-up, 79.3% of eyes maintained a visual acuity between 20/32 and 20/20.[17]

Once disease is established, guidelines for screening and follow-up as recommended by the American Academy of Pediatrics and Southwood should be followed, even though the underlying disease may no longer be active.[47,48]

Diagnostic guidelines for the workup of the more common IEDs have been reviewed in the past.[3] In addition to the conventional risk factors, a recent study seems to suggest that there also might be an association between psychological stress and chronic eye disease.[49]

The most common causes associated with anterior uveitis in adults include seronegative arthritis, followed by vasculitides, Behçet syndrome, VKH syndrome, and arteritis.[50] By contrast, in children the most common underlying cause of chronic uveitis in Europe and North America is JIA, followed by idiopathic uveitis and pars planitis.[6] Risk factors for uveitis in JIA patients include oligoarticular disease, antinuclear antibody (ANA) positivity, and female gender when disease onset occurs before the age of 7 years.[51]

JIA-associated anterior uveitis is typically bilateral, nongranulomatous, and tends to have a chronic relapsing disease course. Children with pauciarticular-onset juvenile arthritis and positive ANA (13%–34%) and children with psoriatic arthritis (8.5%–10%) have the highest prevalence of chronic uveitis. The prevalence is lower in polyarticular, rheumatoid factor–negative JIA (4%–22.5%) and even more rare in the systemic form of JIA (~1%).[1,5,52]

Children with chronic anterior JIA-associated uveitis are often asymptomatic, and may not present to the ophthalmologist or rheumatologist before serious ocular complications and visual impairment have already developed. Uveitis can independently occur at any time during the course of arthritis and can precede arthritis in approximately 10% of patients.[53]

The early onset of uveitis after arthritis has developed has been reported as a predictor of poor visual outcome. The most common complications of JIA-associated anterior uveitis include cataracts, band keratopathy, synechiae, ocular hypertension/hypotension, and maculopathy.[54,55] The presence of these complications at the time of initial visit, with high-density anterior chamber cells and high photometric flare measurements, are risk factors for development of new complications and a poor visual prognosis.[55–57]

SPECIAL DISEASE CONSIDERATIONS
VKH Syndrome

VKH syndrome is a rare bilateral granulomatous panuveitis, often associated with an inflammatory response targeting the meninges, the inner ear, and melanocyte-containing tissues, which leads to sensorineural hearing loss, vitiligo, and poliosis.[58,59] Criteria for the diagnosis of VKH disease were established in 1999, and were refined to include patients with both early- and late-stage disease.[60] VKH is most prevalent in the Middle East, Asia, and South America. It has a female predominance, typically affects patients in their thirties to fifties, and is rare in children.[61–64] Similar to the other forms of IED, the pathogenesis of VKH disease is not well understood. There is a strong genetic association with HLA-DR4 and HLA-DRB1*0405.[20,65] Recent studies suggest that IL-23, through its induction of IL-17–producing CD4$^+$ T cells, is driving the inflammatory response, which is unique to VKH but similar to other autoimmune diseases such as inflammatory bowel disease, psoriasis, multiple sclerosis (MS), and rheumatoid arthritis.[66,67] On the other hand, elevated levels of IL-10 and transforming growth factor β are seen during the remission phase in these patients.[68]

Clinically, patients present with signs of bilateral anterior granulomatous uveitis including large deposits, known as mutton-fat keratic precipitates, which tend to occur in more chronically ill and undertreated patients. In addition, bilateral choroiditis, exudative retinal changes, papillitis, glaucoma, and vitritis can be present.[62] Infectious causes of IED, masquerade syndromes, and other systemic rheumatologic diseases should be ruled out before diagnosing VKH. Although most VKH patients can be diagnosed by clinical examination and slit-lamp examination, additional testing with fluorescein angiography, OCT, electroretinogram, cerebrospinal fluid analysis, brain magnetic resonance imaging, and audiometry can be useful to solidify the diagnosis.[58,59,69]

Therapeutically, VKH requires early initiation of disease-modifying antirheumatic drug (DMARD) therapy, and it has been shown that this treatment approach results in better visual outcomes than no or delayed initiation of DMARD treatment.[70,71] Similar to the other forms of IED, daily high-dose prednisone (1–2 mg/kg/d) or intravenous pulses of solumedrol in conjunction with topical or intraocular steroids are still considered the mainstay of therapy, but should be used sparingly and for a limited time. The long-term use of corticosteroids can have deleterious effects on patients of all ages, but is particularly problematic in children with active bone development.[72]

DMARD options that are primarily used as steroid-sparing agents include cyclosporine, cyclophosphamide, chlorambucil, azathioprine, and mycophenolate mofetil (MMF).[69] On the other hand, there have been very few reports on systemic treatment in children with VKH, especially with the newer immunosuppressive agents or biologics. In 2006, Soheilian and colleagues[73] reported on the clinical course of 10 pediatric VKH patients, who were all treated with topical, intravitreal, or subconjunctival and systemic corticosteroids. Methotrexate (MTX) was started in 6 children who were either intolerant or nonresponsive to corticosteroids or had developed corticosteroid-related side effects. Final corrected visual acuity was 20/200 in 16 eyes. After a mean follow-up of 16.8 months, subretinal neovascularization was observed in 70% of eyes, cataracts in 55%, and glaucoma in 40%.[73] Paredes and colleagues[70] reported on two treatment groups with VKH (age range 9–71 years), one with pro-longed steroid treatment with or without delayed addition of immunomodulatory ther-apy (IMT), including MMF and cyclosporine A, and the second with prompt IMT (including MMF, cyclosporine A, MTX, and azathioprine) with or without steroids. In the steroid group, visual acuity deteriorated in 3 of the 5 patients and improved in 1. The fifth patient showed improvement in visual acuity in one eye, but decreased acuity in the other eye. In the IMT group, 7 of the 8 patients showed improvement in their vi-sual acuity, with deterioration of acuity in only 1 patient. The report did not indicate the stage of VKH with which the patients presented, and the investigators pointed out the limitations of their retrospective analysis, including the small number of patients and a patient selection bias, as all of their cases were referred to a tertiary care facility.

Although biologics have not yet been studied for the treatment of VKH disease as thoroughly as in the other forms of IED, infliximab, rituximab, and adalimumab have been successfully used in treating adults with this condition.[74] In a recent case series in two children with VKH treated with infliximab, improvement was noted in one patient but not in the other.[75]

Lastly, given that IL-23 plays a pivotal and unique role in the inflammatory cascade of VKH disease, other biologics such as ustekinumab targeting the IL-12/IL-23 pathway might provide an additional therapeutic option for this difficult-to-treat con-dition. From the personal experience of the senior author in treating children with VKH, the latter drug is less beneficial than traditional biologics, including TNF inhibitors (A.R., unpublished observation). At present, no specific treatment guidelines exist for the management of pediatric VKH patients.[76,77]

The prognosis of VKH patients depends on the early initiation of aggressive therapy and is, in general, fair, with approximately two-thirds of adult patients maintaining at least 20/40 vision. The prognosis in children with VKH seems to be more variable when compared with adults, in that some have limited inflammation and others have severe inflammation with recurrent episodes and rapid vision loss.[64] However, data are contradictory; Tabbara and colleagues[64] found that ocular complications occur more frequently in children than in adults, and Read and colleagues[77] reported better visual prognosis in patients with a young age at disease onset. Nevertheless, if the disease is recognized too late or remains undertreated, complications including cataracts, vision loss, choroidal neovascularization, and optic atrophy are more common.[78]

Pars Planitis

Pars planitis defines a subset of idiopathic intermediate uveitis that is characterized by snowbanking or snowball formation, in which the vitreous is the primary site of inflammation.[9] It typically affects children and adolescents and favors males, but is rarely associated with a systemic disease.[79,80] Disease onset is usually insidious, and most children with pars planitis are asymptomatic, might complain about floaters, and are often diagnosed during a routine ophthalmologic examination or only after significant visual impairment has occurred. Even though pars planitis pre-sents asymmetrically, most children ultimately have bilateral eye involvement. Typical findings at slit-lamp examination include peripheral corneal edema, anterior segment inflammation, diffuse vitreitis with cells and haze, and inferior snowbanking. Frequent complications include optic disc edema, cataracts, and cystoid macular edema (CME), which is the leading cause of visual impairment. Vitreous hemorrhage caused by neovascularization of the optic disc and inferior peripheral retinoschisis are typical complications of pars planitis during childhood.[81] Similar to VKH and MS, a linkage to HLA-DR2 and HLA-DR15 suggests an immunogenetic predisposition.[82] Treatment of pars planitis is similar to that for other forms of IEDs and usually includes intraocular or systemic steroids, especially for children with CME.[81] However, repeated corticosteroid injections may induce ocular hypertension, therefore DMARD therapy in the form of MTX or cyclosporine may be helpful as steroid-sparing agents. Support for biological treatment with agents such as infliximab is limited but in one retrospective study in 8 children with treatment refractory pars planitis, infliximab controlled the disease in all patients and was successfully discontinued in 2 patients after 7 and 12 infusions.[83]

Despite the high rate of ocular complications in children with pars planitis, which is likely a result of late recognition and treatment of disease, visual prognosis is usually good. In a recent retrospective study in 16 children from Spain (30 eyes, average age at onset 9.2 years), pars planitis had a good prognosis in most cases, with mean initial and final best-corrected visual acuities of 0.640 and 0.840, respectively, despite cataract formation as the most prevalent complication (36.7%). Periocular steroids were used in 33.3% and cryotherapy or laser photocoagulation in 16.7% of the patients. Complications requiring surgical management occurred in 4 eyes (13.3%).[80] By contrast, in the authors' series a significant proportion of patients who required medium to high doses of infliximab were those with pars planitis, who had a substantially poorer outcome than patients with other forms of uveitis.[84] It appears that children younger than 7 years have a poorer visual prognosis and are at higher risk of complications such as cataract, glaucoma, and vitreous hemorrhage.[85,86]

Tubulointerstitial Nephritis and Uveitis Syndrome

Tubulointerstitial nephritis and uveitis (TINU) syndrome describes the concurrence of acute tubulointerstitial nephritis (TIN) and bilateral acute anterior uveitis, a particular form of IED that typically affects male children and adolescents around 15 years of age.[87–89] TINU syndrome is more common in children than in adults, accounting for 1.7% of all adult uveitis cases.[90] Uveitis may precede, but more commonly develops after, the onset of renal disease. TINU syndrome tends to present with systemic symptoms, including fever, arthralgias, weight loss, abdominal and flank pain, and evidence of nephritis with microscopic hematuria and proteinuria. Unlike with other forms of IED, patients often present with eye pain and photophobia. Atypical cases with posterior or panuveitis may occur.[87] Despite a tendency for a chronic disease course, the visual prognosis is generally good and topical corticosteroids are often sufficient to achieve disease control.[91] In a recent retrospective study of 12 Finnish children with TINU syndrome, 4 of 12 (33%) developed chronic uveitis but only 1 patient required anti-TNF treatment for disease control. The prognosis for the renal component of the disease may not be as beneficial.[90]

Behçet Syndrome

Behçet disease (BD), first described by Hulusi Behçet in 1937, is a chronic multisystem disorder characterized by recurrent episodes of uveitis, oral aphthous lesions, genital ulcers, and skin lesions, with underlying vasculitis.[92,93] Although the most frequent initial manifestations are oral and genital ulcerations, the majority of patients present with more severe ocular, joint, gastrointestinal, vascular, or central nervous system involvement.[94] There is no pathognomonic finding or test for BD, therefore the diagnosis remains mostly clinical. Various sets of diagnostic criteria for BD have been suggested, and the criteria of the Japanese Research Committee of BD and 1990 classification of the International Study Group for BD are widely used.[95,96] BD affects males more than females (2–10:1) along the silk route that extends from the Mediterranean region to Japan. However, the male/female ratio is reversed in western Europe and the United States. Epidemiologic studies disclose a prevalence of BD in the range of 0.12 to 420 per 100,000, with the highest rates in Turkey and the lowest in the United States.[97] The average age for the onset of BD is in the second to third decade; it is rare in childhood.[98] In a recent cohort of 3382 patients with BD, only 110 (3.3%) were younger than 16 years[98] and only 10 of these had ocular involvement at the time of referral. In 2004, 8 ophthalmology departments from university clinics in Turkey analyzed the data of their uveitis patients, including in the study a total of 761 patients. The most common cause was BD with 245 cases (32.1%), only 5 of which were in children younger than 16 years.[15]

Ocular manifestations have been reported in 70% to 95% of adult BD cases,[93,98–100] whereas in pediatric series ocular involvement varies between 27.3% and 80%. In most cases, the eyes become involved within 2 to 4 years of disease onset.[98] The mean age at onset of uveitis ranges between 25 and 35 years.[93,101] In 20% of cases, ocular involvement may be the initial manifestation of the disease. The ocular disease may start unilaterally but becomes bilateral in at least 80% of patients within 5 years.[93] Eye involvement, which is reported to be more frequent and more severe in males,[93,100] may lead to severe vision loss in 25% of the cases.[102] The inflammation is typically nongranulomatous, accompanied by necrotizing obstructive vasculitis, and affects the anterior, posterior, or both segments. Anterior uveitis is commonly observed in females, whereas panuveitis is the main type of involvement in males.[93]

The main symptoms of anterior uveitis are blurred vision, redness, periorbital or global pain, photophobia, and tearing. Slit-lamp biomicroscopy discloses conjunctival injection most marked at the perilimbal area, cells and flare in the anterior chamber, fine keratic precipitates, and hypopyon, though not as frequent.[93,99] The anterior uveitis may resolve within 2 to 3 weeks even without therapy; however, it is recurrent and may result in posterior synechiae, iris atrophy, peripheral anterior synechiae, iris bombé due to seclusio pupillae, and secondary glaucoma. Cataract and glaucoma are common serious complications of Behçet uveitis.[93,103] The incidence of secondary glaucoma in 230 eyes of 129 patients with BD was found to be 10.9% (25 eyes).[104]

Involvement of the posterior segment is the most serious ocular manifestation of BD.[105] Patients usually present with decreased visual acuity with floaters. Vitritis and retinal vasculitis are the most prominent features. Another common finding is retinitis characterized by yellow-white solitary or multifocal infiltrates of the inner retina with indistinct margins, giving the retina a cloudy appearance with obscuration of the retinal vessels.[93] These lesions are usually transient and heal without scarring. The most frequent posterior-segment complication is macular edema, reported in up to half of cases. It can either resolve with appropriate treatment or result in chronic structural changes such as scarring, atrophy, or formation of macular holes.[106] Epiretinal membrane, vascular sheathing, occluded vessels, optic atrophy, and retinal detachment are other frequently encountered complications. Subsequently, repeat episodes of posterior segment flare-ups and complications result in end-stage ocular BD characterized by blindness with a clinical picture of optic atrophy, vascular attenuation, sheathing with occluded vessels that look like white cords, and diffuse retinal atrophy with variable chorioretinal pigmentation and scarring.[99]

The latest report on childhood BD disclosed ocular findings in 34 (20 boys, 14 girls) of 110 children (41 boys, 69 girls) examined between 1986 and 2005.[98] Ocular disease was found in 48.7% of males and 20.3% of females. Eye involvement was bilateral in 21 (61.8%) patients. Uveitis was anterior in 18 eyes (32.8%), posterior in 24 eyes (43.6%), and diffuse in 13 eyes (23.6%). Hypopyon was observed in 5 eyes (9%). Rubeosis iritis, posterior synechiae, and cataract were found in 1 eye (1.8%). Optic atrophy was observed in 6 (10.9%), ghost vessels and sheathing of vessels in 5 (9%), swelling of optic nerve head in 2 (3.6%), vitreous hemorrhage due to retinal neovascularization in 1 (1.8%), and phthisis bulbi in 2 (3.6%) eyes. Fluorescein angiography assisted in revealing retinal vasculitis in 10 eyes, disc hyperfluorescence in 5 eyes, and CME in 4 eyes.[98] A previous study on 34 children with uveitis disclosed panuveitis (diffuse uveitis) as the most common form and optic atrophy as the most common posterior-segment complication.[107] Anterior uveitis in children younger than 10 years and panuveitis in those older than 10 years was reported to be more frequent in another study of pediatric Behçet cases.[108] This study revealed frequent family history in younger patients, which was supported by another study from Germany.[109]

Fundus fluorescein angiography (FFA) and OCT are the main imaging techniques used in the evaluation of a Behçet patient with posterior uveitis. FFA demonstrates diffuse fluorescein leakage from retinal vessels, including the capillaries and the optic disc, during acute inflammation. It can reveal fundus changes even in BD patients with normal findings on clinical examination.[110] FFA can better identify macular edema, capillary leakage, retinal vascular leakage and staining, optic disc staining, areas of nonperfusion caused by vascular occlusions resulting from vasculitis in BD, pinpoint leakage, and retinal and optic disc neovascularization. OCT is a new technique for high-resolution cross-sectional imaging of retinal thickness. It is noninvasive, and therefore is ideally suited for the measurement of retinal thickness in the diagnosis and follow-up of patients with CME.[111]

Corticosteroids (topical, periocular, and systemic), colchicine, azathioprine, cyclosporine A, cyclophosphamide, MTX, chlorambucil, and immunomodulatory agents such as IFN-α and TNF-α inhibitors have all been used to treat BD.[94,98,107,108,112] In the past years better immunosuppressive therapy has dramatically improved the overall visual prognosis in BD.[93] As the course of uveitis is more severe in children than in adults, timely and efficient treatment to prevent permanent damage to visual structures is mandatory.[113] The most recent therapeutic modalities for ocular BD are outlined here.

Corticosteroids are used in acute flare-ups of ocular manifestations in BD, but they do not prevent further involvement or progression. High-dose intravenous corticosteroid therapy resulted in decreased inflammatory activity and improved visual acuity in BD patients in 2 recent series.[114,115] Data are not available for pediatric BD cases with ocular inflammation. The authors have grade A evidence for azathioprine in the treatment of ocular involvement in BD.[116] At present, the authors start azathioprine on all BD patients with posterior uveitis.

Lately, triamcinolone acetonide as an intravitreal injection for the treatment of sight-threatening vitritis or uveitic macular edema has been used in BD patients.[117–119] Despite improvement in visual acuity and resolution of macular edema, one should consider that the effect may only last months and that cataracts and increased intraocular pressure may be seen.[107] Intravitreal dexamethasone implants are currently available for the treatment of posterior uveitis and uveitic macular edema. The only report in children revealed clinical control of inflammation and/or resolution of CME in 13 of 14 treated eyes in 11 children with intermediate uveitis, posterior uveitis, or panuveitis.[120] Four eyes relapsed within 6 months at a median time to relapse of 4 months, and 4 eyes developed glaucoma necessitating treatment.

IFN-α has been successfully used in the treatment of adult and pediatric BD uveitis that is resistant to traditional immunosuppressive agents.[121,122] In a pediatric study of 7 patients with corticodependent BD uveitis, a remarkable corticosteroid-sparing effect with remission was achieved in 5 of 7 patients.[123,124] In a study of adult Behçet patients, 75% achieved remission of at least 18.7 months after cessation of IFN therapy.[123]

Evidence is accumulating for the efficacy of new and promising drugs, such as TNF-α inhibitors, in particular clinical situations. Infliximab, a TNF-α blocker, as a single infusion of 5 mg/kg (maximum dose: 400 mg) at day 1, at weeks 2 and 6, and then every 8 weeks, was found to be useful in 4 cases of refractory panuveitis due to BD[125] and at weeks 0, 2, 6, and 14 in 13 male patients with BD in whom uveitis was resistant to combination therapy with corticosteroids, azathioprine, and cyclosporine.[126] In another recent study, the improvement with infliximab was maintained for 2 years in 78% of the patients.[127] Recently intravenous infusions of 5 mg/kg infliximab at weeks 0, 2, 4, and subsequently every 6–8 weeks for up to 2 years were approved in Japan for treatment-refractory BD uveoretinitis.[128] In yet another retrospective analysis of 20 children with uveitis treated with infliximab, a 12-year-old boy with BD panuveitis received 31 infusions over 1 year. At the end of year 1, vision increased from 0.1 to 0.5 with no further flares.[83] Besides the lack of controlled prospective trials, the cost and the need for intravenous infusions are the main barriers to the use of this agent as a first-line treatment. Adalimumab, another monoclonal antibody to TNF, has been used in a few cases of BD uveitis, and preliminary evidence appears promising.[129] It also has the practical advantage of subcutaneous administration. However, to the best of the authors' knowledge, no data exist for pediatric Behçet uveitis.

Cogan Syndrome

First described in 1945, Cogan syndrome (CS) is a rare disease mostly seen in the second and fourth decade of life.[130] It is a vasculitis, mainly affecting the eyes in the form of interstitial keratitis and the audiovestibular system in the form of bilateral hearing loss, tinnitus, and vertigo. Headache, fever, arthritis, arthralgia, myalgia, fatigue, and weight loss are the most common systemic manifestations. Though rare, lymphadenopathy, hepatosplenomegaly, rash, chest or abdominal pain, aortitis, cardiac involvement, and encephalitis have also been reported.[130]

Although the etiology and pathogenesis is unknown, it is thought to be triggered by infections, especially those of upper respiratory tract, resulting in an autoimmune response supported by demonstration of autoantibodies against corneal and inner ear tissues.[131]

Presenting ocular complaints are discomfort, redness, and photophobia. The primary ocular finding is interstitial keratitis with corneal infiltrates more prominent at the periphery. In later stages peripheral corneal vascularization may develop. Although the classic ocular manifestation is interstitial keratitis, conjunctivitis, iritis, episcleritis, scleritis, choroiditis, tendonitis, retinal hemorrhage, papilledema, and exophthalmos have been reported with or without interstitial keratitis.[130] Ocular symptoms can develop before, simultaneously with, or after the onset of audiovestibular symptoms. Manifestations of ocular and auditory involvement usually begin within 1 to 6 months of each other, making the diagnosis particularly challenging when only the ocular or only the audiovestibular manifestations are present.

Diagnosis of CS is often missed or delayed, as it is a rare disease especially in children. The clinical signs at presentation are mostly nonspecific, and there is no confirmatory laboratory test. Ocular examination with slit lamp, audiometric testing, and vestibular studies are essential for the confirmation of diagnosis. Few pediatric cases have been reported in the literature, probably because of underdiagnosis of the disease. In a recent report, Pagnini and colleagues[132] reviewed clinical records of children with CS followed at 2 pediatric rheumatology institutions and those from a database search. Data of 23 children with CS were analyzed, including clinical features at onset, course of the disease, treatment, and outcome. There were 15 males and 8 females with a mean age of 11.4 years (range 4–18 years). Systemic features including fever, arthralgias/arthritis or myalgias, headache, and weight loss were present in 11 children (47.8%) at disease onset. Twenty-one patients (91.3%) had ocular symptoms, mainly in the form of interstitial keratitis, uveitis, or conjunctivitis/episcleritis. Vestibular symptoms observed in 39.1% included vertigo, vomiting, and dizziness. Auditory involvement (65.2%) consisted of sensorineural hearing loss, tinnitus, and deafness. Four patients had cardiac valve involvement and 3 had skin manifestations. After 1 to 16 years (median 2 years) of follow-up, only 30.4% of the patients were in clinical remission. The others had irreversible complications of deafness (21.7%), sensorineural hearing loss (13.0%), vestibular dysfunction (4.3%), and ocular complications in the form of relapsing scleritis, interstitial keratitis or uveitis (13.0%), and cardiac valve damage (17.4%).

Regarding treatment, the ocular component is easier to treat and is often more responsive to therapy than the audiovestibular component.[130] Interstitial keratitis responds well to topical corticosteroids, rarely requiring systemic treatment. However, for audiovestibular involvement, high-dose corticosteroid therapy is the initial and standard therapeutic approach in patients with pediatric CS.[132] However, even though corticosteroids are efficacious for systemic, vestibular, and ocular signs, they may have less effect on hearing loss, as has been reported in adults.[133] In this case, the suggested second-line agent is MTX.[134,135] In refractory cases other immunosuppressants such as cyclophosphamide, MMF, or leflunomide have been recommended.[136,137] Initiation of therapy early in the course of the disease is considered to be essential for the prevention of deafness.[138,139]

LATEST DEVELOPMENTS IN THE TREATMENT OF IED

The treatment of IEDs remains challenging, and can only be successful when the interdisciplinary management between ophthalmologists and rheumatologists is perfectly aligned. At least 50% of children with chronic uveitis require immunosuppressive therapy in addition to topical or intraocular steroids, and pediatric rheumatologists are commonly charged to manage systemic therapy.

Unlike in adults, treatment guidelines for the management of uveitis in the pediatric population have not been published.[76] On the other hand, chronic inflammatory changes and preexisting damage may preclude systemic treatment to reach its full potential. Hence, the paradigm of early, aggressive treatment that has been successful in so many other autoimmune diseases that we treat needs to be applied to the treatment of IEDs and communicated to our ophthalmologic colleagues.

With the introduction of newer DMARDs and biological agents, therapy recommendations for IEDs are still evolving, and need to be tailored to the individual patient and the individual eye disease.

Steroids

Topical corticosteroids, topical nonsteroidal anti-inflammatory drugs, and mydriatics remain the mainstay of short-term therapy, although topical corticosteroids in particular should be limited in duration and dose, and are ineffective in more than one-third of children after 6 months.[140] Because even systemic corticosteroids can leave approximately 30% of children with uveitis uncontrolled,[141] recent research has been focusing on the optimization of subconjunctival, sub-Tenon, transseptal, or retrobulbar injections in the form of surgically implantable depots. In a recent small study evaluating the efficacy and safety of an intravitreal fluocinolone acetonide implant in 4 children with intractable noninfectious posterior uveitis, the inflammation was controlled in all 6 eyes and all patients were successfully weaned off topical steroids. Unfortunately, intraocular steroid injections carry a risk of severe complications such as glaucoma, cataracts, intravitreal hemorrhage, retinal detachment, and infections.[120,142]

DMARDs

Methotrexate
Weekly MTX has become the drug of choice in treating chronic corticosteroid-resistant uveitis. In a recent meta-analysis of articles published between January 1990 and June 2011 on the efficacy of MTX in chronic childhood autoimmune uveitis with MTX doses ranging from 7.5 to 30 mg/m^2, about three-quarters of the patients experienced an improvement in intraocular inflammation.[143] Nevertheless, evidence is limited by the lack of prospective, randomized controlled trials.[144–147] The existing literature seems to suggest that higher weekly doses in the range of 1 mg/kg are required to effectively control ocular inflammation. At these higher doses MTX can achieve detectable aqueous humor levels, despite the absence of detectable serum levels.[148] However, even though MTX may act as a good steroid-sparing agent, many patients do not achieve disease remission, frequently experience early disease relapse, and depending on their type of IED may need to be switched to more aggressive therapy.[149]

Calcineurin inhibitors
Cyclosporine A (CsA) and tacrolimus have been used as alternatives to MTX in corticosteroid-resistant chronic uveitis.[150–154] Since the last review by Gerloni and colleagues[155] in 2001, no larger pediatric studies have been conducted with any of these agents. More recent studies in adults confirmed the steroid-sparing effect but also reemphasized the toxicity risk associated with these drugs.[156] The usual dosing for CsA ranges from 3 to 5 mg/kg/d whereas tacrolimus is used at a dose of about 3 mg/d (serum trough level of ~5 ng/mL). In some studies tacrolimus appears to be more effective as a steroid-sparing agent than CsA, and can also be administered topically.[157]

Mycophenolate mofetil (MMF) and everolimus
MMF is a potent immunomodulatory inhibitor of T- and B-lymphocyte function, which has been successfully used alone or in combination with other immunomodulatory drugs for the treatment of recurrent noninfectious uveitis in adults and children.[158–160] Unlike in adults, however, studies with MMF in pediatric uveitis are limited to smaller case series, and no controlled studies have been performed. In 3 more recent case series with MMF including a total of 109 children (age range 2–14 years) with various forms of uveitis, a steroid-sparing effect was noted in the majority of patients, and vision was preserved or improved in 62% to 94% of the patients. Discontinuation of the drug due to toxicity was rare, and occurred in about 10% to 15% of patients. These results are compatible with recent findings in adult trials.[161–163] In addition, studies in adults seem to suggest that MMF acts faster than MTX in controlling ocular inflammation, and appears safer than azathioprine.[164]

Sirolimus binds to and inhibits the activation of mammalian target of rapamycin (mTOR), a protein promoting cell growth and division thereby suppressing cytokine-driven T-cell proliferation.[165] It has been used in a very limited fashion in ocular inflammatory disease, especially in children, and no dosing recommendations have been established. Sirolimus can be administered orally or intraocularly. In a small prospective study in 8 adult patients, 5 were able to taper or discontinue their concomitant steroids.[166]

Everolimus, another inhibitor of mTOR, is currently approved for children with subependymal giant-cell astrocytomas and other tumors associated with the tuberous sclerosis complex. It has been used as an immunosuppressant to prevent rejection of organ transplants and treatment of renal cell cancer.[167] The use everolimus in the treatment of IEDs appears to be even rarer, and to the authors' knowledge no studies have been conducted in children. In a recent study including 12 adult cyclosporine refractory uveitis patients from Germany, treatment with everolimus resulted in remission in all patients after 3 months, but a disease occurrence was noted in 4 of 12 patients after tapering or withdrawing concomitant cyclosporine, and in 50% of patients after the withdrawal of everolimus.[168]

Historically, other therapeutic agents such as azathioprine, cyclophosphamide, and chlorambucil have been used with variable and usually temporary success, but are limited by their toxicity with long-term use.[11,169,170]

A recent survey of adult uveitis specialists distributed by the American Uveitis Society about the effectiveness, usage, and preferences related to 7 immunomodulatory treatments demonstrated that MTX was the most commonly used initial therapy for anterior, intermediate, and posterior/panuveitis (85%, 57%, and 37%), whereas MMF was the most preferred drug for intermediate (35%) and posterior/panuveitis (42%). Primary reasons not to prescribe azathioprine were lack of efficacy, insufficient safety/tolerability for cyclosporine and cyclophosphamide, and a mixture of cost, safety/tolerability, and difficulty of administration for the biological drugs.[171]

Biologics

Since the introduction of biological agents to pediatric chronic IEDs, this family of drugs has become a frequently used treatment modality in MTX-refractory disease. Adverse effects that are common to the class of anticytokine therapies include infusion reactions, opportunistic infections, latent tuberculosis, malignancies, lupus-like reactions, formation of autoantibodies, and elevated transaminases and lipid levels. However, most of these adverse events are far less common in children than in adults; nevertheless, patients must be screened for hepatitis B and C as well as tuberculosis before the initiation of therapy.[172]

Anti-TNF agents

Although not approved by the Food and Drug Administration (FDA) for this indication, TNF-α inhibitors are the most frequently used agents based on the published literature.

TNF-α has been implicated in the pathogenesis of various forms of uveitis, including JIA-associated uveitis, and has been extensively studied in several animal models of IED.[173,174] An upregulated TNF-α gene expression in the iris/cystoid body and high levels of aqueous humor TNF-α parallel the disease course and contribute to the intraocular inflammation.[175] Dick and colleagues[176] demonstrated more than 17 years ago that the administration of a TNF-α receptor immunoglobulin G (IgG) fusion protein decreased the severity and delayed the onset of uveitis in rats. In the late 1990s the authors' group published the first clinical evidence that TNF inhibitors may be an effective treatment for IED in humans.[177]

Since the publication of this first case series, a multitude of mainly uncontrolled studies have confirmed the utility of the various forms of TNF inhibitors in pediatric IEDs. Unfortunately, the lack of uniformly used clinical outcome parameters such as cell counts, flare readings, intraocular pressure measurements, and visual acuity assessments across studies limit the interpretation of data.[178–187]

Over the last several years a discussion has ensued as to whether there might be a therapeutic advantage of the monoclonal antibodies over the fusion proteins or Fab fragments for the treatment of IEDs. This article does not discuss this further, other than to say that it reviews the scientific evidence rather than echo the often strong "opinions" expressed by some investigators. If one understands the differences in the pharmacokinetic profiles of the various anti-TNF drugs and comprehends the disease state–dependent pathophysiology of the blood-eye barrier during an inflammatory event, one can easily recognize why in certain circumstances monoclonal antibodies seem to have a therapeutic advantage over the other formulations. Patients with more acute disease are usually more responsive to any form of TNF inhibitor than patients with low-grade chronic disease. Serum concentrations of TNF and VEGF parallel disease activity and regulate vascular hyperpermeability, intraocular blood flow, and subsequent intraocular drug concentrations.[188] In summary, differences in the binding affinity and pharmacokinetic ability to achieve higher serum levels (ie, though intravenous administration) among the various TNF-α inhibitors may account for the discrepancies observed in clinical trials.[189]

Over the last few years larger studies and pooled data reviews have added important information about the long-term efficacy and safety of the various anti-TNF agents in the treatment of IED. These drugs specifically include adalimumab and golimumab as the latest edition to the uveitis treatment armamentarium.[183–187,190] Most of these studies enrolled patients who had failed prior steroid and DMARD treatments, which suggests that they already had a partially restored blood-brain barrier. In one of the more recent publications about the long-term efficacy and safety of infliximab and adalimumab, which is representative for most of the recent published studies, 47 of 91 (55.3%) patients with JIA-related uveitis achieved remission while 28 (32.9%) had recurrent disease, and 10 (11.8%) remained irresponsive to treatment. None of the patients experienced serious adverse events.[185] In another study of 17 children (32 eyes) with treatment-refractory noninfectious childhood chronic uveitis from a single center treated with subcutaneous adalimumab, visual acuity improved and intraocular inflammation stabilized in most patients, but did not completely obviate the use of systemic or periocular steroid treatment.[183]

Two recent studies and a literature review expanded on prior reports' rather paradoxic findings of an association of new-onset uveitis, scleritis, and optic neuritis with the use of etanercept.[191,192] In the first study from Israel, 4 children with JIA-associated uveitis (3 girls with oligoarticular JIA, 1 boy with HLA-B27–positive juvenile spondyloarthropathy) treated with etanercept were found to have reduced visual acuity due to optic neuritis and associated vitreitis after a mean follow-up of 10 months (range 2.5–18 months). In 3 of 4 children, the discontinuation of etanercept, together with steroid treatment, resulted in resolution of the inflammation, whereas the fourth patient experienced no further deterioration in visual acuity despite ongoing etanercept treatment. In the second study, 2 children with JIA "developed" uveitis with the initiation of etanercept. Thus far 42 cases of IEDs including 33 cases of uveitis, 8 cases of scleritis, and 1 case of orbital myositis, presumably associated with the use of etanercept, have been reported in the literature, including 10 patients with JIA. A dechallenge was performed in 28 patients, leading to symptom resolution, and a rechallenge in 6 cases resulted in disease reemergence. In all of these studies it was difficult to determine whether etanercept was truly involved in the pathogenesis of the eye disease or rather was not potent enough to suppress it.[193]

Emerging knowledge from summarizing the more recent literature about the use of anti-TNF agents in IEDs seems to suggest that:

- Anti-TNF agents are safe and effective in IEDs even when used over longer periods of time
- No clear superiority of any of the anti-TNF drugs can be established, although studies in treatment-refractory patients favor the monoclonal antibodies
- Higher doses of infliximab and frequent dosing intervals are often required to achieve disease control in some patients, and doses as high as 20 mg/kg have been used especially in patients with VKH and pars planitis
- About one-third of patients do not respond to treatment with anti-TNF inhibitors even when higher doses are used
- Paradoxic emergence of IED may occur in patients treated with etanercept

Because many patients require higher doses of intravenous infliximab to achieve disease control, several older small case series reported the use of intravitreally administered infliximab and adalimumab, with mixed results. Two recent smaller studies expanded on these reports and the administration of intraocular infliximab in IED.[194,195] In the first study in 15 adult patients with BD, a single intravitreal injection of infliximab (1 mg/0.05 mL) was given, with subsequent significant improvement in several clinical parameters in most of the patients. In another study from Iran, 7 adult patients with noninfectious uveitis were intravitreally injected with 1.5 mg of infliximab and followed for 6 months. Even though the investigators observed improved vision and decreases in macular edema in some patients, they concluded that the effect was temporary and that repeated injections would be needed to sustain the treatment effect. These 2 studies also demonstrate again that treatment effects observed in patients with BD are not necessarily translatable to other forms of uveitis.

Anti–IL-1 therapies
Until recently, evidence for the use of anti–IL-1 therapies was limited to studies in rodents, when Lim and colleagues[196] demonstrated that anakinra suppressed immune-mediated experimental autoimmune uveitis in mice.

However, several recent studies in adult patients with DMARD and steroid-refractory BD have reported successful outcomes in acute posterior uveitis, panuveitis, and/or retinal vasculitis with monoclonal antibodies against IL-1.[197,198] Furthermore, a recent case report about the successful treatment of severe uveitis in a 4-year old patient with Blau syndrome with canakinumab, a monoclonal anti–IL-1 antibody, suggests that anti–IL-1 therapy may also be effective for children with uveitis.[199] Because IL-1 is an important cytokine for the maintenance of intraocular inflammation, anti–IL-1 therapeutics may become an important component of uveitis therapy, especially in patients with anti–TNF-refractory disease.

Anti–IL-2 therapies
IL-2 is a cytokine that is primarily synthesized by activated T cells, and plays an essential role in the cellular immune response by promoting proliferation and differentiation of T-helper cells. The clinical experience with the 2 commercially available antibodies targeting IL-2, daclizumab (humanized anti–IL-2 receptor monoclonal antibody) and basiliximab (chimeric human-murine anti–IL-2 receptor monoclonal antibody) in the treatment of IEDs have been summarized in previous reviews.[3,200] Since the withdrawal of daclizumab from the market by the manufacturer in early 2009 and the

lack of efficacy with basiliximab in IED studies due to antibody formation against the drug, no further studies with these agents have been published.

Anti–IL-6 therapies
Tocilizumab (TCZ) is a humanized monoclonal antibody that targets the IL-6 receptor and is FDA-approved for the treatment of rheumatoid arthritis, polyarticular juvenile arthritis and systemic juvenile arthritis.[201,202] Most patients with arthritis require intravenous TCZ at 8 to 12 mg/kg body weight at 2- or 4-weekly intervals, with beneficial outcome and acceptable safety profile.

In 2 small case series including 5 adult patients with treatment-refractory chronic uveitis, treatment with intravenous TCZ at 8 mg/kg either as a single infusion or at 4-weekly intervals, resulted in an improvement in anterior chamber cells, visual acuity, and central retinal thickness by optical coherence tomography in 4 of 5 patients. No adverse events related to TCZ were observed.[203,204] To date, no experience with this drug in pediatric IEDs has been published. Similar to IL-1, IL-6 is an important cytokine for the maintenance of intraocular inflammation, and TCZ may become an important component of uveitis therapy, especially in patients with anti–TNF-refractory disease.

Anti–IL-17 therapies
IL-17 is a proinflammatory cytokine that is produced by T-helper cells and is induced by IL-23. IL-17 acts synergistically with TNF and IL-1 as potent mediator in delayed-type reactions by increasing chemokine production and recruiting monocytes and neutrophils to sites of inflammation. IL-17 has been implicated in the pathogenesis of several forms of IED.[205,206] Although initial phase II trial data appeared promising, 3 very recent multicenter, randomized, double-blind, placebo-controlled studies with secukinumab, a fully human monoclonal antibody against IL-17A enrolling 274 patients with various forms of noninfectious IED, demonstrated no statistically significant differences in uveitis recurrence between secukinumab and placebo. Of note, analysis of secondary efficacy data from these studies suggested a beneficial effect of secukinumab in reducing concomitant DMARD and steroid use.[207] Inhibitors against IL-17 are currently being explored in the treatment of psoriasis.

Abatacept
Abatacept is a selective costimulatory molecule inhibitor consisting of the extracellular domain of the human cytotoxic T-lymphocyte antigen 4 (CTLA4) fused to the FC domain of human IgG$_1$. Abatacept interferes with antigen presentation by binding to CD80/CD86 on antigen-presenting cells, leading to the interruption of the CD28 costimulatory signal and inactivation of T cells.[208] Marketed under the trade name Orencia, abatacept is FDA-approved for the treatment of polyarticular JIA and rheumatoid arthritis.[209,210] In several recent small, mainly retrospective case series including 12 children with treatment-refractory JIA-associated uveitis, abatacept appeared to be a promising alternative treatment in refractory cases of JIA uveitis with a surprisingly high success rate and steroid-sparing capacity, even though the concomitant joint disease remained uncontrolled.[211–214] In his own fairly large pediatric IED practice, the senior author has been unable to replicate the success rates with Orencia reported in the literature.

Anti–B-cell therapies
Rituximab Rituximab is a chimeric monoclonal antibody against CD20, a surface marker primarily found on B cells. Rituximab lyses B cells, and is therefore used to treat lymphomas, leukemias, transplant rejection, and autoimmune disorders. In

autoimmunity, rituximab is FDA-approved for rheumatoid arthritis, granulomatosis with polyangiitis (Wegener granulomatosis), and microscopic polyangiitis.[215] Growing evidence in the ophthalmology literature suggests that rituximab may be useful for the treatment of IEDs.[216–218] Similar to the other non–anti-TNF biological agents, evidence is limited to smaller adult and pediatric uveitis case series in patients with treatment-refractory uveitis, scleritis, and peripheral ulcerative keratitis. In a recent literature review on the efficacy of rituximab in 8 children with severe and long-standing uveitis who had failed anti-TNF therapy, all patients showed improvement in disease activity and were able to reduce concomitant corticosteroids and immunosuppressants after a mean of 14.87 months. No serious adverse events were observed.[217] In another case series in 10 children with treatment-refractory JIA-associated uveitis who had failed topical/systemic steroids, immunosuppressives, and at least 1 TNF-α inhibitor, 7 of 10 children achieved remission after a mean of 11 months and were able to discontinue some or all of their concomitant medications. However, 4 children relapsed between 6 and 9 months, and 3 of 4 were recaptured with another treatment course. Most children in this study only received a single course of 2 rituximab infusions at 375 mg/m^2 body surface at 2-week intervals with some intravenous methylprednisolone. Similar to the previous study, no serious adverse events were observed.[218]

Further studies are needed to assess the efficacy of rituximab in the treatment of IEDs, but this drug should be considered in patients with severe disease refractory to conventional DMARDs and other biological agents.

Alemtuzumab Alemtuzumab (Campath) is a chimeric monoclonal antibody against CD52, a surface marker primarily found on B cells and mature lymphocytes, but not on stem cells, and is used in the treatment of chronic lymphocytic leukemia, cutaneous T-cell lymphoma, and T-cell lymphoma. It is also used for the treatment of a variety of autoimmune diseases including IEDs. The evidence for alemtuzumab in the treatment of IEDs has been reviewed in prior articles.[3,219] Since the publication of the early case series in the mid-1990s, no articles have been published on extending the use of alemtuzumab in IEDs.

Anti-VEGF therapy

Monoclonal antibodies or Fab fragments against VEGF such as bevacizumab (Avastin) and ranibizumab (Lucentis) have been used individually or in combination with other medications in the treatment of IEDs.[220] Originally designed and FDA-approved for the treatment of age-related macular degeneration and colorectal cancer, these 2 compounds seem to be particularly effective for uveitis with cystic macular edema (CME). The author often combines these agents with anti-TNF therapy in children with treatment-refractory IED and CME (unpublished observations).

FUTURE TREATMENTS

Similar to studies in other autoimmune diseases such as arthritis and Crohn disease, approximately 20% to 30% of patients with IED do not respond to first-line biological therapies such as anti-TNF agents. As a result, intense research is focusing on treatment alternatives for these devastating diseases.[221]

In a recent study, a novel genetically engineered IL27p28/IL12p40 heterodimeric cytokine (p28/p40), which antagonizes signaling downstream of the gp130 receptor, was successfully explored in the EAU model, suggesting that cytokines comprising unique IL-12 α- and β-subunit pairing may exist in nature and may constitute a new class of therapeutic cytokines.[222] In another recent study by Lennikov and colleagues,[223] a novel IκB kinase β inhibitor was successful in ameliorating acute uveitis in an endotoxin-induced uveitis mouse model, suggesting that small molecule inhibitors will potentially become future treatments for IED.

Another interesting approach is Optiquel, a natural product that contains B27PD, a small protein decoy, mimicking autoantigenic intraocular proteins that may induce tolerance. This peptide is currently being tested as a steroid-sparing therapy in 60 adult patients with chronic autoimmune uveitis (ClinicalTrials.gov identifier: NCT01195948).

Lastly, ESBA-105 is a topical anti-TNFα single-chain antibody for the treatment of uveitis, diabetic retinopathy, and age-related macular degeneration, which aims to replace systemic anti-TNFα administration, if it can achieve sufficient penetration and drug concentration after passing the cornea.[224]

OUTCOMES

Overall, outcomes of children with IED remain variable. Some of the individual prognoses have already been discussed above. The long-term impact of biological therapy on the overall outcome of these diseases still remains to be seen. In the authors' experience the prognosis of most IEDs depends less on the individual treatment choice than on early diagnosis and the implementation of early and aggressive treatment. The ocular condition at the first visit is the most significant predictor of visual outcome.[225] This notion is also supported by more recent studies in childhood IEDs suggesting that the visual prognosis of pediatric uveitis is improving as a result of earlier diagnosis and treatment.[51,226]

In a summary of 35 long-term follow-up studies including 5300 children with various forms of IEDs and an average 5-year follow-up, cataract formation was observed in 27%, band keratopathies in 30%, glaucoma in 20%, synechiae in 35%, and decreased vision of 20/40 or worse in 30% of the children. Sixty percent had a relapsing disease course, and bilateral eye involvement was noted in 70% of the patients within 1 year.[3] These results represent a slight improvement over the findings of Cabral and colleagues[227] in 1994. Permanent blindness is still seen in approximately 10% of children, but was as high as 27% in a recent study by Gregory and colleagues.[228]

Posterior uveitis and panuveitis appear to have a worse prognosis, and Hispanic ethnicity appears to be associated with a higher prevalence of infectious uveitis and vision loss at baseline.[12,229] Damage accrued during childhood can have long-term consequences into adulthood, with a significant impact on employability and quality of life. A recent study from the United Kingdom demonstrated that chronic uveitis, even if well controlled, can have substantial effects on a patient's social and psychological health, and can lead to significant work disability.[230] It is estimated that the various forms of IED cause approximately 30,000 new cases of blindness among children and adults at an incidence of 20 to 52 cases per 100,000 person-years.[18,231,232]

SUMMARY

Vision-threatening complications of pediatric uveitis are significant. Even though IEDs are less common in children than in adults, their diagnosis and management can be particularly challenging and the causes are different from those in adults. Young children are often asymptomatic, due to their inability to express complaints or because of the truly asymptomatic nature of their disease. Even in advanced cases, parents may not be aware of any visual impairment until the development of visible changes such as band keratopathy, strabismus, or cataracts. Therefore, the diagnosis is often delayed, and severe complications may already be present at the time of the initial visit with the ophthalmologist. In children who present with amblyopia or strabismus, a careful examination is required to rule out uveitis as an underlying cause. There are unique forms of uveitis and masquerade syndromes that are specific to the pediatric age group, while some entities commonly encountered in adults are rare in children. A prompt referral to a rheumatologist with sufficient expertise in the management of these diseases should be made because very few ophthalmologists treat these patients with anything other than steroids, which have limited therapeutic value especially in the later stages of these disorders. Prospective studies using standard outcome measures in clearly defined diseases instead of mixing a variety of IEDs are clearly needed to identify children most at risk and to define the best treatment strategies for each type of IED. Even though therapeutic options for the treatment of childhood IEDs have expanded over the last 30 years outcomes remain fair to poor. DMARDs are associated with significant toxicity and often offer limited efficacy and less success in inducing remission in comparison with adult patients. Although it is too early to say with certainty, biological agents may become first-line treatment in IEDs, but they should be used early and aggressively to be maximally efficient. Prior experience with biologics from other pediatric rheumatologic diseases has demonstrated that the risk/benefit ratio clearly favors the drug over the devastating impact of permanent vision loss. Future treatments will also require better delivery systems to provide targeted treatment with minimal side effects and reduced cost.

REFERENCES

1. Pivetti-Pezzi P. Uveitis in children. Eur J Ophthalmol 1996;6:293–8.
2. Gery I, Nussenblatt RB, Chan CC, et al. Autoimmune diseases of the eye. In: Theofilopoulos AN, Bona CA, editors. The molecular pathology of autoimmune diseases. New York: Taylor and Francis; 2002. p. 978–98.
3. Reiff A. Ocular complication in childhood rheumatologic diseases: uveitis [review]. Curr Rheumatol Rep 2006;6(8):459–68.
4. Reiff A. Ocular complication in child hood rheumatologic diseases: non uveitic disorders [review]. Curr Rheumatol Rep 2009;11(3):226–32.
5. Heinz C, Heiligenhaus A, Kümmerle-Deschner J, et al. Uveitis in juvenile idiopathic arthritis. Z Rheumatol 2010;69(5):411–8.
6. Tugal-Tutkun I, Havrlikova K, Power WJ, et al. Changing patterns in uveitis of childhood. Ophthalmology 1996;103:375–83.
7. Petty RE, Smith JR, Rosenbaum JT. Arthritis and uveitis in children: a pediatric rheumatology perspective. Am J Ophthalmol 2003;135:879–84.
8. Khairallah M. Are the Standardization of the Uveitis Nomenclature (SUN) Working Group criteria for codifying the site of inflammation appropriate for all uveitis problems? Limitations of the SUN Working Group Classification. Ocul Immunol Inflamm 2010;18(1):2–4.
9. Jabs DA, Nussenblatt RB, Rosenbaum JT, Standardization of Uveitis Nomenclature (SUN) Working Group. Standardization of uveitis nomenclature for reporting clinical data. Results of the First International Workshop. Am J Ophthalmol 2005; 140(3):509–16.
10. Edelsten C, Reddy MA, Stanford MR, et al. Visual loss associated with pediatric uveitis in English primary and referral centers. Am J Ophthalmol 2003;135:676–80.
11. Becker MD, Smith JR, Max R, et al. Management of sight-threatening uveitis: new therapeutic options. Drugs 2005;65:497–519.
12. Smith JA, Mackensen F, Sen HN, et al. Epidemiology and course of disease in childhood uveitis. Ophthalmology 2009;116:1544–51.

13. BenEzra D, Cohen E, Maftzir G. Uveitis in children and adolescents. Br J Ophthalmol 2005;89:444–8.
14. Rathinam SR, Namperumalsamy P. Global variation and pattern changes in epidemiology of uveitis. Indian J Ophthalmol 2007;55:173–83.
15. Kazokoglu H, Onal S, Tugal-Tutkun I, et al. Demographic and clinical features of uveitis in tertiary centers in Turkey. Ophthalmic Epidemiol 2008;15:285–93.
16. Paivönsalo-Hietanen T, Tuominen J, Saari KM. Uveitis in children: population-based study in Finland. Acta Ophthalmol Scand 2000;78:84–8.
17. Paroli MP, Spinucci G, Liverani M, et al. Uveitis in childhood: an Italian clinical and epidemiological study. Ocul Immunol Inflamm 2009;17:238–42.
18. Gritz DC, Wong IG. Incidence and prevalence of uveitis in Northern California; the Northern California Epidemiology of Uveitis Study. Ophthalmology 2004;111:491–500.
19. Liu B, Sen HN, Nussenblatt R. Susceptibility genes and pharmacogenetics in ocular inflammatory disorders. Ocul Immunol Inflamm 2012;20(5):315–23.
20. Davis JL, Mittal KK, Freidlin V, et al. HLA associations and ancestry in Vogt-Koyanagi-Harada disease and sympathetic ophthalmia. Ophthalmology 1990;97(9):1137–42.
21. Gasparin F, Takahashi BS, Scolari MR, et al. Experimental models of autoimmune inflammatory ocular diseases [review]. Arq Bras Oftalmol 2012;75(2):143–7.
22. Bora NS, Sohn JH, Kang SG, et al. Type I collagen is the autoantigen in experimental anterior uveitis. J Immunol 2004;172:7086–94.
23. Caspi RR. A look at autoimmunity and inflammation in the eye. J Clin Invest 2010;120(9):3073–83.
24. Takeuchi M, Yokoi H, Tsukahara R, et al. Differentiation of Th1 and Th2 cells in lymph nodes and spleens of mice during experimental autoimmune uveoretinitis. Jpn J Ophthalmol 2001;45:463–9.
25. Sun M, Yang P, Du L, et al. Contribution of CD4+CD25+ T cells to the regression phase of experimental autoimmune uveoretinitis. Invest Ophthalmol Vis Sci 2010;51:383–9.
26. Pennesi G, Mattapallil MJ, Sun SH, et al. A humanized model of experimental autoimmune uveitis in HLA class II transgenic mice. J Clin Invest 2003;111(8):1171–80.
27. Ruggieri S, Frassanito MA, Dammacco R, et al. Treg lymphocytes in autoimmune uveitis. Ocul Immunol Inflamm 2012;20(4):255–61.
28. Lacomba MS, Martin CM, Gallardo Galera JM, et al. Aqueous humor and serum tumor necrosis factor-alpha in clinical uveitis. Ophthalmic Res 2001;33:251–5.
29. Noma H, Funatsu H, Yamasaki M, et al. Pathogenesis of macular edema with branch retinal vein occlusion and intraocular levels of vascular endothelial growth factor and interleukin-6. Am J Ophthalmol 2005;140:256–61.
30. Chan CC, Caspi RR, Ni M, et al. Pathology of experimental autoimmune uveoretinitis in mice. J Autoimmun 1990;3:247–55.
31. Caspi RR, Chan CC, Wiggert B, et al. The mouse as a model of experimental autoimmune uveoretinitis (EAU). Curr Eye Res 1990;9:169.
32. Jiang HR, Lumsden L, Forrester JV. Macrophages and dendritic cells in IRBP-induced experimental autoimmune uveoretinitis in B10.RIII mice. Invest Ophthalmol Vis Sci 1999;40:3177–85.
33. Zhang Z, Zhong W, Hall MJ, et al. CXCR4 but not CXCR7 is mainly implicated in ocular leukocyte trafficking during ovalbumin-induced acute uveitis. Invest Ophthalmol Vis Sci 2012;53(8):4668–75.

34. Mochizuki M, Sugita S, Kamoi K. Immunological homeostasis of the eye. Prog Retin Eye Res 2013;33:10–27.

35. Lacomba MS, Martin CM, Chamond RR, et al. Aqueous and serum interferon gamma, interleukin (IL) 2, IL-4, and IL-10 in patients with uveitis. Arch Ophthalmol 2000;118:768–72.

36. El-Shabrawi Y, Livir-Rallatos C, Christen W, et al. High levels of interleukin-12 in the aqueous humor and vitreous of patients with uveitis. Ophthalmology 1998; 105:1659–63.

37. de Boer JH, Hack CE, Verhoeven AJ, et al. Chemoattractant and neutrophil degranulation activities related to interleukin-8 in vitreous fluid in uveitis and vitreo-retinal disorders. Invest Ophthalmol Vis Sci 1993;34:3376–85.

38. Perez VL, Papaliodis GN, Chu D, et al. Elevated levels of interleukin 6 in the vitreous fluid of patients with pars planitis and posterior uveitis: the Massachusetts eye & ear experience and review of previous studies. Ocul Immunol Inflamm 2004;12:193–201.

39. Franks WA, Limb GA, Stanford MR, et al. Cytokines in human intraocular inflammation. Curr Eye Res 1992;11(Suppl):187–91.

40. Hooks JJ, Chan CC, Detrick B. Identification of the lymphokines, interferon-gamma and interleukin-2, in inflammatory eye diseases. Invest Ophthalmol Vis Sci 1988;29:1444–51.

41. Norose K, Yano A, Wang XC, et al. Dominance of activated T cells and interleukin-6 in aqueous humor in Vogt-Koyanagi-Harada disease. Invest Ophthalmol Vis Sci 1994;35:33–9.

42. Zierhut M, Michels H, Stubiger N, et al. Uveitis in children. Int Ophthalmol Clin 2005;45:135–56.

43. Shulman S, Goldenberg D, Habot-Wilner Z, et al. Optical coherence tomography characteristics of eyes with acute anterior uveitis. Methods Mol Biol 2012; 900:443–69.

44. Cauduro RS, Ferraz Cdo A, Morales MS, et al. Application of anterior segment optical coherence tomography in pediatric ophthalmology. J Ophthalmol 2012; 2012:313120.

45. Ducos de Lahitte G, Terrada C, Tran TH, et al. Maculopathy in uveitis of juvenile idiopathic arthritis: an optical coherence tomography study. Br J Ophthalmol 2008;92:64–9.

46. JTuran-Vural E, Torun Acar B, Sevim MS, et al. Corneal biomechanical properties in patients with recurrent anterior uveitis. Biol Chem 2012;287(43): 36012–21.

47. Reininga JK, Los LI, Wulffraat NM, et al. The evaluation of uveitis in juvenile idiopathic arthritis (JIA) patients: are current ophthalmologic screening guidelines adequate? Clin Exp Rheumatol 2008;26(2):367–72, Int Ophthalmol 2009;29(1): 33–7.

48. Cassidy J, Kivlin J, Lindsley C, et al, Section on Rheumatology, Section on Ophthalmology. Ophthalmologic examinations in children with juvenile rheumatoid arthritis. Pediatrics 2006;117:1843–5.

49. Khanfer R, Wallace G, Keane PA, et al. Uveitis and psychological stress. Ocul Immunol Inflamm 2012;20(5):349–53.

50. Kanski JJ, Shun-Shin GA. Systemic uveitis syndromes in childhood: an analysis of 340 cases. Ophthalmology 1984;91:1247–52.

51. Saurenmann RK, Levin AV, Feldman BM, et al. Risk factors for development of uveitis differ between girls and boys with juvenile idiopathic arthritis. Insight 2012;37(2):11–6.

52. Heiligenhaus A, Niewerth M, Ganser G, et al, German Uveitis in Childhood Study Group. Prevalence and complications of uveitis in juvenile idiopathic arthritis in a population-based nation-wide study in Germany: suggested modification of the current screening guidelines. Rheumatol Oxf 2007;46(6):1015–9.
53. Kanski JJ. Anterior uveitis in juvenile rheumatoid arthritis. Arch Ophthalmol 1977;95(10):1794–7.
54. Kump LI, Cervantes-Castaneda RA, Androudi SN, et al. Analysis of pediatric cases at a tertiary referral center. Ophthalmology 2005;112:1287–92.
55. Thorne JE, Woreta F, Kedhar SR, et al. Juvenile idiopathic arthritis-associated uveitis: incidence of ocular complications and visual acuity loss. Am J Ophthalmol 2007;143:840–6.
56. Davis JL, Dacanay LM, Holland GN, et al. Laser flare photometry and complications of chronic uveitis in children. Am J Ophthalmol 2003;135:763–71.
57. Holland GN. A reconsideration of anterior chamber flare and its clinical relevance for children with chronic anterior uveitis (an American Ophthalmological Society thesis). Trans Am Ophthalmol Soc 2007;105:344–64.
58. Damico F, Bezerra FT, Silva GC, et al. New insights into Vogt-Koyanagi-Harada disease. Arq Bras Oftalmol 2009;72(3):413–20.
59. Fang W, Yang P. Vogt-Koyanagi-Harada Syndrome Mini Review. Curr Eye Res 2008;33:517–23.
60. da Silva FT, Damico FM, Marin ML, et al. Revised diagnostic criteria for Vogt-Koyanagi-Harada disease: considerations on the different disease categories. Am J Ophthalmol 2009;147(2):339–45.
61. El-Asrar AM, Al-Kharashi AS, Aldibhi H, et al. Vogt-Koyanagi-Harada disease in children. Eye 2008;22:1124–31.
62. Damico FM, Kiss S, Young LH. Vogt-Koyanagi-Harada disease. Semin Ophthalmol 2005;20(3):183–90.
63. Garcia LA, Carroll MO, Garza León MA. Vogt-Koyanagi-Harada syndrome in childhood. Int Ophthalmol Clin 2008;48(3):107–17.
64. Tabbara KF, Chavis PS, Freeman WR. Vogt-Koyanagi-Harada syndrome in children compared to adults. Acta Ophthalmol Scand 1998;76(6):723–6.
65. Shindo Y, Inoko H, Yamamoto T, et al. HLA-DRB1 typing of Vogt-Koyanagi-Harada's disease by PCR-RFLP and the strong association with DRB1*0405 and DRB1*0410. Br J Ophthalmol 1994;78(3):223–6.
66. Chi W, Yang P, Li B, et al. IL-23 promotes CD4+ T cells to produce IL-17 in Vogt-Koyanagi-Harada disease. J Allergy Clin Immunol 2007;119(5):1218–24.
67. Wang C, Tian Y, Lei B, et al. Decreased IL-27 expression in association with an increased Th17 response in Vogt-Koyanagi-Harada disease. Invest Ophthalmol Vis Sci 2012;53(8):4668–75.
68. Commodaro AG, Bueno V, Belfort R Jr, et al. Autoimmune uveitis: the associated proinflammatory molecules and the search for immunoregulation. Autoimmun Rev 2011;10(4):205–9.
69. Moorthy RS, Inomata H, Rao NA. Vogt-Koyanagi-Harada syndrome. Surv Ophthalmol 1995;39(4):265–92.
70. Paredes I, Ahmed M, Foster CS. Immunomodulatory therapy for Vogt-Koyanagi-Harada patients as first-line therapy. Ocul Immunol Inflamm 2006;14(2):87–90.
71. Andreoli CM, Foster CS. Vogt-Koyanagi-Harada disease. Int Ophthalmol Clin 2006;46(2):111–22.
72. Perente I, Utine CA, Cakir H, et al. Management of ocular complications of Vogt-Koyanagi-Harada syndrome. J Pediatr Ophthalmol Strabismus 2007;44(5):288–93.

73. Soheilian M, Aletaha M, Yazdani S, et al. Management of paediatric Vogt-Koyanagi-Harada (VKH)-associated panuveitis. Ocul Immunol Inflamm 2006; 14:91–8.

74. Michalova K, Lim L. Biologic agents in the management of inflammatory eye diseases. Curr Allergy Asthma Rep 2008;8(4):339–47.

75. Khalifa YM, Bailony MR, Acharya NR. Treatment of pediatric Vogt-Koyanagi-Harada syndrome with infliximab. Ocul Immunol Inflamm 2010;18(3): 218–22.

76. Jabs DA, Rosenbaum JT, Foster CS, et al. Guidelines for the use of immunosuppressive drugs in patients with ocular inflammatory disorders: recommendations of an expert panel. Am J Ophthalmol 2000;130:492–513.

77. Read RW, Yu F, Accorinti M, et al. Evaluation of the effect on outcomes of the route of administration of corticosteroids in acute Vogt-Koyanagi-Harada disease. Am J Ophthalmol 2006;142(1):119–24.

78. Al-Kharashi AS, Aldibhi H, Al-Fraykh H, et al. Prognostic factors in Vogt-Koyanagi-Harada disease. Int Ophthalmol 2007;27(2–3):201–10.

79. Guest S, Funkhouser E, Lightman S. Pars planitis: a comparison of childhood onset and adult onset disease. Clin Experiment Ophthalmol 2001;29:81–4.

80. Romero R, Peralta J, Sendagorta E, et al. Pars planitis in children: epidemiologic, clinical, and therapeutic characteristics. J Pediatr Ophthalmol Strabismus 2007;44:288–93.

81. de Boer J, Berendschot TT, van der Does P, et al. Long-term follow-up of intermediate uveitis in children. Am J Ophthalmol 2006;141(4):616–21.

82. Tang WM, Pulido JS, Eckels DD, et al. The association of HLA-DR15 and intermediate uveitis. Am J Ophthalmol 1997;123(1):70–5.

83. Tugal-Tutkun I, Ayranci O, Kasapcopur O, et al. Retrospective analysis of children with uveitis treated with infliximab. J AAPOS 2008;12(6):611–3.

84. Sukumaran S, Marzan K, Reiff A. High dose infliximab in the treatment of refractory uveitis: does dose really matter? ISRN Rheumatol 2012;2012:765380.

85. Kalinina Ayuso V, ten Cate HA, van den Does P, et al. Young age as a risk factor for complicated course and visual outcome in intermediate uveitis in children. Br J Ophthalmol 2011;95(5):646–51.

86. Paroli MP, Spinucci G, Monte R, et al. Intermediate uveitis in a pediatric Italian population. Arthritis Rheum 2010;62(6):1824–8.

87. Mandeville JT, Levinson RD, Holland GN. The tubulointerstitial nephritis and uveitis syndrome. Surv Ophthalmol 2001;46(3):195–208.

88. Levinson R. Tubulointerstitial nephritis and uveitis syndrome. Int Ophthalmol Clin 2008;48(3):51–9.

89. Mackensen F, Billing H. Tubulointerstitial nephritis and uveitis syndrome. Curr Opin Ophthalmol 2009;20(6):525–31.

90. Jahnukainen T, Ala-Houhala M, Karikoski R, et al. Clinical outcome and occurrence of uveitis in children with idiopathic tubulointerstitial nephritis. Pediatr Nephrol 2011;26(2):291–9.

91. Mackensen F, Smith JR, Rosenbaum JT. Enhanced recognition, treatment, and prognosis of tubulointerstitial nephritis and uveitis syndrome. Ophthalmology 2007;114(5):995–9.

92. Behçet H. Uber rezidivierende Aphthose, durch ein Virus verursachte Geschwure am Mund, am Auge und an den Genitalien. Dermatol Wochenschr 1937; 105:1152–7.

93. Tugal-Tutkun I, Onal S, Altan-Yaycioglu R, et al. Uveitis in Behçet disease: an analysis of 880 patients. Am J Ophthalmol 2004;138:373–80.

94. Kansu T, Kadayifcilar S. Visual aspects of Behçet's disease. Curr Neurol Neurosci Rep 2005;5:382–8.
95. Behçet's Disease Research Committee. Clinical research section recommendations. Jpn J Ophthalmol 1974;18:291–4.
96. International Study Group for Behçet's disease. Criteria for diagnosis of Behçet's disease. Lancet 1990;335:1078–80.
97. Kneifel CE, Köhler AK, Altenburg A, et al. Epidemiology of ocular involvement in Adamantiades-Behçets disease. Ophthalmologe 2012;109:542–7.
98. Atmaca L, Boyvat A, Yalçındağ FN, et al. Behçet disease in children. Ocul Immunol Inflamm 2011;19:103–7.
99. Evereklioğlu C. Current concepts in the etiology and treatment of Behçet's disease. Surv Ophthalmol 2005;50:297–350.
100. Masuda K, Inaba G, Mizushima H, et al. A nation-wide survey of Behçet's disease in Japan. Jpn J Ophthalmol 1975;19:278–85.
101. Colvard DM, Robertson DM, O'Duffy JD. The ocular manifestations in Behçet's disease. Arch Ophthalmol 1977;95:1813–7.
102. Hazleman BL. Rheumatic disorders of the eye and the various structures involved. Br J Rheumatol 1996;35:258–68.
103. Kadayifcilar S, Gedik S, Eldem B, et al. Cataract surgery in patients with Behçet's disease. J Cataract Refract Surg 2002;28:316–20.
104. Elgin U, Berker N, Batman A. Incidence of secondary glaucoma in Behçet's disease. J Glaucoma 2004;13:441–4.
105. Ozdal PC, Ortac S, Taskintuna I, et al. Posterior segment involvement in ocular Behçet's disease. Eur J Ophthalmol 2002;12:424–31.
106. Kadayıfçılar S, Eldem B. Full thickness macular holes associated with Behçet's disease. VIIth International Congress of International Ocular Inflammation Society. Padua, 2003, Abstract Book. p. 102.
107. Citirik M, Berker N, Songur MS, et al. Ocular findings in childhood-onset Behçets disease. J AAPOS 2009;13:391–5.
108. Sungur GK, Hazirolan D, Yalvac I, et al. Clinical and demographic evaluation of Behçets disease among different paediatric age groups. Br J Ophthalmol 2009; 93:83–7.
109. Altenburg Ai Mahr A, Maldini C, Kneifel CE, et al. Epidemiology and clinical aspects of Adamantiades—Behçet disease in Germany. Current data. Ophthalmologe 2012;109:531–41 [in German].
110. Atmaca LS. Fundus changes associated with Behçet's disease. Graefes Arch Clin Exp Ophthalmol 1989;227:340–4.
111. Tugal-Tutkun I. Imaging in the diagnosis and management of Behçet's disease. Int Ophthalmol Clin 2012;52:183–90.
112. Ozen S. Pediatric onset Behçet disease. Curr Opin Rheumatol 2010;22:585–9.
113. Tugal-Tutkun I, Urgancioglu M. Childhood-onset uveitis in Behçet disease: a descriptive study of 36 cases. Am J Ophthalmol 2003;136:1114–9.
114. Toker E, Kazokoglu H, Acar N. High dose intravitreal steroid therapy for severe posterior segment uveitis in Behçet's disease. Br J Ophthalmol 2002;86:321–3.
115. Yalçındag FN, Can E, Ozdemir O. Intravenous methylprednisolone pulse therapy for acute posterior segment uveitis attacks in Behçet's disease. Ann Ophthalmol 2007;39:194–7.
116. Hatemi G, Silman A, Bang D. Management of Behçet disease: a systematic literature review for the European League Against Rheumatism evidence-based recommendations for the management of Behçet disease. Ann Rheum Dis 2009;68:1528–34.

117. Kramer M, Ehrlich R, Snir M, et al. Intravitreal injection of triamcinolone aceto-nide for severe vitritis in patients with incomplete Behçet's disease. Am J Oph-thalmol 2004;138:666–7.
118. Tuncer S, Yilmaz S, Urgancioglu M, et al. Results of intravitreal triamcinolone acetonide (IVTA) injection for the treatment of panuveitis attacks in patients with Behçet disease. J Ocul Pharmacol Ther 2007;23:395–401.
119. Atmaca LS, Yalçındağ FN, Ozdemir O. Intravitreal triamcinolone acetonide in the management of cystoid macular edema in Behçet's disease. Graefes Arch Clin Exp Ophthalmol 2007;245:451–6.
120. Taylor SR, Tomkins-Netzer O, Joshi L, et al. Dexamethasone implant in pediatric uveitis. Ophthalmology 2012;119:2412.
121. Kotter I, Zierhut M, Eckstein AK, et al. Human recombinant interferon-α2a for the treatment of Behçet's disease with sight threatening posterior or panuveitis. Br J Ophthalmol 2003;87:423–31.
122. Tugal Tutkun I, Guney Tefekli E, Urgancioglu M. Results of interferon alfa therapy in patients with Behçet uveitis. Graefes Arch Clin Exp Ophthalmol 2006;244:1692–5.
123. Guillaume-Czitrom S, Berger C, Pajot C, et al. Efficacy and safety of interferon-α in the treatment of corticodependent uveitis of pediatric Behçet's disease. Rheu-matology 2007;46:1570–3.
124. Deuter CM, Zierhut M, Mohle A, et al. Long-term remission after cessation of interferon-alpha treatment in patients with severe uveitis due to Behçet's dis-ease. Arthritis Rheum 2010;62:2796–805.
125. Wechsler B, Sable-Fourtassou R, Bodaghi B, et al. Infliximab in refractory uveitis due to Behçet's disease. Clin Exp Rheumatol 2004;22:14–6.
126. Tugal Tutkun I, Mudun A, Urgancioglu M. Efficacy of infliximab in the treatment of uveitis that is resistant to treatment with the combination of azathioprine, cyclo-sporine, and corticosteroids in Behçet's disease: an open-label trial. Arthritis Rheum 2005;52:2478–84.
127. Niccoli L, Nannini C, Benucci M, et al. Long term efficacy of infliximab in refrac-tory posterior uveitis of Behçet's disease: a 24 month follow up study. Rheuma-tology 2007;46:1161–4.
128. Sfikakis PP, Markomichelakis NM, Alpsoy E, et al. Anti TNF therapy in the man-agement of Behçet's disease-review and basis for recommendations. Rheuma-tology 2007;46:736–41.
129. Neri P, Zucchi M, Allegri P, et al. Adalimumab (HumiraTM): a promising mono-clonal anti-tumor necrosis factor alpha in ophthalmology. Int Ophthalmol 2011;31:165–73.
130. Mazlumzadeh M, Matteson EL. Cogan's syndrome: an audio vestibular, ocular, and systemic autoimmune disease. Rheum Dis Clin North Am 2007;33:855–74.
131. Lunardi C, Bason C, Leandri M, et al. Autoantibodies to inner ear and endothe-lial antigens in Cogan's Syndrome. Lancet 2002;360:915–21.
132. Pagnini I, Zannin ME, Vittadello F, et al. Clinical features and outcome of Cogan syndrome. J Pediatr 2012;160:303–7.
133. Chynn EW, Jakobiec FA. Cogan's syndrome: ophthalmic, audio vestibular and systemic manifestations and therapy. Int Ophtalmol Clin 1996;36:61–72.
134. Riente L, Taglone E, Berrettini S. Efficacy of methotrexate in Cogan's syndrome. J Rheumatol 1996;23:1830–1.
135. Richardson B. Methotrexate therapy for hearing loss in Cogan's syndrome. Arthritis Rheum 1994;37:1559–61.

136. Watanabe K, Nishimaki T, Yoshida M, et al. Atypical Cogan's syndrome success-fully treated with glucocorticoids and pulse cyclophosphamide therapy. Fukush-ima J Med Sci 2000;46:49–54.
137. Xie L, Cai Y, Bao X, et al. Leflunomide for the successful management of juvenile Cogan's syndrome. Clin Rheumatol 2009;28:1453–5.
138. Orsoni JG, Zavota L, Vincenti V, et al. Cogan syndrome in children: early diag-nosis and treatment is critical to prognosis. Am J Ophthalmol 2004;137:757–8.
139. Edelsten C, Lee V, Bentley CR, et al. An evaluation of baseline risk factors pre-dicting severity in juvenile idiopathic arthritis associated uveitis and other chronic anterior uveitis in early childhood. Br J Ophthalmol 2002;86(1):51–6.
140. Chylack LT Jr. The ocular manifestations of juvenile rheumatoid arthritis. Arthritis Rheum 1977;20:217–23.
141. Nguyen QD, Foster CS. Saving the vision of children with juvenile rheumatoid arthritis-associated uveitis. JAMA 1998;280:1133–4.
142. Patel CC, Mandava N, Oliver SC, et al. Treatment of intractable posterior uveitis in pediatric patients with the fluocinolone acetonide intravitreal implant (Reti-sert). Retina 2012;32(3):537–42.
143. Simonini G, Paudyal P, Jones GT, et al. Current evidence of methotrexate effi-cacy in childhood chronic uveitis: a systematic review and meta-analysis approach. Rheumatology (Oxford) 2013;52(5):825–31.
144. Samson CM, Waheed N, Baltatzis S, et al. Methotrexate therapy for chronic noninfectious uveitis: analysis of a case series of 160 patients. Ophthalmology 2001;108:1134–9.
145. Weiss AH, Wallace CA, Sherry DD. Methotrexate for resistant chronic uveitis in children with juvenile rheumatoid arthritis. J Pediatr 1998;133:266–8.
146. Malik AR, Pavesio C. The use of low dose methotrexate in children with chronic anterior and intermediate uveitis. Br J Ophthalmol 2005;89:806–8.
147. Foeldvari I, Wierk A. Methotrexate is an effective treatment for chronic uveitis associated with juvenile idiopathic arthritis. J Rheumatol 2005;32:362–5.
148. Puchta J, Hattenbach LO, Baatz H. Intraocular levels of methotrexate after oral low-dose treatment in chronic uveitis. Ophthalmologica 2005;219:54–5.
149. Kalinina Ayuso V, van de Winkel EL, Rothova A, et al. Relapse rate of uveitis post-methotrexate treatment in juvenile idiopathic arthritis. Am J Ophthalmol 2011;151(2):217–22.
150. Kilmartin DJ, Forrester JV, Dick AD. Cyclosporin A therapy in refractory non-infectious childhood uveitis. Br J Ophthalmol 1998;82:737–42.
151. Thorne JE, Jabs DA, Qazi FA, et al. Rescue therapy with mycophenolate mofetil in refractory uveitis. Lancet 1998;352:35–6.
152. Lau CH, Comer M, Lightman S. Long-term efficacy of mycophenolate mofetil in the control of severe intraocular inflammation. Clin Experiment Ophthalmol 2003;31:487–91.
153. Kilmartin DJ, Forrester JV, Dick AD. Tacrolimus (FK506) in failed cyclosporin A therapy in endogenous posterior uveitis. Ocul Immunol Inflamm 1998;6:101–9.
154. Mochizuki M, Masuda K, Sakane T, et al. A clinical trial of FK506 in refractory uveitis. Am J Ophthalmol 1993;115:763–9.
155. Gerloni V, Cimaz R, Gattinara M, et al. Efficacy and safety profile of cyclosporin A in the treatment of juvenile chronic (idiopathic) arthritis. Results of a 10-year prospective study. Rheumatology 2001;40:907–13.
156. Lee SH, Chung H, Yu HG. Clinical outcomes of cyclosporine treatment for nonin-fectious uveitis. Korean J Ophthalmol 2012;26(1):21–5.

157. Taddio A, Cimaz R, Caputo R, et al. Childhood chronic anterior uveitis associated with vernal keratoconjunctivitis (VKC): successful treatment with topical tacrolimus. Case series. Pediatr Rheumatol Online J 2011;9(1):34.
158. Doycheva D, Zierhut M, Blumenstock G, et al. Long-term results of therapy with mycophenolate mofetil in chronic non-infectious uveitis. Graefes Arch Clin Exp Ophthalmol 2011;249(8):1235–43.
159. Daniel E, Thorne JE, Newcomb CW, et al. Mycophenolate mofetil for ocular inflammation. Am J Ophthalmol 2010;149(3):423–32.
160. Teoh SC, Hogan AC, Dick AD, et al. Mycophenolate mofetil for the treatment of uveitis. Am J Ophthalmol 2008;146(5):752–60.
161. Doycheva D, Deuter C, Stuebiger N, et al. Mycophenolate mofetil in the treatment of uveitis in children. Br J Ophthalmol 2007;91(2):180–4.
162. Chang PY, Giuliari GP, Shaikh M, et al. Mycophenolate mofetil monotherapy in the management of paediatric uveitis. Eye (Lond) 2011;25(4):427–35.
163. Schatz CS, Uzel JL, Leininger L, et al. Immunosuppressants used in a steroid-sparing strategy for childhood uveitis. J Pediatr Ophthalmol Strabismus 2007;44(1):28–34.
164. Galor A, Jabs DA, Leder HA, et al. Comparison of antimetabolite drugs as corticosteroid-sparing therapy for noninfectious ocular inflammation. Ophthalmology 2008;115(10):1826–32.
165. Nussenblatt RB, Coleman H, Jirawuthiworavong G, et al. The treatment of multifocal choroiditis associated choroidal neovascularization with sirolimus (rapamycin). Acta Ophthalmol Scand 2007;85(2):230–1.
166. Shanmuganathan VA, Casely EM, Raj D, et al. The efficacy of sirolimus in the treatment of patients with refractory uveitis. Br J Ophthalmol 2005;89(6):666–9.
167. Gurk-Turner C, Manitpisitkul W, Cooper M. A comprehensive review of everolimus clinical reports: a new mammalian target of rapamycin inhibitor. Transplantation 2012;94(7):659–68.
168. Heiligenhaus A, Zurek-Imhoff B, Roesel M, et al. Everolimus for the treatment of uveitis refractory to cyclosporine A: a pilot study. Graefes Arch Clin Exp Ophthalmol 2013;251(1):143–52.
169. Ramadan A, Nussenblatt R. Cytotoxic agents in ocular inflammation. Ophthalmol Clin North Am 1997;10:377–87.
170. Andrasch RH, Pirofsky B, Burns RP. Immunosuppressive therapy for severe chronic uveitis. Arch Ophthalmol 1978;96:247–51.
171. Esterberg E, Acharya NR. Corticosteroid-sparing therapy: practice patterns among uveitis specialists. J Ophthalmic Inflamm Infect 2012;2(1):21–8.
172. Ungar WJ, Costa V, Burnett HF, et al. The use of biologic response modifiers in polyarticular-course juvenile idiopathic arthritis: a systematic review. Semin Arthritis Rheum 2013;42(6):597–618.
173. Nakamura S, Yamakawa T, Sugita M, et al. The role of tumor necrosis factor-alpha in the induction of experimental autoimmune uveoretinitis in mice. Invest Ophthalmol Vis Sci 1994;35:3884–9.
174. Okada AA, Sakai J, Usui M, et al. Intraocular cytokine quantification of experimental autoimmune uveoretinitis in rats. Ocul Immunol Inflamm 1998;6:111–20.
175. De Vos AF, Klaren VN, Kijlstra A. Expression of multiple cytokines and IL-1RA in the uvea and retina during endotoxin-induced uveitis in the rat. Invest Ophthalmol Vis Sci 1994;35:3873–83.
176. Dick AD, McMenamin PG, Korner H, et al. Inhibition of tumor necrosis factor activity minimizes target organ damage in experimental autoimmune uveoretinitis

despite quantitatively normal activated T cell traffic to the retina. Eur J Immunol 1996;26:1018–25.

177. Reiff A, Takei S, Sadeghi S, et al. Etanercept therapy in children with treatment-resistant uveitis. Arthritis Rheum 2001;44:1411–5.

178. Mackensen F, Lutz T. Therapy for childhood uveitis: biologics: too often—too late? Ophthalmologe 2011;108(3):213–21.

179. Tynjälä P, Lindahl P, Honkanen V, et al. Infliximab and etanercept in the treatment of chronic uveitis associated with refractory juvenile idiopathic arthritis. Ann Rheum Dis 2007;66(4):548–50.

180. Gallagher M, Quinones K, Cervantes-Castañeda RA, et al. Biological response modifier therapy for refractory childhood uveitis. Br J Ophthalmol 2007;91(10): 1341–4.

181. Foeldvari I, Nielsen S, Kümmerle-Deschner J, et al. Tumor necrosis factor-alpha blocker in treatment of juvenile idiopathic arthritis-associated uveitis refractory to second-line agents: results of a multinational survey. J Rheumatol 2007; 34(5):1146–50.

182. Ardoin SP, Kredich D, Rabinovich E, et al. Infliximab to treat chronic noninfectious uveitis in children: retrospective case series with long-term follow-up. Am J Ophthalmol 2007;144(6):844–9.

183. Sen ES, Sharma S, Hinchcliffe A, et al. Use of adalimumab in refractory non-infectious childhood chronic uveitis: efficacy in ocular disease—a case cohort interventional study. Rheumatology (Oxford) 2012;51(12):2199–203.

184. Díaz-Llopis M, Salom D, Garcia-de-Vicuña C, et al. Treatment of refractory uveitis with adalimumab: a prospective multicenter study of 131 patients. Ophthalmology 2012;119(8):1575–81.

185. Zannin ME, Birolo C, Gerloni VM, et al. Safety and efficacy of infliximab and adalimumab for refractory uveitis in juvenile idiopathic arthritis: 1-year followup data from the Italian Registry. J Rheumatol 2013;40(1):74–9.

186. Miserocchi E, Modorati G, Pontikaki I, et al. Golimumab treatment for complicated uveitis. Clin Exp Rheumatol 2013;31(2):320–1.

187. William M, Faez S, Papaliodis GN, et al. Golimumab for the treatment of refractory juvenile idiopathic arthritis-associated uveitis. J Ophthalmic Inflamm Infect 2012;2(4):231–3.

188. Vinores SA, Chan CC, Vinores MA, et al. Increased vascular endothelial growth factor (VEGF) and transforming growth factor beta (TGF-beta) in experimental autoimmune uveoretinitis upregulation of VEGF without neovascularization. J Neuroimmunol 1998;89:43–50.

189. Wallis RS, Ehlers S. Tumor necrosis factor and granuloma biology: explaining the differential infection risk of etanercept. Semin Arthritis Rheum 2005; 34(5 Suppl 1):34–8.

190. Cordero-Coma M, Yilmaz T, Onal S. Systematic review of anti-tumor necrosis factor-alpha therapy for treatment of immune-mediated uveitis. Ocul Immunol Inflamm 2013;21(1):12–20.

191. Tauber T, Turetz J, Barash J, et al. Optic neuritis associated with etanercept therapy for juvenile arthritis. J AAPOS 2006;10(1):26–9.

192. Wendling D, Paccou J, Berthelot JM, et al, CRI. New onset of uveitis during anti-tumor necrosis factor treatment for rheumatic diseases. Semin Arthritis Rheum 2011;41(3):503–10.

193. Gaujoux-Viala C, Giampietro C, Gaujoux T, et al. Scleritis: a paradoxical effect of etanercept? Etanercept-associated inflammatory eye disease. J Rheumatol 2012;39(2):233–9.

194. Markomichelakis N, Delicha E, Masselos S, et al. Intravitreal infliximab for sight-threatening relapsing uveitis in Behçet disease: a pilot study in 15 patients. Am J Ophthalmol 2012;154(3):534–41.

195. Farvardin M, Afarid M, Shahrzad S. Long-term effects of intravitreal infliximab for treatment of sight threatening chronic noninfectious uveitis. J Ocul Pharmacol Ther 2012;28(6):628–31.

196. Lim WK, Fujimoto C, Ursea R, et al. Suppression of immune-mediated ocular inflammation in mice by interleukin 1 receptor antagonist administration. Arch Ophthalmol 2005;123:957–63.

197. Gül A, Tugal-Tutkun I, Dinarello CA, et al. Interleukin-1β-regulating antibody XOMA 052 (gevokizumab) in the treatment of acute exacerbations of resistant uveitis of Behçet's disease: an open-label pilot study. Ann Rheum Dis 2012; 71(4):563–6.

198. Ugurlu S, Ucar D, Seyahi E, et al. Canakinumab in a patient with juvenile Behçet's syndrome with refractory eye disease. Ann Rheum Dis 2012;71(9): 1589–91.

199. Simonini G, Xu Z, Caputo R, et al. Clinical and transcriptomic response to the long-acting IL-1 blocker canakinumab in Blau syndrome-related uveitis. Antiin-flamm Antiallergy Agents Med Chem 2012;11(2):113–20.

200. Bhat P, Castañeda-Cervantes RA, Doctor PP, et al. Intravenous daclizumab for recalcitrant ocular inflammatory disease. Graefes Arch Clin Exp Ophthalmol 2009;247(5):687–92.

201. Smolen JS, Schoels MM, Nishimoto N, et al. Consensus statement on blocking the effects of interleukin-6 and in particular by interleukin-6 receptor inhibition in rheumatoid arthritis and other inflammatory conditions. Ann Rheum Dis 2013; 72(4):482–92. http://dx.doi.org/10.1136/annrheumdis-2012-202469.

202. De Benedetti F. Tocilizumab for systemic juvenile idiopathic arthritis. N Engl J Med 2013;368(13):1256–7.

203. Tappeiner C, Heinz C, Ganser G, et al. Is tocilizumab an effective option for treatment of refractory uveitis associated with juvenile idiopathic arthritis? J Rheumatol 2012;39(6):1294–5.

204. Muselier A, Bielefeld P, Bidot S, et al. Efficacy of tocilizumab in two patients with anti-TNF-alpha refractory uveitis. Ocul Immunol Inflamm 2011;19(5):382–3.

205. Shen H, Xia L, Lu J. Elevated levels of interleukin-27 and effect on production of interferon-γ and interleukin-17 in patients with Behçet's disease. Scand J Rheu-matol 2013;42(1):48–51.

206. Yang Y, Xiao X, Li F, et al. Increased IL-7 expression in Vogt-Koyanagi-Harada disease. Invest Ophthalmol Vis Sci 2012;53(2):1012–7.

207. Dick AD, Tugal-Tutkun I, Foster S, et al. Secukinumab in the treatment of nonin-fectious uveitis: results of three randomized, controlled clinical trials. Ophthal-mology 2013;120(4):777–87.

208. Herrero-Beaumont G, Martínez Calatrava MJ, Castañeda S. Abatacept mechanism of action: concordance with its clinical profile. Reumatol Clin 2012;8(2):78–83.

209. Weinblatt ME, Moreland LW, Westhovens R, et al. Safety of abatacept admin-istered intravenously in treatment of rheumatoid arthritis: integrated analyses of up to 8 years of treatment from the Abatacept Clinical Trial Program. J Rheumatol 2013;40(6):787–97.

210. Ruperto N, Lovell DJ, Quartier P, et al, Paediatric Rheumatology International Tri-als Organization and the Pediatric Rheumatology Collaborative Study Group. Long-term safety and efficacy of abatacept in children with juvenile idiopathic arthritis. Arthritis Rheum 2010;62(6):1792–802.

211. Kenawy N, Cleary G, Mewar D, et al. Abatacept: a potential therapy in refractory cases of juvenile idiopathic arthritis-associated uveitis. Graefes Arch Clin Exp Ophthalmol 2011;249(2):297–300.

212. Angeles-Han S, Flynn T, Lehman T. Abatacept for refractory juvenile idiopathic arthritis-associated uveitis- a case report. J Rheumatol 2008;35(9):1897–8.

213. Elhai M, Deslandre CJ, Kahan A. Abatacept for refractory juvenile idiopathic arthritis-associated uveitis: two new cases. Comment on the article by Zulian et al. Arthritis Care Res (Hoboken) 2011;63(2):307–8 [author reply: 308].

214. Zulian F, Balzarin M, Falcini F, et al. Abatacept for severe anti-tumor necrosis factor alpha refractory juvenile idiopathic arthritis-related uveitis. Arthritis Care Res (Hoboken) 2010;62(6):821–5.

215. Boross P, Leusen JH. Mechanisms of action of CD20 antibodies. Am J Cancer Res 2012;2(6):676–90.

216. Miserocchi E, Modorati G. Rituximab for noninfectious uveitis. Dev Ophthalmol 2012;51:98–109.

217. Miserocchi E, Pontikaki I, Modorati G, et al. Anti-CD 20 monoclonal antibody (rituximab) treatment for inflammatory ocular diseases. Autoimmun Rev 2011; 11(1):35–9.

218. Heiligenhaus A, Miserocchi E, Heinz C, et al. Treatment of severe uveitis associated with juvenile idiopathic arthritis with anti-CD20 monoclonal antibody (rituximab). Rheumatology (Oxford) 2011;50(8):1390–4.

219. Isaacs JD, Hale G, Waldmann H, et al. Monoclonal antibody therapy of chronic intraocular inflammation using Campath-1H. Br J Ophthalmol 1995;79(11): 1054–5.

220. Larson T, Nussenblatt RB, Sen HN. Emerging drugs for uveitis. Expert Opin Emerg Drugs 2011;16(2):309–22.

221. Liu B, Chan CC, Nussenblatt RB. Application of small molecules/macromolecules in ocular inflammatory diseases. Ophthalmology 2012;119(11):2412.

222. Wang RX, Yu CR, Mahdi RM, et al. Novel IL27p28/IL12p40 cytokine suppressed experimental autoimmune uveitis by inhibiting autoreactive Th1/Th17 cells and promoting expansion of regulatory T cells. Exp Eye Res 2009;89(4):522–31.

223. Lennikov A, Kitaichi N, Noda K, et al. Amelioration of endotoxin-induced uveitis treated with an IκB kinase β inhibitor in rats. Mol Vis 2012;18:2586–97.

224. Ottiger M, Thiel MA, Feige U, et al. Efficient intraocular penetration of topical anti-TNF-alpha single-chain antibody (ESBA105) to anterior and posterior segment without penetration enhancer. Invest Ophthalmol Vis Sci 2009;50(2): 779–86.

225. Tugal-Tutkun I. Pediatric uveitis. J Ophthalmic Vis Res 2011;6(4):259–69.

226. Carvounis PE, Herman DC, Cha S, et al. Incidence and outcomes of uveitis in juvenile rheumatoid arthritis, a synthesis of the literature. Graefes Arch Clin Exp Ophthalmol 2006;244(3):281–90.

227. Cabral DA, Petty RE, Malleson PN, et al. Visual prognosis in children with chronic anterior uveitis and arthritis. J Rheumatol 1994;21(12):2370–5.

228. Gregory AC 2nd, Kempen JH, Daniel E, et al, Systemic Immunosuppressive Therapy for Eye Diseases Cohort Study Research Group. Risk factors for loss of visual acuity among patients with uveitis associated with juvenile idiopathic arthritis: the Systemic Immunosuppressive Therapy for Eye Diseases Study. Ophthalmology 2013;120(1):186–92.

229. Heiligenhaus A, Niewerth M, Mingels A, et al. Epidemiology of uveitis in juvenile idiopathic arthritis from a national paediatric rheumatologic and ophthalmologic database. Klin Monbl Augenheilkd 2005;222(12):993–1001 [in German].

230. Jalil A, Yin K, Coyle L, et al. Vision-related quality of life and employment status in patients with uveitis of working age: a prospective study. Ocul Immunol Inflamm 2012;20(4):262–5.
231. Nussenblatt RB. The natural history of uveitis. Int Ophthalmol 1990;14(5–6): 303–8.
232. Darrell RW, Wagener HP, Kurland LT. Epidemiology of uveitis. Incidence and prevalence in a small urban community. Arch Ophthalmol 1962;68:502–14.

Biomarkers and Updates on Pediatrics Lupus Nephritis

Michael Bennett, PhD[a], Hermine I. Brunner, MD, MSc[b],*

KEYWORDS

- Biomarkers • Lupus nephritis • Systemic lupus erythematosus
- Childhood-onset SLE • Treatment

KEY POINTS

- Lupus nephritis is frequently diagnosed in children with systemic lupus erythematosus and warrants close medical attention to avoid progression to end-stage renal disease.
- Diagnosis of lupus nephritis requires at present a kidney biopsy.
- Current laboratory tests used to monitor lupus nephritis lack accuracy, making appropriate management difficult.
- Novel urine biomarkers hold promise for improving the approach to the surveillance of lupus nephritis and interpretation of patient response to therapy.
- Despite the lack of adequately powered clinical trials, standardized approaches to the therapy for children and adolescents with lupus nephritis are now available.

INTRODUCTION

Systemic lupus erythematosus (SLE) is a multiorgan autoimmune disease with increasing mortality that often targets young women and children of United States minorities. Childhood-onset SLE (cSLE)[1] has manifestations similar to those of SLE in adults, but earlier disease onset is accompanied by more severe multiorgan involvement, including lupus nephritis (LN) in up to 80% of pediatric patients. Treatment of LN in children continues to lack support from large randomized clinical trials.

Funding Sources: H.I.B. is supported by research grants from the National Institutes of Health, including 2P60AR047784, U01AR059509 and UL1 TR000077-04; M.B. is supported by a research grant from the National Institutes of Health, P50 DK096418 and two translational research grants from the Cincinnati Children's Hospital Medical Center/University of Cincinnati Joint Center for Clinical and Translational Science and Training.
Conflict of Interest: Nil.
[a] Division of Nephrology and Hypertension, Cincinnati Children's Hospital Medical Center, University of Cincinnati, MC 7022, 3333 Burnet Avenue, Cincinnati, OH 45229, USA; [b] Division of Rheumatology, Cincinnati Children's Hospital Medical Center, University of Cincinnati, MC 4010, 3333 Burnet Avenue, Cincinnati, OH 45229, USA
* Corresponding author.
E-mail address: Hermine.brunner@cchmc.org

Rheum Dis Clin N Am 39 (2013) 833–853
http://dx.doi.org/10.1016/j.rdc.2013.05.001
0889-857X/13/$ – see front matter © 2013 Elsevier Inc. All rights reserved.

Instead, medication regimens for pediatric LN are deduced from studies in adult SLE and pediatric solid-organ transplants, or are based on consensus reached by associations of health care providers.

The criterion standard for the diagnosis and monitoring of LN remains histologic evidence from a kidney biopsy. Conversely, to reduce cost and avoid invasive procedures, monitoring of LN in clinics is achieved by measures that consider changes in certain blood and urine tests. Because such traditional testing for LN has limited responsiveness to change, it is ill suited to capture worsening or improvement of LN in a timely manner. Recently, promising LN biomarkers have been discovered that accurately reflect LN activity and chronicity as seen on kidney biopsy, and can forecast LN flares. In the future, such biomarkers are expected to facilitate the monitoring of LN in daily clinical care and the conduct of research studies in support of evidence-based therapies for LN in children.

EPIDEMIOLOGY, COURSE, AND ECONOMIC IMPACT

Given the phenotypic differences of cSLE around the world, the prevalence of kidney involvement with cSLE likely also varies with racial background and environmental exposures. The incidence of SLE is thought to have increased 10-fold during the preceding 50 years in industrialized Western countries,[2] which could indicate that cSLE in general, and LN in children in particular, also are becoming more frequent. Using information available in administrative databases and an algorithm that correctly identifies 80% of LN cases, Hiraki and colleagues[3] report that in the United States 37% of children with cSLE and who are enrolled in Medicaid have renal disease. Based on this study, the risk of developing LN is independent of gender but is higher among teens than younger children. Compared with Caucasians, Asians have almost 5 times and African Americans a nearly 3 times higher risks of developing LN. Overall, the annual incidence of LN is 0.72 cases per 100,000 children in the United States. This figure may be a conservative estimate of the frequency of LN, as higher estimates are reported by population-based studies from tertiary pediatric rheumatology centers and a recent meta-analysis.[4,5]

Recent 5-year renal survival rates in children with cSLE have ranged from 77% to 93%,[6–8] with marked improvement over the preceding decades.[9] Nonetheless, adults with LN have an 8-times higher mortality and children with LN a 19-times higher risk of dying compared with age-matched general populations.[6,7,10] The poor prognosis of children with end-stage renal disease from LN is particularly troublesome. There is 22% mortality during the 5-year period since the initiation of renal replacement therapy, with cardiopulmonary compromise and infections accounting for 47% of all causes of death.[6]

Associated with the higher mortality is the need of more intensive therapy for LN in children. Among the almost 7400 cSLE-related hospitalizations in the United States in 2006, 57% noted the presence of LN[11] with an average charge of $43,100 per admission.[11] Based on this and an earlier study, LN accounts for 11% to 28% of cSLE-associated medical costs in the United States.[12] Taken together, the cost of therapy for LN in children likely exceeds $350 million annually in the United States.[3,11–13]

DIAGNOSIS OF LN AND CLASSIFICATION

Kidney biopsies are required to establish the diagnosis of LN. Despite considerable variation in practice, there is consensus that reproducible daily proteinuria of at least 0.5 g, especially in the setting of an active urinary sediment, warrants a kidney biopsy in a child with cSLE who has not yet been diagnosed with LN.[14,15] Although clinically relevant biopsy findings are more common in the presence of significant proteinuria, the current approach results in at least 50% of newly diagnosed patients already being found to have proliferative LN, rendering them at a higher risk of end-stage renal disease.[16–19] A lower threshold for performing a kidney biopsy arguably is warranted in cSLE patients, including those with persistent isolated glomerular hematuria and new-onset low-grade proteinuria.

When interpreting a kidney biopsy specimen it is important to ensure that an adequate sample with sufficient numbers of glomeruli is available, namely, a minimum of 8 glomeruli that can be examined under light microscopy.[20,21] The International Society of Nephrology/Renal Pathology Society (ISN/RPS) Classification replaced in 2004 the previously used World Health Organization (WHO) Classification for LN.[20] The ISN/RPS Classification is based on light microscopy, rather than electron microscopy, as a tool for interpreting LN histology, even though it has been shown that electron microscopy greatly enhances the interpretation and classification of kidney biopsies.[20]

The ISN/RPS Classification was introduced to standardize and clarify the interpretation of LN histology findings.[20] Six classes of LN are described with focus on changes concerning the renal glomeruli, and the National Institutes of Health (NIH) Histology Score is often used to quantify the degree of LN activity and chronicity (**Table 1**).[22] The maximum score of the NIH-AI (activity index) and the NIH-CI (chronicity index) is 24 and 12, respectively, because scores from "(fibro)cellular crescents" and "fibrinoid necrosis/karyorrhexis" are given a weight of 2 in the NIH-AI

Table 1
Classification and interpretation of lupus nephritis biopsy findings

ISN/RPS Lupus Nephritis Classification Criteria	
Class I	Minimal mesangial lupus nephritis
Class II	Mesangial proliferative lupus nephritis
Class III	Focal lupus nephritis[a]
Class IV	Diffuse segmental (IV-S) or global (IV-G) lupus nephritis[b]
Class V	Membranous lupus nephritis[c]
Class VI	Advanced sclerosing lupus nephritis

NIH Activity and Chronicity Index[d]	
Active Lesions	**Chronic Lesions**
1. Endocapillary hypercellularity, with or without leukocyte infiltration and with substantial luminal reduction	1. Glomerular sclerosis (segmental, global)
2. Karyorrhexis (fibrinoid necrosis)[e]	2. Fibrous adhesions
3. Rupture of glomerular basement membrane	3. Fibrous crescents
4. Crescents (cellular or fibrocellular)[e]	4. Tubular atrophy
5. Subendothelial deposits identifiable by light microscopy (wireloops)	
6. Intraluminal immune aggregates (hyaline thrombi)	
NIH Activity Index 0–24	NIH Chronicity Index 0–12

[a] Indicates the proportion of glomeruli with active and with sclerotic lesions.
[b] Indicates the proportion of glomeruli with fibrinoid necrosis and cellular crescents.
[c] Class V may occur in combination with class III or IV, in which case both will be diagnosed.
[d] Each item scored from 0 to 3 depending on degree of involvement: 0 = no lesions; 1 = <25% of glomeruli; 2 = 25%–50% of glomeruli; 3 = >50% of glomeruli.
[e] These items scores have a weight of 2.

(see **Table 1**). Pathologic changes of the kidney interstitium, are not well considered in the ISN/RPS Classification, although they are considered critical for the course of LN.[23] However, it is recommended to report the extent, severity, and type of tubulointerstitial (tubular atrophy, interstitial inflammation, and fibrosis) and vascular disease (vascular deposits, thrombi, vasculitis, sclerosis).[20]

RISK FACTORS TO POOR OUTCOME OF LN

Clinical research has identified, albeit inconsistently, several risk factors for poor LN outcome[3,6,16,24–33]; these include male gender, non-Caucasian race, nonadherence to treatment, presence of antiphospholipid or anti-dsDNA antibodies, persistent hypocomplementemia or proteinuria, nephrotic syndrome at presentation, failure to adequately respond to therapy by 3 months,[34] flare of LN,[35] or diagnosis with proliferative LN, especially in the setting of a high degree of histologic activity and damage. Given the multitude of the proposed risk factors for LN, close monitoring of any child patient with LN seems to be warranted in achieving the best possible control of LN.[15,34]

MONITORING OF LN IN CLINICAL CARE

There are no studies that directly compare the clinical features of the various classes of LN between children and adults with SLE. However, the presentation of children with LN varies considerably, ranging from mild abnormalities on urinalysis, to anasarca caused by marked proteinuria, to posterior reversible encephalopathy owing to uncontrolled hypertension with nephritic syndrome.[36]

Proteinuria

Abnormally elevated excretions of albumin and total protein in the urine are highly sensitive indicators of glomerular disease. Albumin is a small-sized molecule, and one of the first proteins able to pass through the kidneys. The value of monitoring microalbuminuria for the early diagnosis of LN has not been well established, and mesangial LN can be present without proteinuria.[37] A prompt and significant decrease in proteinuria after 3 and 6 months of therapy is an important prognostic factor for good long-term renal outcome.[38] Proteinuria furthers the development of tubulointerstitial inflammation and injury, and thereby a decline in renal function in the long term.[39]

Traditionally proteinuria is quantified by a 24-hour urine collection. Conversely, and despite its common use, urine dipstick is poorly suited to quantify the degree of proteinuria.[40] There is now sufficient evidence that the protein-to-creatinine ratio in a random urine specimen, best from first morning urine,[41–43] is adequate to estimate daily proteinuria in cSLE. Whether 12-hour overnight urine collection is more accurate than estimation of proteinuria using spot urine will need further study.[44]

Urine Sediment

The presence of cellular casts on urine-sediment examinations, for example, the microscopic examination of the cellular components at casts seen in centrifuged urine, is supportive of glomerulonephritis. Accuracy of urine-sediment interpretation requires timely processing of the urine, as lysis of leukocytes and erythrocytes occurs even within the first hour after collection, especially when low specific gravity and high urine pH are present. Presence of mucus in the urine can entrap both cells and casts, and sometimes repeated assessment of urine sediment is necessary to detect cellular casts.[45]

Glomerular Filtration Rate

The reference method for assessing the "true" glomerular filtration rate (GFR) is to measure the renal clearance of inulin, ethylenediaminetetraacetic acid, and iohexol; that is, markers freely filtered through the glomerulus, neither secreted nor reabsorbed by the tubule. Because such techniques are complex and costly to perform, alternative means to estimate the GFR in a clinical setting have been developed.[46] In pediatrics, the 2009 modification of the Schwartz Formula and serum cystatin C–based methods seem reasonably accurate and easy to use in a clinical setting (**Table 2**).[46] Despite its appeal, the use of serum cystatin C to estimate the GFR of patients with LN will need further evaluation, as levels of cystatin C seem positively correlated with general SLE activity, even in the absence of LN or changes in renal function.[47,48]

SHORTCOMINGS OF TRADITIONAL MEASURES OF LN

Whereas blood urea nitrogen and creatinine often stay in the normal range in cSLE, even if with profound histologic pathology, the urinary sediment and urinalysis are generally abnormal in untreated LN. Conversely, in pretreated patients only minor abnormalities on urinalysis, including mild proteinuria or hematuria, may be present in patients with severely active biopsy-proven LN. This finding is supported by the research of Christopher-Stine and colleagues,[49] who reviewed 25 LN patients undergoing serial kidney biopsies. At diagnosis proteinuria, hematuria, hypoalbuminemia, and hypertension were all associated with a worse LN class. By contrast, none of these parameters correlated with the LN class on follow-up biopsy, raising the possibility that normal urinalyses do not necessarily ensure the absence of active LN.[49]

With LN, there is a balance between complement activation via the classical pathway, which facilitates the removal of immune complexes, and activation of the

Table 2
Estimation of GFR (eGFR) in children in comparison with the reference standard of inulin clearance (iGFR)

Comparators	Modified Schwartz Formula[a]	Le Bricon[b]
	eGFR = 36.5 × Height (cm)/Cr	eGFR = (78/Cys) + 4
eGFR means ± SD (mL/min per 1.73 m²)	109 ± 44[c]	99 ± 26
iGFR-eGFR means ± SD (mL/min per 1.73 m²)	−8 ± 29	2 ± 19
Accuracy 10% (%)[d]	38	46
Accuracy 30% (%)	84	90
Accuracy 50% (%)	96	98
Correlation between eGFR and iGFR	0.779[e]	0.784[e]

[a] Schwartz GJ, Muñoz A, Schneider MF, et al. New equations to estimate GFR in children with CKD. J Am Soc Nephrol 2009;20:629–37.
[b] Le Bricon T, Thervet E, Froissart M, et al. Plasma cystatin C is superior to 24-h creatinine clearance and plasma creatinine for estimation of glomerular filtration rate 3 months after kidney transplantation. Clin Chem 2000;46;1206–7.
[c] $P<.05$, Wilcoxon paired test, in comparison with inulin clearance.
[d] Interpretation: 38% of the patient's eGFR is within 10% of the reference standard, ie, inulin clearance.
[e] $P<.001$; Spearman correlation coefficient.

alternative pathway, which promotes kidney injury.[50] The literature is inconsistent at best as to whether the concentration of complement and anti-dsDNA antibodies can serve as useful markers of concurrent SLE activity or future flares.[51] In 98 patients who experienced 146 flares, Ho and colleagues[52] showed that hypocomplementemia and anti-dsDNA antibodies accompanied SLE relapse in only 54% and 27% of patients, respectively.

Research in adults with LN suggests that less than 25% of LN patients with low C3, C4, or anti-dsDNA levels have a concurrent flare of LN, and only 50% of LN flares are preceded by a drop in the levels of C3 and C4 or an increase in anti-dsDNA antibodies, respectively.[51,53] In other words, these tests are not much better than the flip of a coin in helping clinicians anticipate LN flare. These reports from adults with LN have been confirmed in children with LN.[54]

Like the immunologic markers C3, C4, and anti-dsDNA antibodies that are traditionally used to assess the course of LN, kidney biopsies have their pitfalls. In a recent study, 5 experienced nephropathologists rated 126 renal biopsy specimens of 87 patients with proliferative LN.[55] These experts demonstrated significant variation in agreement when rating the various histologic aspects of biopsy specimens as part of the ISN/RPS Classification. Excellent agreement (>60%) was reached only for the number of glomeruli seen in the biopsy, the overall activity index score, and the presence of proliferative features. Conversely, agreement was less than 40% (interclass correlation coefficient <0.4) for the presence of mesangial proliferation, tubular necrosis, and, notably, the overall ISN-RPS class designation.[55]

The aforementioned shortcomings of kidney biopsies, as well as the limitations of currently available urine and blood laboratory tests, support a need for potent biomarkers to help accurately diagnose LN and to determine the response of LN to therapy in a clinical setting.

BIOMARKERS AND ASSESSMENT OF THEIR QUALITY

In its simplest definition, a biomarker is anything that can be measured to extract information about a biological state or process. The NIH Biomarkers Definitions Working Group has defined a biological marker (biomarker) as "A characteristic that is objectively measured and evaluated as an indicator of normal biological processes, pathogenic processes, or pharmacologic responses to a therapeutic intervention."[56] Biomarkers are the essential tools for the implementation of personalized medicine. The biomarker development process, also sometimes referred to as biomarker qualification, has typically been divided into 5 phases,[57] as shown in **Table 3**. In recent years, the ready availability of powerful tools to scan both the genome and the proteome of an organism have revolutionized and greatly accelerated biomarker discovery.

For biomarker discovery, microarrays are used to screen messenger RNA (mRNA) levels. This approach has yielded several biomarkers of kidney disease, such as neutrophil gelatinase-associated lipocalin (NGAL). Microarrays can be combined with other techniques, such as laser-capture microdissection, to target specific areas of diseased tissue to give mechanistic clues not possible just a decade ago. Even with this level of specificity, a daunting amount of biomarker candidates will be identified with these approaches, and the usefulness of such candidates must be sifted through for relevance. Another shortcoming of transcriptomic profiling approaches is that direct measurement in biological fluids is not possible and that mRNA levels do not always correlate with protein levels or enzyme activity. Hence, larger validation studies are necessary that measure protein levels to confirm the biological relevance of mRNA biomarkers.

Table 3
Phases of biomarker discovery, translation, and validation

Phase	Terminology	Action Steps
Phase 1	Preclinical discovery	Discover biomarkers in tissues or body fluids Confirm and prioritize promising candidates
Phase 2	Assay development	Develop and optimize clinically useful assay Test on existing samples of established disease
Phase 3	Retrospective study	Test biomarker in completed clinical trial Test if biomarker detects the disease early Evaluate sensitivity, specificity, receiver-operating characteristic
Phase 4	Prospective screening	Use biomarker to screen population Identify extent and characteristics of disease Identify false referral rate
Phase 5	Disease control	Determine impact of screening on reducing disease burden

From Devarajan P. Proteomics for biomarker discovery in acute kidney injury. Semin Nephrol 2007;27(6):637–51; with permission.

Focusing on peptides and actual proteins, proteomics allow one to go beyond simple translation of mRNA into protein. Instead protein regulation, posttranslational modifications such as glycosylation and methylation, and even disease-specific fragmentation of proteins are assessed. Proteomic techniques are capable of identifying and quantifying proteins and peptides in exceedingly large numbers.[58] The urinary proteome itself is quite large, with laboratories having identified more than 1500 proteins to date.[59,60] The blood proteome is even larger, with more than 3000 nonredundant proteins identified in the plasma alone.[61–63] Adding the proteome of the cellular component of blood will yield thousands more.[64,65] To this end, we have entered what has been termed an "open loop,"[66] or unbiased, approach to biomarker discovery, in stark contrast to the hypothesis-driven approach of our past. With such a vast pool of potential biomarkers from readily available, noninvasive sources, one must take care to plan and design the proper experimental approach to ensure parsimony.

There are universal characteristics important for any biomarker: (1) they should be noninvasive, easily measured, inexpensive, and produce rapid results; (2) they should be from readily available sources, such as blood or urine; (3) they should have a high sensitivity, allowing early detection, and no overlap in values between diseased patients and healthy controls; (4) they should have a high specificity, being greatly upregulated (or downregulated) specifically in the diseased samples and unaffected by comorbid conditions; (5) their levels should vary rapidly in response to treatment; (6) their levels should aid in risk stratification and possess prognostic value in terms of real outcomes; and (7) they should be biologically plausible and provide insight into the underlying disease mechanism.[56,57]

The most readily available sources of biomarkers are urine and blood. Urine is an excellent source of biomarkers produced in the kidney,[67] and thus may give better mechanistic insight into specific renal abnormalities. Urine is less complex than serum, and thus is easier to screen for potential biomarkers. Urinary biomarker studies typically adjust for urine creatinine to account for differences in urine concentration resulting from hydration status and medications such as diuretics. However, the utility of urine creatinine in biomarker correction has been questioned because of its variable excretion throughout the day and its dependence on normal renal function.

Serum biomarkers are considered more stable, as they are less prone than urine biomarkers to bacterial contamination. However, serum biomarkers are more likely to represent a systemic response to disease, rather than an organ response. There are exceptions, such as the troponins in cardiac disease. The real problem with serum as a source of biomarkers lies in the discovery phase. Serum has a wide range of protein concentrations across several orders of magnitude, with a small number of proteins (such as albumin) accounting for a large percentage of the volume; this can be akin to trying to spot a single strand of cotton in a large tapestry. Although assays do exist to remove these high-abundance proteins from serum, many potential biomarkers have been shown to bind to albumin.[68] Thus, albumin depletion to help identify relevant biomarkers risks erroneous removal of proteins relevant to LN.

The sensitivity and specificity of a biomarker go hand in hand. The receiver-operating characteristic (ROC) curve is a binary classification test, based on the sensitivity and specificity of a biomarker at certain cutoff points. ROC curves are often used to determine the clinical diagnostic value of a biomarker.[57,69] The area under the ROC curve (AUC_{ROC}) is a common statistic derived from ROC curves. An AUC_{ROC} of 1.0 represents a perfect biomarker, whereas an AUC_{ROC} of 0.5 is a result that is no better than expected by chance. An AUC_{ROC} of 0.75 or greater is generally considered a good biomarker while an AUC_{ROC} of 0.90 is considered an excellent biomarker.[57] However, even a sensitive biomarker with what experimentally would be considered an excellent specificity of 90% would still yield a false-positive rate of 10%, which may be unacceptably high for clinical use as a stand-alone marker.[66] As a result, the best approach clinically may be to find multiple biomarkers that can be combined as part of a panel to achieve even higher specificity.

TYPES OF LN BIOMARKERS

Traditional measures of LN have limited responsiveness to change, and are unsuited to capture worsening or improvement of LN in a timely manner. This lack of early response measures to verify the effectiveness of LN therapies hinders clinical care, requires clinical trials of new medications for LN to study large populations and follow them over several years, and increases the risk of negative trials. In addition, traditional measures of kidney function, such as creatinine clearance or protein-to-creatinine ratio, reflect significant loss of kidney function such that major renal damage can occur before it is detected by these traditional methods. Thus, novel biomarkers that can rapidly detect lupus renal involvement and severity, predict flares, and monitor treatment response and disease progression are greatly needed, and have been the subject of intense research.

The advent of new technologies to rapidly screen the genome and proteome over the last few decades has led to an explosion in the identification of novel biomarkers for many disease states. Ann immense number of biomarkers has been investigated in recent years, far too many to discuss in this article. The authors therefore focus the discussion on the most promising investigational biomarkers for LN discovered over the last several years.

Urine MCP-1

Monocyte chemoattractant protein-1 (MCP-1) is a leukocyte chemotactic protein involved in the mediation of inflammation and renal injury in LN.[70] Animal models of LN have demonstrated direct involvement of MCP-1 in renal abnormality, as blockade of MCP-1 through the use of an antagonist or an RNA oligonucleotide specifically designed to bind to and sequester MCP-1 (also known as a spiegelmer) led to marked improvement in LN and lupus-like inflammatory skin lesions.[71,72] Several cross-sectional studies have demonstrated that urine MCP-1 levels are concurrently higher in those patients with active LN than with nonactive LN.[73–75] The AUC_{ROC} of MCP-1 for distinguishing active LN from inactive LN[76] or nonrenal flares is 0.76.[77] Urine MCP-1 also seems to have promise in helping to distinguish certain classes of LN. Urine MCP-1 levels are significantly higher with ISN/RPS Classes III and IV than with other classes of LN ($P = .01$).[78,79] Both children and adults with Class IV LN have the highest glomerular expression of MCP-1.[46] There are some differing findings regarding the potential of urine MCP-1 to predict renal flares. A study by Rovin and colleagues[73] reported increases in urine MCP-1 as early as 2 to 4 months before the clinical diagnosis of a renal flare. However, a similar study by Tian and colleagues,[80] while demonstrating elevated MCP-1 during renal flares, did not find MCP-1 levels to be an independent predictor of flare.

Similar results were found by Chan and colleagues[81] when examining chemokine mRNA from urine sediment of LN patients. MCP-1 mRNA levels were elevated during active LN in comparison with inactive LN and healthy controls. However, in this study urine MCP-1 mRNA levels were found not to be useful predictors of LN flares. It should be noted that the best use for MCP-1 as it relates to SLE is as part of a broader panel of markers, as elevated urine MCP-1 can also signal chronic fibrosis[82,83] and has presented in other glomerular disorders.[84] Thus a combinatorial approach may lead to additional specificity for LN.

Urine NGAL

NGAL is expressed in several cell types, including neutrophils, specific epithelia, and renal tubular cells. NGAL is markedly upregulated in the distal tubules in response to many types of kidney injury. It has garnered significant attention as a promising early marker for acute kidney injury,[85–91] but recent studies have also shed light on NGAL's potential as a biomarker for chronic kidney disease, such as diabetic nephropathy[92,93] and focal segmental glomerulosclerosis,[94] as well as LN.[95,96] Two cross-sectional studies investigated NGAL as a biomarker for LN in pediatric patients[95] and adults.[97] In children, elevated urine NGAL levels had a high sensitivity and specificity for active biopsy-proven LN (AUC_{ROC} 0.94). In adults the specificity was still high (91%), but sensitivity was lower (50%) for LN. This thread is a common one in biomarker studies, as adults typically have more concurrent confounding physiologic conditions, which leads to higher variability in biomarker measurements. NGAL was not correlated with extrarenal SLE disease activity in either population. More recent longitudinal studies in the pediatric population have shown that urine NGAL as well as plasma NGAL levels are significantly higher in SLE patients than those with juvenile idiopathic arthritis (JIA) or healthy controls, unrelated to physiologic factors such as height, weight, and age.[98] Levels of urine NGAL, but not plasma NGAL, correlated well with LN activity scores.[96,98] Urine NGAL rose 3 to 6 months before worsening renal disease activity, demonstrating value in predicting flares.[96,98] One study demonstrated a lesser, though significant, increase in plasma NGAL as early as 3 months before flare.[96] In addition, in patients with a biopsy, urine NGAL levels were greater in patients with diffuse proliferative than membranous nephropathy, indicating, along with MCP-1, the possible use of NGAL in a panel to distinguish LN classes.[98] Similar to MCP-1, urine NGAL is not specific to LN and thus must be used in a context-specific setting.

Hepcidin

Hepcidin is a small peptide hormone mainly produced in the liver, and has a role in iron homeostastis. Hepcidin is upregulated in response to high iron levels and inflammation, and decreases during anemia and iron deficiency. Proteomic evaluation by surface-enhanced laser desorption-ionization time-of-flight mass spectrometry (SELDI) revealed the 25- and 20-amino-acid isoforms of hepcidin as potential biomarkers for LN.[79] Zhang and colleagues[79] prospectively analyzed 24 LN flare cycles in 19 patients, and demonstrated an increase in hepcidin-20 4 months before flare, which then decreased to baseline levels by 4 months after flare. An opposing pattern was discovered for hepcidin-25, which decreased during renal activity then returned to baseline along with hepcidin-20 after flare. It will be interesting in future studies to evaluate the physiologic role of hepcidin in LN because it is regulated in part by inflammatory cytokines, such as interferon-α and interleukin (IL)-6, which are known to play a role in modulating tissue damage in SLE,[99,100] and have been shown experimentally to induce monocyte expression of hepcidin in vitro.[101] It has been speculated that monocyte infiltration of the kidney may be the source of urine hepcidin in LN.

Urine Protein Signature

Also using SELDI, Suzuki and colleagues[102] discovered and subsequently validated[54] a protein signature that identified active LN in children. After removal of 4 albumin fragments from the signature, the panel included transferrin (Tf), orosomucoid (or α-1 acid glycoprotein [AGP]), ceruloplasmin (CP), and lipocalin-type prostaglandin D synthase (L-PDGS, or β-trace protein). Using enzyme-linked immunosorbent assay or immuno-nephelometry, all 4 proteins were found to be significantly higher in patients with active LN than in those with nonrenal SLE or JIA controls. Urine L-PDGS, AGP, and Tf all increased as early as 3 months before renal flare, but Tf did so most consistently, demonstrating increased sensitivity to renal changes in SLE in comparison with L-PDGS or AGP. Urine CP did not demonstrate the ability to predict flares. Combining this panel with other markers such as NGAL and MCP-1 may demonstrate enhanced predictive and diagnostic value in comparison with individual markers alone.

Complement Component C4d

C4d is a breakdown product of the activated complement factor C4b, a critical component of the C5 convertase. In a controversial pilot study using an alternative approach, Batal and colleagues[103] evaluated cellular deposition of the immune complex C4d on circulating erythrocytes, reticulocytes, and platelets as a potential biomarker for LN activity. Previous studies had linked peritubular capillary and glomerular staining of C4d with severity of LN and development of renal thrombotic microangiopathy, respectively.[104,105] The investigators found higher circulating levels of erythrocyte-bound C4d (EC4d) and reticulocyte-bound C4d (RC4d) in LN patients than in both nonrenal SLE patients and patients with renal disease without SLE. Moreover, EC4d levels correlated with the NIH renal activity index. There has been some level of skepticism[106] regarding the ability of these markers to distinguish renal from nonrenal SLE, as higher levels can also observed in SLE patients without LN,[107,108] and there have been no scientific findings to date that dispute the results. An additional study lends credence to the finding in this study, indicating higher levels of certain C4d-positive circulating T cells in LN patients than in those without LN.[109] Further prospective investigations of circulating C4d are needed for it to rise to the levels of the previously discussed biomarkers for LN, but the novel approach warranted mention in this review.

TWEAK

Tumor necrosis factor–like weak inducer of apoptosis (TWEAK) is a member of the tumor necrosis factor (TNF) superfamily, and is involved in modulating cell survival and induction of several proinflammatory chemokines through its receptor fibroblast growth factor–inducible protein 14 (Fn14).[110] In human kidney, TWEAK acts on multiple Fn14-expressing cells types, including podocytes, tubular cells, and mesangial cells, and is responsible for induction of several mediators of inflammation, including MCP-1, interferon-γ–inducible protein 10 (IP-10), intercellular cell adhesion molecule 1, vascular cell adhesion molecule 1 (VCAM-1), matrix metalloproteinases 1 and 9, and macrophage inflammatory protein α.[111,112] During periods of inflammation, Fn14 expression is upregulated, which lends itself to enhancing a positive feedback loop. The major source of TWEAK in LN is thought to be infiltrating monocytes and macrophages. Cross-sectionally, urinary TWEAK levels are significantly higher in active LN; levels are significantly higher in patients with LN flare than in those with stable disease.[113,114] In a multicenter longitudinal analysis, Schwartz and colleagues[115] discovered that whereas urinary TWEAK levels peaked at the height of renal flare, urinary TWEAK was significantly elevated 4 to 6 months before and following renal flare. Performance of urinary TWEAK in distinguishing LN patients from SLE patients without kidney involvement was better than that of anti-dsDNA levels and complement C3 or C4 levels. The study also demonstrated a strong association between urinary TWEAK levels and LN activity over time. Conversely, serum levels of TWEAK were not associated with LN activity. TWEAK is intriguing as a biomarker for LN, and has a biologically plausible role in LN pathology.

Other Chemokines, Receptors, and Adhesion Molecules

Space does not permit in-depth discussion of all biomarkers under investigation for LN, but several cytokines, chemokines, and their receptors deserve some mention. Chemokine C-X-C motif ligand 10 (CXCL10, also known as IP-10) and its receptor CXCR3 promote T-cell migration to areas of inflammation and are upregulated in SLE.[116,117] CXCL10 and CXCR3 mRNA levels collected from urine sediment were highly specific for identifying Class IV LN (AUC_{ROC} 0.89 for CXCL10 and 0.79 for CXCR3), and also demonstrated reduction in response to successful treatment signified by clinical remission.[118] FOXP3 (forkhead box P3) mRNA collected from urine sediment of LN patients has been found to be significantly higher in LN patients,[119] despite FOXP3 levels in regulatory T cells having been found to be lower in patients with active lupus than in healthy controls.[120] Research has also shown that a reduced number of circulating FOXP3[+] T cells and serum transforming growth factor β levels inversely correlated with LN activity as measured by SLE disease activity index renal domain score ($P = .0013$ and 0.0005, respectively).[109] Collection of mRNA from urine sediment presents several technical difficulties, such as stability, which may limit the clinical utility of urine mRNAs as biomarkers. So although there may be a link between FOXP3 and LN, additional study must be completed to solidify its role and usefulness as a biomarker for LN.

VCAM-1 demonstrates reliability as an indicator of renal disease activity in LN. VCAM-1 has been shown to be induced in mice by inflammatory cytokines such as IL-1 and TNF.[121] VCAM-1 plays a role in tethering leukocytes, which are drawn to sites of inflammation, to endothelial cells.[122] Urinary VCAM-1 has been shown in several studies of human disease to be strongly correlated with LN activity and severity[77,123,124] in LN. Serum levels of VCAM have previously been shown to correlate with the severity of LN, being highest in WHO Class III and IV, versus inactive or mild nephritis (WHO Class I or II),[125] and levels diminished with treatment. Singh and colleagues[126] compared urine levels of VCAM-1, MCP-1, and CXCL16 (another potential LN biomarker) with pathologic features of LN on biopsy collected concurrently with the urine sample. Urine VCAM and MCP-1 were highly predictive of LN when compared with healthy controls (AUC_{ROC} 0.92 and 0.89, respectively). Surprisingly, urine MCP-1 was also significantly higher in African American subjects than in persons of other ethnic origins. Of the 3 markers, urine VCAM-1 was most highly correlated with LN activity, with none shown by CXCL16. CXCL16 and urine VCAM-1 were significantly higher in patients with WHO Class IV LN compared with other Classes, as determined by concurrent biopsy analysis. It should be noted that this association with Class IV proliferative nephritis may not be specific to pathology, but a may be a result of these patients having a high degree of renal disease activity. These findings provide a great deal of support for urine VCAM-1 as a biomarker for LN, but these studies have all been cross-sectional. Longitudinal studies are needed to determine the utility of VCAM-1 in monitoring disease progression and detecting flares. It should also be noted that, like NGAL and MCP-1, elevated VCAM-1 is not exclusive to LN. Increased levels of VCAM-1 have been found in other glomerular diseases such as membranous nephropathy and focal segmental glomerulosclerosis.[126]

CURRENT TREATMENT OF LUPUS NEPHRITIS IN CHILDREN

The novel biomarkers introduced in the preceding sections are not used to support efficacy in clinical trials at present, although validation studies are ongoing to achieve biomarker qualification by regulatory bodies. Qualification would allow for the use of biomarkers in clinical care and research.[127,128] In addition, there is no known biomarker at present that a priori would support the choice of therapeutics for the treatment of LN. However, it seems reasonable to assume that novel biomarkers will become available for clinical use within the next 5 to 7 years.

No medication has likely improved the prognosis of LN more than systemic glucocorticoids (GC), especially if combined with immunosuppressive medications. Nonetheless, use of GC is a concern, given the often devastating short-term and long-term side effects. There is a lack of systematic studies in support of the most appropriate dose of GC in patients with LN. Based on consensus among pediatric rheumatologists in the United States, three GC dosing regimens for the treatment of proliferative LN in children have been proposed,[129] but data are lacking to determine which regimen is the most appropriate for a given patient. Of note, the Joint European League Against Rheumatism and the American College of Rheumatology consider much lower GC exposure sufficient for mainly adults with LN.[14,130]

Unless commanded by cSLE activity in other organ systems, hydroxychloroquine and GC are considered sufficient for the treatment of ISN/RPS Class I and, often, Class II LN.[14,131] For proliferative LN Class III or IV with or without membranous features, treatment with cyclophosphamide or mycophenolate mofetil (MMF) for induction therapy, and maintenance therapy using MMF or azathioprine are proposed.[14,129] Based on a Cochrane review of studies of adults with LN,[132,133] compared with intravenous cyclophosphamide, MMF was as effective in achieving stable kidney function and complete remission of proteinuria. No differences in mortality or major infections were observed. In maintenance therapy, the risk of LN flare was significantly higher with azathioprine or cyclophosphamide compared with MMF. Based on small studies, children and adolescents have a response to MMF and cyclophosphamide similar to that of adults with LN.[134] Whether MMF is as effective in children as it is in adults[135] or whether cyclophosphamide might have a better risk/benefit profile in children than in adults owing to lower frequency of clinically relevant ovarian injury and lower risk of nonadherence is not supported by high-level scientific evidence.[129] In addition, the pediatric correlate of the "Euro Lupus Regimen" for the dosing of intravenous cyclophosphamide has not been developed or systematically studied.[14]

There is mounting evidence that individualized dosing of MMF based on pharmaco-kinetic profiling will increase the likelihood of achieving remission of LN.[136,137] Target exposure between 60 and 90 mg/h/L is more often associated with LN improvement, with the highest exposures being reserved for the most severe cases because of the increased frequency of adverse effects.[136] Given high interindividual differences, weight-based or body-surface–based dosing of MMF does not suffice to reliably achieve such a target exposure.[138]

Pure membranous lupus glomerulonephritis (ISN/RPS Class V) seems rarely the initially diagnosed type of LN, and typically the other forms of LN develop into Class V over time. Treatment of Class V probably should not differ from that of idiopathic membranous nephropathy. Depending on the degree of proteinuria, only angiotensin-inhibiting medications, or GC with MMF or other immunosuppressives are the preferred initial therapy.[139]

Despite favorable reports mostly from observational studies,[140–144] the clinical trial of the anti-CD20 antibody rituximab (Rituxan, Mabthera) failed to show clinically relevant improvement of LN.[145] The anti–B-lymphocyte stimulator antibody belimumab (Benlysta) has recently been approved for the treatment of active SLE,[146,147] but its benefit or detrimental effects on LN will require further study.

There are currently several ongoing studies of LN, some including younger patients, which explore the efficacy of various combination therapies of GC with regimens including various combinations of cyclophosphamide, cyclosporin, azathioprine, tacrolimus, MMF, fludarabine, azathioprine, rituximab, abatacept, etanercept, and leflunomide, as well as mesenchymal stem cells. It is hoped that these studies consider the genetic differences of patients and include potent LN biomarkers when assessing the benefits of these therapies under investigation.

It is plausible to assume that the use of novel biomarkers will yield better stratification of patient populations for the purpose of clinical trials, and enable researchers to determine the response to LN therapy earlier and more accurately. This approach would necessitate smaller sample sizes for clinical trials, and ultimately make possible adequately powered studies in children with LN.

REFERENCES

1. Silva CA, Avcin T, Brunner HI. Taxonomy for systemic lupus erythematosus with onset before adulthood. Arthritis Care Res (Hoboken) 2012;64(12):1787–93.
2. Danchenko N, Satia JA, Anthony MS. Epidemiology of systemic lupus erythematosus: a comparison of worldwide disease burden. Lupus 2006;15(5):308–18.
3. Hiraki LT, Feldman CH, Liu J, et al. Prevalence, incidence, and demographics of systemic lupus erythematosus and lupus nephritis from 2000 to 2004 among children in the US Medicaid beneficiary population. Arthritis Rheum 2012; 64(8):2669–76.
4. Aletaha D, Landewe R, Karonitsch T, et al. Reporting disease activity in clinical trials of patients with rheumatoid arthritis: EULAR/ACR collaborative recommendations. Arthritis Rheum 2008;59(10):1371–7.
5. Livingston B, Bonner A, Pope J. Differences in clinical manifestations between childhood-onset lupus and adult-onset lupus: a meta-analysis. Lupus 2011; 20(13):1345–55.
6. Hiraki LT, Lu B, Alexander SR, et al. End-stage renal disease due to lupus nephritis among children in the US, 1995-2006. Arthritis Rheum 2011;63(7):1988–97.
7. Bernatsky S, Boivin JF, Joseph L, et al. Mortality in systemic lupus erythematosus. Arthritis Rheum 2006;54(8):2550–7.

8. Lionaki S, Kapitsinou PP, Iniotaki A, et al. Kidney transplantation in lupus patients: a case-control study from a single centre. Lupus 2008;17(7):670–5.

9. Pereira T, Abitbol CL, Seeherunvong W, et al. Three decades of progress in treating childhood-onset lupus nephritis. Clin J Am Soc Nephrol 2011;6(9): 2192–9.

10. Costenbader KH, Desai A, Alarcon GS, et al. Trends in the incidence, demographics, and outcomes of end-stage renal disease due to lupus nephritis in the US from 1995 to 2006. Arthritis Rheum 2011;63(6):1681–8.

11. Tanzer M, Tran C, Messer KL, et al. Inpatient health care utilization by children and adolescents with systemic lupus erythematosus and kidney involvement. Arthritis Care Res (Hoboken) 2013;65(3):382–90.

12. Brunner HI, Sherrard TM, Klein-Gitelman MS. Cost of treatment of childhood-onset systemic lupus erythematosus. Arthritis Rheum 2006;55(2):184–8.

13. NAPRTCS. North American Pediatric Renal Trials and Collaborative Studies Annual Report. 2011. Available at: https://web.emmes.com/study/ped/annlrept/annualrept2011.pdf.

14. Bertsias GK, Tektonidou M, Amoura Z, et al. Joint European League Against Rheumatism and European Renal Association-European Dialysis and Transplant Association (EULAR/ERA-EDTA) recommendations for the management of adult and paediatric lupus nephritis. Ann Rheum Dis 2012;71(11):1771–82.

15. Hollander MC, Sage JM, Greenler AJ, et al. International consensus for provisions of quality-driven care in childhood-onset systemic lupus erythematosus. Arthritis Care Res (Hoboken) 2013. [Epub ahead of print].

16. Marks SD, Sebire NJ, Pilkington C, et al. Clinicopathological correlations of paediatric lupus nephritis. Pediatr Nephrol 2007;22(1):77–83.

17. Brunner HI, Gladman DD, Ibanez D, et al. Difference in disease features between childhood-onset and adult-onset systemic lupus erythematosus. Arthritis Rheum 2008;58(2):556–62.

18. Hiraki LT, Benseler SM, Tyrrell PN, et al. Clinical and laboratory characteristics and long-term outcome of pediatric systemic lupus erythematosus: a longitudinal study. J Pediatr 2008;152(4):550–6.

19. Ruggiero B, Vivarelli M, Gianviti A, et al. Lupus nephritis in children and adolescents: results of the Italian Collaborative Study. Nephrol Dial Transplant 2013; 28(6):1487–96.

20. Weening JJ, D'Agati VD, Schwartz MM, et al. The classification of glomerulonephritis in systemic lupus erythematosus revisited. J Am Soc Nephrol 2004;15(2): 241–50.

21. Corwin HL, Schwartz MM, Lewis EJ. The importance of sample size in the interpretation of the renal biopsy. Am J Nephrol 1988;8(2):85–9.

22. Austin HA 3rd, Muenz LR, Joyce KM, et al. Diffuse proliferative lupus nephritis: identification of specific pathologic features affecting renal outcome. Kidney Int 1984;25(4):689–95.

23. Hsieh C, Chang A, Brandt D, et al. Predicting outcomes of lupus nephritis with tubulointerstitial inflammation and scarring. Arthritis Care Res (Hoboken) 2011; 63(6):865–74.

24. Cortes-Hernandez J, Ordi-Ros J, Labrador M, et al. Predictors of poor renal outcome in patients with lupus nephritis treated with combined pulses of cyclophosphamide and methylprednisolone. Lupus 2003;12(4):287–96.

25. Zappitelli M, Duffy C, Bernard C, et al. Clinicopathological study of the WHO classification in childhood lupus nephritis. Pediatr Nephrol 2004;19(5): 503–10.

26. Lee BS, Cho HY, Kim EJ, et al. Clinical outcomes of childhood lupus nephritis: a single center's experience. Pediatr Nephrol 2007;22(2):222–31.
27. Demircin G, Oner A, Erdogan O, et al. Long-term efficacy and safety of quadruple therapy in childhood diffuse proliferative lupus nephritis. Ren Fail 2008;30(6):603–9.
28. Hagelberg S, Lee Y, Bargman J, et al. Longterm followup of childhood lupus nephritis. J Rheumatol 2002;29(12):2635–42.
29. Vachvanichsanong P, Dissaneewate P, McNeil E. Diffuse proliferative glomerulo-nephritis does not determine the worst outcome in childhood onset lupus nephritis: a 23-year experience in a single centre. Nephrol Dial Transplant 2009;24(9):2729–34.
30. Hersh AO, von Scheven E, Yazdany J, et al. Differences in long-term disease activity and treatment of adult patients with childhood- and adult-onset systemic lupus erythematosus. Arthritis Rheum 2009;61(1):13–20.
31. Zappitelli M, Duffy CM, Bernard C, et al. Evaluation of activity, chronicity and tubulointerstitial indices for childhood lupus nephritis. Pediatr Nephrol 2008; 23(1):83–91.
32. Chrysochou C, Randhawa H, Reeve R, et al. Determinants of renal functional outcome in lupus nephritis: a single centre retrospective study. QJM 2008; 101(4):313–6.
33. Contreras G, Pardo V, Cely C, et al. Factors associated with poor outcomes in patients with lupus nephritis. Lupus 2005;14(11):890–5.
34. Houssiau FA. Therapy of lupus nephritis: lessons learned from clinical research and daily care of patients. Arthritis Res Ther 2012;14(1):202.
35. Mok CC, Ying KY, Tang S, et al. Predictors and outcome of renal flares after successful cyclophosphamide treatment for diffuse proliferative lupus glomeru-lonephritis. Arthritis Rheum 2004;50(8):2559–68.
36. Punaro M, Abou-Jaoude P, Cimaz R, et al. Unusual neurologic manifestations (II): posterior reversible encephalopathy syndrome (PRES) in the context of juvenile systemic lupus erythematosus. Lupus 2007;16(8):576–9.
37. Valente de Almeida R, Rocha de Carvalho JG, de Azevedo VF, et al. Microalbu-minuria and renal morphology in the evaluation of subclinical lupus nephritis. Clin Nephrol 1999;52(4):218–29.
38. Houssiau FA, Vasconcelos C, D'Cruz D, et al. Early response to immunosup-pressive therapy predicts good renal outcome in lupus nephritis: lessons from long-term followup of patients in the Euro-Lupus Nephritis Trial. Arthritis Rheum 2004;50(12):3934–40.
39. Eddy AA, Giachelli CM. Renal expression of genes that promote interstitial inflammation and fibrosis in rats with protein-overload proteinuria. Kidney Int 1995;47(6):1546–57.
40. Siedner MJ, Gelber AC, Rovin BH, et al. Diagnostic accuracy study of urine dipstick in relation to 24-hour measurement as a screening tool for proteinuria in lupus nephritis. J Rheumatol 2008;35(1):84–90.
41. Hebert LA, Birmingham DJ, Shidham G, et al. Random spot urine protein/creatinine ratio is unreliable for estimating 24-hour proteinuria in individual systemic lupus erythematosus nephritis patients. Nephron Clin Pract 2009;113(3):c177–82.
42. KDOQI. KDOQI clinical practice guidelines and clinical practice recommen-dations for diabetes and chronic kidney disease. Am J Kidney Dis 2007; 49(2 Suppl 2):S12–154.
43. Renal Disease Subcommittee of the American College of Rheumatology Ad Hoc Committee on Systemic Lupus Erythematosus Response Criteria. The American

College of Rheumatology response criteria for proliferative and membranous renal disease in systemic lupus erythematosus clinical trials. Arthritis Rheum 2006;54(2):421–32.

44. Fine DM, Ziegenbein M, Petri M, et al. A prospective study of protein excretion using short-interval timed urine collections in patients with lupus nephritis. Kidney Int 2009;76(12):1284–8.

45. Fogazzi GB, Garigali G. The clinical art and science of urine microscopy. Curr Opin Nephrol Hypertens 2003;12(6):625–32.

46. Bacchetta J, Cochat P, Rognant N, et al. Which creatinine and cystatin C equations can be reliably used in children? Clin J Am Soc Nephrol 2011;6(3):552–60.

47. Lertnawapan R, Bian A, Rho YH, et al. Cystatin C is associated with inflammation but not atherosclerosis in systemic lupus erythematosus. Lupus 2012;21(3):279–87.

48. Chew C, Pemberton PW, Husain AA, et al. Serum cystatin C is independently associated with renal impairment and high sensitivity C-reactive protein in systemic lupus erythematosus. Clin Exp Rheumatol 2013;31(2):251–5.

49. Christopher-Stine L, Siedner M, Lin J, et al. Renal biopsy in lupus patients with low levels of proteinuria. J Rheumatol 2007;34(2):332–5.

50. Vernon KA, Cook HT. Complement in glomerular disease. Adv Chronic Kidney Dis 2012;19(2):84–92.

51. Rovin BH, Birmingham DJ, Nagaraja HN, et al. Biomarker discovery in human SLE nephritis. Bull N Y U Hosp Jt Dis 2007;65(3):187–93.

52. Ho A, Barr SG, Magder LS, et al. A decrease in complement is associated with increased renal and hematologic activity in patients with systemic lupus erythematosus. Arthritis Rheum 2001;44(10):2350–7.

53. Esdaile JM, Abrahamowicz M, Joseph L, et al. Laboratory tests as predictors of disease exacerbations in systemic lupus erythematosus. Why some tests fail. Arthritis Rheum 1996;39(3):370–8.

54. Suzuki M, Wiers K, Brooks EB, et al. Initial validation of a novel protein biomarker panel for active pediatric lupus nephritis. Pediatr Res 2009;65(5):530–6.

55. Grootscholten C, Bajema IM, Florquin S, et al. Interobserver agreement of scoring of histopathological characteristics and classification of lupus nephritis. Nephrol Dial Transplant 2008;23(1):223–30.

56. Biomarkers Definitions Working Group. Biomarkers and surrogate endpoints: preferred definitions and conceptual framework. Clin Pharmacol Ther 2001; 69(3):89–95.

57. Devarajan P. Proteomics for biomarker discovery in acute kidney injury. Semin Nephrol 2007;27(6):637–51.

58. Knepper MA. Proteomics and the kidney. J Am Soc Nephrol 2002;13(5): 1398–408.

59. Thongboonkerd V, McLeish KR, Arthur JM, et al. Proteomic analysis of normal human urinary proteins isolated by acetone precipitation or ultracentrifugation. Kidney Int 2002;62(4):1461–9.

60. Adachi J, Kumar C, Zhang Y, et al. The human urinary proteome contains more than 1500 proteins, including a large proportion of membrane proteins. Genome Biol 2006;7(9):R80.

61. Omenn GS. Exploring the human plasma proteome. Proteomics 2005;5(13): 3223–5.

62. Omenn GS, States DJ, Adamski M, et al. Overview of the HUPO Plasma Proteome Project: results from the pilot phase with 35 collaborating laboratories and multiple analytical groups, generating a core dataset of 3020 proteins and a publicly-available database. Proteomics 2005;5(13):3226–45.

63. States DJ, Omenn GS, Blackwell TW, et al. Challenges in deriving high-confidence protein identifications from data gathered by a HUPO plasma proteome collaborative study. Nat Biotechnol 2006;24(3):333–8.

64. D'Alessandro A, Righetti PG, Zolla L. The Red Blood Cell proteome and interactome: an update. J Proteome Res 2010;9(1):144–63.

65. van Gestel RA, van Solinge WW, van der Toorn HW, et al. Quantitative erythrocyte membrane proteome analysis with Blue-Native/SDS PAGE. J Proteomics 2010;73(3):456–65.

66. Knepper MA. Common sense approaches to urinary biomarker study design. J Am Soc Nephrol 2009;20(6):1175–8.

67. Hewitt SM, Dear J, Star RA. Discovery of protein biomarkers for renal diseases. J Am Soc Nephrol 2004;15(7):1677–89.

68. Dos Remedios CG, Liew CC, Allen PD, et al. Genomics, proteomics and bioinformatics of human heart failure. J Muscle Res Cell Motil 2003;24(4–6):251–60.

69. Zweig MH, Campbell G. Receiver-operating characteristic (ROC) plots: a fundamental evaluation tool in clinical medicine. Clin Chem 1993;39(4):561–77.

70. Rovin BH. The chemokine network in systemic lupus erythematous nephritis. Front Biosci 2008;13:904–22.

71. Hasegawa H, Kohno M, Sasaki M, et al. Antagonist of monocyte chemoattractant protein 1 ameliorates the initiation and progression of lupus nephritis and renal vasculitis in MRL/lpr mice. Arthritis Rheum 2003;48(9):2555–66.

72. Kulkarni O, Pawar RD, Purschke W, et al. Spiegelmer inhibition of CCL2/MCP-1 ameliorates lupus nephritis in MRL-(Fas)lpr mice. J Am Soc Nephrol 2007;18(8): 2350–8.

73. Rovin BH, Song H, Birmingham DJ, et al. Urine chemokines as biomarkers of human systemic lupus erythematosus activity. J Am Soc Nephrol 2005;16(2):467–73.

74. Kiani AN, Johnson K, Chen C, et al. Urine osteoprotegerin and monocyte chemoattractant protein-1 in lupus nephritis. J Rheumatol 2009;36(10):2224–30.

75. Tucci M, Barnes EV, Sobel ES, et al. Strong association of a functional polymorphism in the monocyte chemoattractant protein 1 promoter gene with lupus nephritis. Arthritis Rheum 2004;50(6):1842–9.

76. Watson L, Midgley A, Pilkington C, et al. Urinary monocyte chemoattractant protein 1 and alpha 1 acid glycoprotein as biomarkers of renal disease activity in juvenile-onset systemic lupus erythematosus. Lupus 2012;21(5):496–501.

77. Wu T, Xie C, Wang HW, et al. Elevated urinary VCAM-1, P-selectin, soluble TNF receptor-1, and CXC chemokine ligand 16 in multiple murine lupus strains and human lupus nephritis. J Immunol 2007;179(10):7166–75.

78. Graves DT, Alsulaimani F, Ding Y, et al. Developmentally regulated monocyte recruitment and bone resorption are modulated by functional deletion of the monocytic chemoattractant protein-1 gene. Bone 2002;31(2):282–7.

79. Zhang X, Jin M, Wu H, et al. Biomarkers of lupus nephritis determined by serial urine proteomics. Kidney Int 2008;74(6):799–807.

80. Tian S, Li J, Wang L, et al. Urinary levels of RANTES and M-CSF are predictors of lupus nephritis flare. Inflamm Res 2007;56(7):304–10.

81. Chan RW, Lai FM, Li EK, et al. The effect of immunosuppressive therapy on the messenger RNA expression of target genes in the urinary sediment of patients with active lupus nephritis. Nephrol Dial Transplant 2006;21(6):1534–40.

82. Gharaee-Kermani M, Denholm EM, Phan SH. Costimulation of fibroblast collagen and transforming growth factor beta1 gene expression by monocyte chemoattractant protein-1 via specific receptors. J Biol Chem 1996;271(30): 17779–84.

83. Sakai N, Wada T, Furuichi K, et al. MCP-1/CCR2-dependent loop for fibrogenesis in human peripheral CD14-positive monocytes. J Leukoc Biol 2006;79(3):555–63.

84. Rovin BH. Chemokines as therapeutic targets in renal inflammation. Am J Kidney Dis 1999;34(4):761–4 [discussion: 765–7].

85. Mishra J, Dent C, Tarabishi R, et al. Neutrophil gelatinase-associated lipocalin (NGAL) as a biomarker for acute renal injury after cardiac surgery. Lancet 2005;365(9466):1231–8.

86. Mishra J, Ma Q, Kelly C, et al. Kidney NGAL is a novel early marker of acute injury following transplantation. Pediatr Nephrol (Berlin, Germany) 2006;21(6): 856–63.

87. Mishra J, Mori K, Ma Q, et al. Neutrophil gelatinase-associated lipocalin: a novel early urinary biomarker for cisplatin nephrotoxicity. Am J Nephrol 2004;24(3): 307–15.

88. Bennett M, Dent CL, Ma Q, et al. Urine NGAL predicts severity of acute kidney injury after cardiac surgery: a prospective study. Clin J Am Soc Nephrol 2008; 3(3):665–73.

89. Haase M, Bellomo R, Devarajan P, et al. Novel biomarkers early predict the severity of acute kidney injury after cardiac surgery in adults. Ann Thorac Surg 2009;88(1):124–30.

90. Krawczeski CD, Goldstein SL, Woo JG, et al. Temporal relationship and predictive value of urinary acute kidney injury biomarkers after pediatric cardiopulmonary bypass. J Am Coll Cardiol 2011;58(22):2301–9.

91. Krawczeski CD, Woo JG, Wang Y, et al. Neutrophil gelatinase-associated lipocalin concentrations predict development of acute kidney injury in neonates and children after cardiopulmonary bypass. J Pediatr 2011;5:5.

92. Bolignano D, Lacquaniti A, Coppolino G, et al. Neutrophil gelatinase-associated lipocalin as an early biomarker of nephropathy in diabetic patients. Kidney Blood Press Res 2009;32(2):91–8.

93. Bolignano D, Lacquaniti A, Coppolino G, et al. Neutrophil gelatinase-associated lipocalin (NGAL) and progression of chronic kidney disease. Clin J Am Soc Nephrol 2009;4(2):337–44.

94. Bennett MR, Piyaphanee N, Czech K, et al. NGAL distinguishes steroid sensitivity in idiopathic nephrotic syndrome. Pediatr Nephrol (Berlin, Germany) 2012;27(5):807–12.

95. Brunner HI, Mueller M, Rutherford C, et al. Urinary neutrophil gelatinase-associated lipocalin as a biomarker of nephritis in childhood-onset systemic lupus erythematosus. Arthritis Rheum 2006;54(8):2577–84.

96. Hinze CH, Suzuki M, Klein-Gitelman M, et al. Neutrophil gelatinase-associated lipocalin is a predictor of the course of global and renal childhood-onset systemic lupus erythematosus disease activity. Arthritis Rheum 2009;60(9): 2772–81.

97. Pitashny M, Schwartz N, Qing X, et al. Urinary lipocalin-2 is associated with renal disease activity in human lupus nephritis. Arthritis Rheum 2007;56(6):1894–903.

98. Suzuki M, Wiers KM, Klein-Gitelman MS, et al. Neutrophil gelatinase-associated lipocalin as a biomarker of disease activity in pediatric lupus nephritis. Pediatr Nephrol 2008;23(3):403–12.

99. Ivashkiv LB. Type I interferon modulation of cellular responses to cytokines and infectious pathogens: potential role in SLE pathogenesis. Autoimmunity 2003; 36(8):473–9.

100. Tackey E, Lipsky PE, Illei GG. Rationale for interleukin-6 blockade in systemic lupus erythematosus. Lupus 2004;13(5):339–43.

101. Zhang X, Rovin BH. Hepcidin expression by human monocytes in response to adhesion and pro-inflammatory cytokines. Biochim Biophys Acta 2010; 1800(12):1262–7.
102. Suzuki M, Ross GF, Wiers K, et al. Identification of a urinary proteomic signature for lupus nephritis in children. Pediatr Nephrol 2007;22(12):2047–57.
103. Batal I, Liang K, Bastacky S, et al. Prospective assessment of C4d deposits on circulating cells and renal tissues in lupus nephritis: a pilot study. Lupus 2012; 21(1):13–26.
104. Li SJ, Liu ZH, Zen CH, et al. Peritubular capillary C4d deposition in lupus nephritis different from antibody-mediated renal rejection. Lupus 2007;16(11): 875–80.
105. Cohen D, Koopmans M, Kremer Hovinga IC, et al. Potential for glomerular C4d as an indicator of thrombotic microangiopathy in lupus nephritis. Arthritis Rheum 2008;58(8):2460–9.
106. Dhir V. Is cellular C4d a good biomarker for SLE nephritis? Lupus 2012;21(9):1036.
107. Liu CC, Manzi S, Kao AH, et al. Reticulocytes bearing C4d as biomarkers of disease activity for systemic lupus erythematosus. Arthritis Rheum 2005; 52(10):3087–99.
108. Navratil JS, Manzi S, Kao AH, et al. Platelet C4d is highly specific for systemic lupus erythematosus. Arthritis Rheum 2006;54(2):670–4.
109. Edelbauer M, Kshirsagar S, Riedl M, et al. Activity of childhood lupus nephritis is linked to altered T cell and cytokine homeostasis. J Clin Immunol 2012;32(3): 477–87.
110. Campbell S, Michaelson J, Burkly L, et al. The role of TWEAK/Fn14 in the pathogenesis of inflammation and systemic autoimmunity. Front Biosci 2004;9: 2273–84.
111. Campbell S, Burkly LC, Gao HX, et al. Proinflammatory effects of TWEAK/Fn14 interactions in glomerular mesangial cells. J Immunol 2006;176(3):1889–98.
112. Reyes-Thomas J, Blanco I, Putterman C. Urinary biomarkers in lupus nephritis. Clin Rev Allergy Immunol 2011;40(3):138–50.
113. Schwartz N, Michaelson JS, Putterman C. Lipocalin-2, TWEAK, and other cytokines as urinary biomarkers for lupus nephritis. Ann N Y Acad Sci 2007;1109: 265–74.
114. Schwartz N, Su L, Burkly LC, et al. Urinary TWEAK and the activity of lupus nephritis. J Autoimmun 2006;27(4):242–50.
115. Schwartz N, Rubinstein T, Burkly LC, et al. Urinary TWEAK as a biomarker of lupus nephritis: a multicenter cohort study. Arthritis Res Ther 2009;11(5):R143.
116. Luster AD. Chemokines—chemotactic cytokines that mediate inflammation. N Engl J Med 1998;338(7):436–45.
117. Bauer JW, Baechler EC, Petri M, et al. Elevated serum levels of interferon-regulated chemokines are biomarkers for active human systemic lupus erythematosus. PLoS Med 2006;3(12):e491.
118. Avihingsanon Y, Phumesin P, Benjachat T, et al. Measurement of urinary chemokine and growth factor messenger RNAs: a noninvasive monitoring in lupus nephritis. Kidney Int 2006;69(4):747–53.
119. Wang G, Lai FM, Tam LS, et al. Urinary FOXP3 mRNA in patients with lupus nephritis—relation with disease activity and treatment response. Rheumatology (Oxford) 2009;48(7):755–60.
120. Valencia X, Yarboro C, Illei G, et al. Deficient CD4+CD25 high T regulatory cell function in patients with active systemic lupus erythematosus. J Immunol 2007; 178(4):2579–88.

121. McHale JF, Harari OA, Marshall D, et al. TNF-alpha and IL-1 sequentially induce endothelial ICAM-1 and VCAM-1 expression in MRL/lpr lupus-prone mice. J Immunol 1999;163(7):3993–4000.

122. Alon R, Kassner PD, Carr MW, et al. The integrin VLA-4 supports tethering and rolling in flow on VCAM-1. J Cell Biol 1995;128(6):1243–53.

123. Kiani AN, Wu T, Fang H, et al. Urinary vascular cell adhesion molecule, but not neutrophil gelatinase-associated lipocalin, is associated with lupus nephritis. J Rheumatol 2012;39(6):1231–7.

124. Abd-Elkareem MI, Al Tamimy HM, Khamis OA, et al. Increased urinary levels of the leukocyte adhesion molecules ICAM-1 and VCAM-1 in human lupus nephritis with advanced renal histological changes: preliminary findings. Clin Exp Nephrol 2010;14(6):548–57.

125. Ikeda Y, Fujimoto T, Ameno M, et al. Relationship between lupus nephritis activity and the serum level of soluble VCAM-1. Lupus 1998;7(5):347–54.

126. Singh S, Wu T, Xie C, et al. Urine VCAM-1 as a marker of renal pathology activity index in lupus nephritis. Arthritis Res Ther 2012;14(4):R164.

127. Goodsaid F, Frueh F. Biomarker qualification pilot process at the US Food and Drug Administration. AAPS J 2007;9(1):E105–8.

128. Goodsaid FM, Frueh FW, Mattes W. Strategic paths for biomarker qualification. Toxicology 2008;245(3):219–23.

129. Mina R, von Scheven E, Ardoin SP, et al. Consensus treatment plans for induction therapy of newly diagnosed proliferative lupus nephritis in juvenile systemic lupus erythematosus. Arthritis Care Res (Hoboken) 2012;64(3): 375–83.

130. Ad Hoc Working Group on Steroid-Sparing Criteria in Lupus. Criteria for steroid-sparing ability of interventions in systemic lupus erythematosus: report of a consensus meeting. Arthritis Rheum 2004;50(11):3427–31.

131. Pons-Estel GJ, Alarcon GS, McGwin G Jr, et al. Protective effect of hydroxychloroquine on renal damage in patients with lupus nephritis: LXV, data from a multiethnic US cohort. Arthritis Rheum 2009;61(6):830–9.

132. Henderson L, Masson P, Craig JC, et al. Treatment for lupus nephritis. Cochrane Database Syst Rev 2012;(12):CD002922.

133. Henderson LK, Masson P, Craig JC, et al. Induction and maintenance treatment of proliferative lupus nephritis: a meta-analysis of randomized controlled trials. Am J Kidney Dis 2013;61(1):74–87.

134. Sundel R, Solomons N, Lisk L. Efficacy of mycophenolate mofetil in adolescent patients with lupus nephritis: evidence from a two-phase, prospective randomized trial. Lupus 2012;21(13):1433–43.

135. Lehman TJ, Sherry DD, Wagner-Weiner L, et al. Intermittent intravenous cyclophosphamide therapy for lupus nephritis. J Pediatr 1989;114(6):1055–60.

136. Daleboudt GM, Reinders ME, den Hartigh J, et al. Concentration-controlled treatment of lupus nephritis with mycophenolate mofetil. Lupus 2013;22(2): 171–9.

137. Sagcal-Gironella AC, Fukuda T, Wiers K, et al. Pharmacokinetics and pharmacodynamics of mycophenolic acid and their relation to response to therapy of childhood-onset systemic lupus erythematosus. Semin Arthritis Rheum 2011; 40(4):307–13.

138. Sherwin CM, Fukuda T, Brunner HI, et al. The evolution of population pharmacokinetic models to describe the enterohepatic recycling of mycophenolic acid in solid organ transplantation and autoimmune disease. Clin Pharmacokinet 2011; 50(1):1–24.

139. Swan JT, Riche DM, Riche KD, et al. Systematic review and meta-analysis of immunosuppressant therapy clinical trials in membranous lupus nephritis. J Investig Med 2011;59(2):246–58.

140. Gunnarsson I, Sundelin B, Jonsdottir T, et al. Histopathologic and clinical outcome of rituximab treatment in patients with cyclophosphamide-resistant proliferative lupus nephritis. Arthritis Rheum 2007;56(4):1263–72.

141. Vigna-Perez M, Hernandez-Castro B, Paredes-Saharopulos O, et al. Clinical and immunological effects of rituximab in patients with lupus nephritis refractory to conventional therapy: a pilot study. Arthritis Res Ther 2006;8(3):R83.

142. van Vollenhoven RF, Gunnarsson I, Welin-Henriksson E, et al. Biopsy-verified response of severe lupus nephritis to treatment with rituximab (anti-CD20 monoclonal antibody) plus cyclophosphamide after biopsy-documented failure to respond to cyclophosphamide alone. Scand J Rheumatol 2004;33(6):423–7.

143. Fra GP, Avanzi GC, Bartoli E. Remission of refractory lupus nephritis with a protocol including rituximab. Lupus 2003;12(10):783–7.

144. Jonsdottir T, Zickert A, Sundelin B, et al. Long-term follow-up in lupus nephritis patients treated with rituximab—clinical and histopathological response. Rheumatology (Oxford) 2013;52(5):847–55.

145. Rovin BH, Furie R, Latinis K, et al. Efficacy and safety of rituximab in patients with active proliferative lupus nephritis: the Lupus Nephritis Assessment with Rituximab study. Arthritis Rheum 2012;64(4):1215–26.

146. Manzi S, Sanchez-Guerrero J, Merrill JT, et al. Effects of belimumab, a B lymphocyte stimulator-specific inhibitor, on disease activity across multiple organ domains in patients with systemic lupus erythematosus: combined results from two phase III trials. Ann Rheum Dis 2012;71(11):1833–8.

147. Dhaun N, Kluth DC. Belimumab for systemic lupus erythematosus. Lancet 2011; 377(9783):2079–80 [author reply: 2080–1].

Developments in Large and Midsize Vasculitis

Maria Teresa Terreri, PhD, MD*, Gleice Clemente, MD

KEYWORDS

- Vasculitis • Childhood • Adolescents • Kawasaki • Coronary artery
- Takayasu's arteritis • Hypertension • Imaging

KEY POINTS

- The diagnosis of KD is based on well-known criteria; however, diagnosis is often quite difficult because the clinical presentation may be incomplete.
- Some factors are associated with unfavorable prognosis and should prompt earlier treatment or the initial introduction of corticosteroids in combination with immunoglobulin.
- There is a delay in the diagnosis in childhood due to the lack of specific symptoms at the beginning of the disease.
- Takayasu arteritis must be ruled out in the presence of hypertension and an increased ESR.
- Clinical manifestations and markers of inflammatory activity are parameters that are helpful to monitor the therapeutic response but disease activity is difficult to assess.

INTRODUCTION

Childhood vasculitis is a complex and fascinating area in pediatric rheumatology that has experienced an unprecedented surge in research, leading to new knowledge over the past several years. Vasculitis is defined as the presence of inflammatory cell infiltration in blood vessel walls, usually with multisystemic involvement. Some forms of vasculitis have an abrupt onset, whereas others are very insidious leading to delayed diagnosis. Some vascular lesions can cause aneurysm formation, whereas others can cause stenosis or occlusion, resulting in ischemia, infarction, hemorrhage, and organ failure.

Vasculitis is difficult to classify and the most acceptable childhood vasculitis classification defines the type of vasculitis according to the size of the vessel affected.[1]

The pathogenic mechanisms of the different forms of vasculitis include presence of circulating immune complexes, disturbance in humoral immune response manifested by the presence of antibodies, antineutrophil cytoplasmic autoantibodies (ANCA), and

Department of Pediatrics, Universidade Federal de São Paulo, Rua Borges Lagoa 802, CEP 04038-001, São Paulo, Brazil
* Corresponding author.
E-mail address: teterreri@terra.com.br

Rheum Dis Clin N Am 39 (2013) 855–875
http://dx.doi.org/10.1016/j.rdc.2013.08.002
0889-857X/13/$ – see front matter © 2013 Elsevier Inc. All rights reserved.

antiendothelial cells; antibodies against antigens in vessel walls; and disturbance in cellular immune response with T-cell reactivity. Complement, cytokines, cell adhesion molecules, chemokines, growth factors, and neutrophils are involved in the immuno-logic processes of the systemic vasculitis.[2] Host susceptibility and environmental triggers play a role in these diseases.

Clinical features suggesting vasculitis include constitutional symptoms, such as fever, weight loss, fatigue, skin lesions, neurologic manifestations, arthralgia, arthritis, myalgia, myositis, serositis, arterial hypertension, and lung and renal involvement with infiltration and hemorrhage. High acute-phase reactants, anemia, leukocytosis with eosinophilia, antibodies, such as antineutrophil cytoplasmic antibodies, and altered urinary sediment are common laboratory features in vasculitis. Because of the nonspecific features, some forms of vasculitis are not recognized and their prevalence might be underestimated.

Diagnosis can be difficult, evaluating disease activity is problematic, and outcome in some cases can be poor.

The most frequent forms of vasculitis in childhood are the small-size vasculitides, of which Henoch-Schoenlein Purpura (HSP) and other leucocytoclastic vasculitis are the best examples, followed by Kawasaki disease, a midsize vasculitis, and Takayasu arteritis, a large-size vasculitis, both of which are topics in this article. Other forms of vasculitis include midsize vasculitis, such as polyarteritis nodosa (PAN), small-size vasculitis, subdivided into granulomatous disease (granulomatosis with polyangii-tis [GPA] or Wegener granulomatosis and eosinophilic granulomatosis with polyangiitis [EGPA], or Churg-Strauss syndrome) and nongranulomatous disease (microscopic polyangiitis [MPA]) and vasculitis affecting various-sized vessels like Behçet disease.

HSP is an IgA immune complex–mediated vasculitis that affects small vessels, with the main characteristics of purpuric rash, followed by arthralgia/arthritis, abdominal pain, and nephritis. The typical histopathologic feature in the acute inflammatory lesions is perivascular accumulation of neutrophils, known as leucocytoclastic vasculitis.[3] HSP is often a self-limited condition that involves skin, joint, and gut, but approximately 40% of patients develop nephritis within 4 to 6 weeks after the skin involvement, and depend-ing on severity may lead to poor disease outcome.[4] Disturbance in the immune system, including elevations in serum levels of immunoglobulin (Ig)A1 and IgA1-containing circulating immune complexes have been detected in patients with HSP.[5] Although the pathogenetic mechanisms are still not fully delineated, several studies suggest that galactose-deficient IgA1 (Gd-IgA1), which is increased in patients with HSP with nephritis, is recognized by antiglycan antibodies, leading to the formation of the circu-lating immune complexes and their mesangial deposition, resulting in renal injury.[6,7] Furthermore, serum levels of alpha–smooth muscle actin and C-Met were found to be higher in patients with HSP than those in the immunoglobulin-A nephropathy and healthy control groups and correlated with blood urea nitrogen levels, serum creatinine levels, hematuria, and proteinuria and may be associated with disease severity.[7]

Polyarteritis nodosa (PAN) is a chronic vasculitis that rarely occurs in childhood, although in some studies it appears to be the third-most common form of vasculitis after HSP and KD.[8] It is a necrotizing form of vasculitis associated with aneurysmal nodules along the walls of the medium-sized muscular vessels, which can be divided into systemic PAN, involving the skin and the gastrointestinal, renal, and central ner-vous systems, and in cutaneous PAN, a form limited to the skin. The main clinical fea-tures of systemic PAN are malaise, fever, weight loss, skin lesions, myalgia, arthropathy, abdominal pain, and testicular involvement, which are often associated with hypertension, proteinuria, and hematuria, secondary to renal artery involvement.[9] Neurologic features, such as focal defects, mononeuritis multiplex, and psychosis may be present.[9] The skin lesions are variable and may range from erythematous rash to necrotic lesions with peripheral gangrene, but livedo reticularis and nodules overlying affected arteries are characteristic features of this disease. Cutaneous PAN is characterized by the presence of painful subcutaneous nodules with or without other lesions, and no systemic involvement, except for myalgia, arthralgia, and nonerosive arthritis.[1] In this type of PAN, serologic or microbiological evidence of streptococcal infection is common.[1] There is controversy as to whether this is a separate entity or part of the systemic PAN spectrum. High acute-phase reactants are usually present in the active phase of both types. Positive hepatitis B serology is an unusual association with PAN in children. In a single-center retrospective study, gastrointestinal involvement was associated with increased risk of relapse, whereas longer time to induce remission and an increased cumulative cyclophosphamide dose were associated with lower risk of relapse.[10] To make a diagnosis for patients whose symptoms suggest cutaneous PAN, a skin biopsy demonstrating necrotizing nongranulomatous medium-sized and small-sized vessel vasculitis is necessary. Patients with symptoms of systemic PAN require an angiogram, which typically shows aneurysms or stenoses/occlusions in medium-sized arteries or a biopsy of the affected organ.[11] Although prognosis has dramatically improved, PAN remains a life-threatening form of systemic vasculitis and late morbidity can occur years after childhood onset from chronic vascular injury.[12]

ANCAs are a heterogeneous group of autoantibodies associated with certain forms of vasculitis characterized by necrotizing inflammation with a paucity of immunoglobulin in the vessel wall detectable by immunohistologic methods. The genesis of the ANCA autoimmune response is a multifactorial process that includes genetic predisposition, environmental factors, an initiating antigen, and failure of T-cell regulation.[13] ANCAs activate primed neutrophils and monocytes by binding to certain antigens expressed on the surface of neutrophils.[13] ANCA-associated vasculitis (AAV) predominantly affects small vessels in any organ of the body, and most patients with AAV have systemic disease that can be classified on the basis of clinical and pathologic features as MPA, GPA, or EGPA.[13] GPA is the most frequent AAV in childhood, characterized by the hallmark triad of granulomatous inflammation of upper and lower respiratory tracts and necrotizing pauci-immune glomerulonephritis.[14] In a cohort of 117 children with GPA and other ANCA-associated vasculitides, most children presented with GPA and the most frequent clinical features were constitutional; ear, nose, and throat; pulmonary; and renal involvement.[14] Almost all patients present with cytoplasmic immunofluorescence staining pattern and positive antiproteinase 3 (PR-3). The diagnosis is based on the combination of pulmonary and renal vasculitis, presence of serologic markers, especially antibodies to PR-3, and characteristic histopathologic findings, like pauci-immune granulomatous inflammation of predominantly small-vessel or pauci-immune glomerulonephritis.[12] At onset, nonspecific complaints of fever, malaise, and weight loss are very common. Prognosis depends in part on the stage of disease at diagnosis and at least 50% of patients relapse within 5 years despite treatment.[12] EGPA, a rare disease in children, is characterized by a nonvasculitic prodrome of asthma and eosinophilic inflammation, such as eosinophilic pneumonia, followed by small-vessel vasculitis and glomerulonephritis. Peripheral eosinophilia is typical and most commonly antimyeloperoxidase ANCA is found in a minority of patients.[15] This diagnosis is suspected in patients with chronic asthma, fever, and eosinophilia and is confirmed by skin, renal, or lung biopsy showing eosinophilic infiltration of granuloma and vasculitis.[12]

MPA is a pauci-immune necrotizing vasculitis that predominantly affects small vessels and is characterized by pulmonary alveolar capillaritis and glomerulonephritis, seen in almost all patients. Other manifestations, such as purpuric rash, arthralgia/arthritis, and abdominal pain, are also common in pediatric patients.[16] Most patients have antimyeloperoxidase ANCA. To make a diagnosis of MPA, GPA or EGPA should be ruled out.[13]

KAWASAKI DISEASE

Kawasaki disease (KD) is a necrotizing arteritis that affects small-size and medium-size arteries. KD is the second-most common systemic vasculitis in childhood and is an important cause of acquired heart disease. The disease is acute and self-limiting and occurs most commonly in children younger than 5 (peak incidence between 6 and 12 months), in males, and individuals of Asian descent.

Pathogenesis

KD occurs more frequently during the winter and spring seasons. The acute and self-limiting nature of KD, its seasonal incidence, its geographic distribution in the pattern of "outbreaks," the increased susceptibility of children between 1 and 5 years old, and the similarity of its clinical manifestations with infectious diseases, such as scarlet fever and toxic shock syndrome, suggest that microorganisms may be the trigger of the immunologic response underlying KD.[17] However, the pathogenesis of KD remains unknown. A yet-unidentified infectious agent is thought to trigger KD in genetically predisposed individuals. Viruses, bacteria, bacterial superantigens, and genetic polymorphisms have been implicated in the etiology of KD.[18] Mechanisms involved in the regulation of disease susceptibility and its evolution are not well understood.

Studies have demonstrated that the vascular injury in KD is associated with the activation of endothelial cells and leukocyte adhesion molecules accompanying the infiltration of CD4+ cells, CD8+ cells, and macrophages. Increased numbers of activated T and B cells in the peripheral blood in conjunction with the increased production of tumor necrosis factor α (TNF-α), interleukin-6 (IL-6), soluble IL-2 receptors, interferon-γ (IFN-γ), IL-1, and CD23 are observed during the acute phase of the disease.[17] Another observation in relation to the immune system involvement is the presence of circulating antibodies with cytotoxic activity against endothelial cells previously stimulated by IL-1β, TNF-α, or IFN-γ but not against nonstimulated cells.[19,20]

Clinical Presentation

Generally, the onset of KD is acute and can be divided into 3 phases: acute (febrile, 10 days), subacute (2–4 weeks, ending with the normalization of platelet counts), and chronic or convalescent (months).

The fever is usually high, persistent, and lasts for at least 5 days. The fever does not respond to antibiotics but may respond partially to antipyretics. If untreated, the febrile phase lasts 5 to 20 days, averaging 10 days, followed by a spontaneous resolution even in the absence of specific treatment.

A skin rash usually accompanies the fever throughout the acute phase of the disease. The rash is polymorphic, nonitchy, and can vary over time. Typically, the rash is localized to the trunk but can also involve the extremities and perineum. The rash can be scarlatiform, macular, papular, multiform, or purpuric. The lesions in the extremities include red purpuric erythema on the palms and soles, usually accompanied by painful soft tissue swelling of the dorsum of the hands and feet. The typical peeling ("glove finger") starts at the fingertips and toes and spreads across the entire palm or sole and can also occur in the perineum (**Fig. 1**). Such changes are more evident after 15 days and can last for weeks.

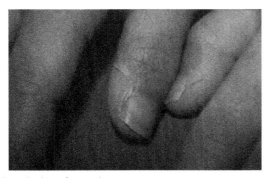

Fig. 1. Typical peeling ("glove finger").

The mucosal changes occur during the febrile period and include labial and oropha-ryngeal erythema, sometimes with strawberry tongue (**Fig. 2**). The most common changes are red, shiny, swollen, and cracked lips. Nonpurulent bilateral conjunctivitis is also quite characteristic (**Fig. 3**). Nail changes (Beau lines) can occur 1 to 2 days after the fever onset.

Cervical lymphadenopathy, usually unilateral and greater than 1.5 cm in diameter, is the least characteristic and most infrequent clinical manifestation (**Fig. 4**).

Compromised cardiac function is the most serious manifestation of KD and is the main cause of mortality and morbidity. Congestive heart failure may occur secondary to myocarditis or myocardial infarction, in addition to pericarditis, endocarditis, or arrhythmias. Aneurysms or coronary artery ectasia are often clinically silent and can be diagnosed years after the acute phase of the disease when the patient presents with myocardial infarction or sudden death. Arterial thrombosis with vessel occlusion can also occur. The coronary aneurysms require echocardiography or angiography for

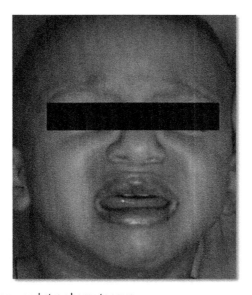

Fig. 2. Labial erythema and strawberry tongue.

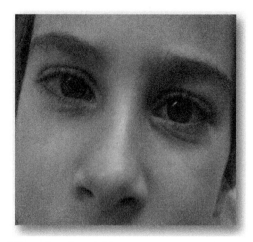

Fig. 3. Nonpurulent bilateral conjunctivitis.

diagnosis. Brachial, axillary, iliac, femoral, and renal artery aneurysms can be observed by angiography.

In addition to these findings, symptoms of KD can include the following: arthralgia/arthritis, aseptic meningitis, facial nerve paralysis, irritability, sensorineural hearing loss, otitis media, interstitial pneumonitis, gastroenteritis, hydropic gallbladder, dysuria and urethritis, Raynaud phenomenon, peripheral gangrene, anterior uveitis, and abdominal pain. Changes in the Bacillus Calmette–Guérin (BCG) vaccine scar with local induration are suggestive of the disease.[21] Younger children tend to exhibit atypical presentations and develop aneurysms more frequently.

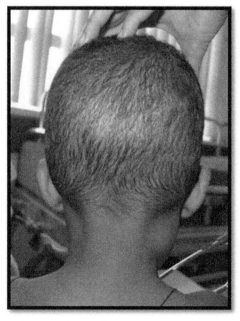

Fig. 4. Cervical unilateral lymphadenopathy.

Diagnostics

There is no specific laboratory diagnostic test for KD. The complete blood count reveals normocytic-normochromic anemia, leukocytosis with neutrophilia and a left shift, and thrombocytosis after the first week of illness. There is an unspecific increase in acute-phase reactants, transaminases and bilirubin, and sterile leucocituria. The analysis of cerebrospinal fluid is positive for leucocytosis with a predominance of lymphocytes. Hyponatremia, hypoalbuminemia, and thrombocytopenia in the acute phase are signs of an unfavorable prognosis.

Antinuclear antibodies and rheumatoid factor are typically negative, whereas ANCAs are detected in 36% of patients.[22]

An electrocardiogram is indicated to look for arrhythmias, conduction disorders, and signs of myocarditis.

Echocardiography should be performed as soon as the diagnosis is established and again at 2 weeks, between 6 and 8 weeks, and at 6 months. Perivascular changes and coronary artery ectasias can be observed early (within 10 days), whereas coronary aneurysms, typical of the disease, are rarely detected in the early stages. Other changes include a reduction in left ventricular contractility, mild mitral or aortic regurgitation, and pericardial effusion.

Compromised coronary function is detected by cardiac catheterization, and these symptoms include dilation, rupture, small and fusiform aneurysms ($\leq$8 mm coronary lumen diameter), and giant aneurysms (>8 mm) that may occur in up to 5% of patients who are treated appropriately and in a timely manner and in 30% of patients who are treated inadequately. Aneurysms may regress in size and disappear over a period of 5 years, but giant aneurysms rarely improve and often become stenotic, leading to myocardial ischemia over time.

Diagnosis

The accurate and timely diagnosis of KD remains essential for a favorable prognosis.

The diagnosis of KD is based on well-known criteria (**Box 1**). However, diagnosis is often quite difficult because the clinical presentation may be incomplete (especially in children younger than 1 year or older than 9 years) or similar to common childhood infectious diseases, such as scarlet fever. However, in incomplete cases that are difficult to diagnose, coronary changes occur as frequently as or even more frequently than in typical cases. An incomplete presentation occurs in 10% of cases and is characterized by a fever lasting at least 5 days, at least 2 of the clinical criteria, the lack of

---

Box 1
Classification criteria for Kawasaki disease

Fever persisting for at least 5 days (required criteria), plus 4 of the following:

Changes in the extremities or perineum

Polymorphic rash

Conjunctivitis

Changes in the lips and/or oral cavity

Cervical lymphadenopathy

In the presence of fever and compromised coronary function detected by echocardiography, Kawasaki disease may be diagnosed based on fewer than 4 of the 5 remaining criteria.
Data from Ozen S, Ruperto N, Dillon MJ, et al. EULAR/PReS endorsed consensus criteria for the classification of childhood vasculitides. Ann Rheum Dis 2006;65:936–41.

other apparent causes, and the presence of systemic inflammatory activity in laboratory tests.

The American Heart Association guidelines state that if the typical clinical findings are present but the fever lasts for fewer than 5 days or if there are 3 classic manifestations and coronary changes in echocardiography, the diagnosis of KD still can be made, and treatment should be initiated. In patients with a fever lasting longer than 5 days and with 2 or 3 classic symptoms of the disease, the erythrocyte sedimentation rate and C-reactive protein levels should be measured. If these values are high, albumin and transaminase measurements, a complete blood count, and a urinalysis should be performed.[23] After the publication of these guidelines, diagnoses of incomplete KD and laboratory use increased while the rate of coronary artery involvement remained stable.[24]

Differential Diagnosis

Many clinical manifestations of KD may be present in other diseases; thus, these diseases must be excluded for a definitive diagnosis. Febrile rash illnesses should be excluded, especially adenovirus infections, infectious mononucleosis, scarlet fever, measles, toxic shock syndrome, serum sickness, and hypersensitivity reactions to drugs. The presence of bacterial conjunctivitis, purulent tonsillitis, vesicular rash, or generalized lymphadenopathy excludes a diagnosis of KD.

Treatment

In the acute phase, the main goal of treatment is to control myocarditis and vasculitis of the coronary arteries as well as to prevent coronary thrombosis. The recommended treatment in the acute phase is the administration of intravenous immunoglobulin as a single dose (2 g/kg/dose) until the 10th day of fever, preferably between the 5th and 7th day, which dramatically reduces the systemic inflammatory process in most patients and is able to prevent the formation of coronary aneurysms. The late administration of immunoglobulin therapy is justified in any period of the disease in the presence of persistent fever, increased acute-phase reactants, or aneurysms. Immunoglobulin therapy alters the erythrocyte sedimentation rate; therefore, the determination of C-reactive protein levels is more accurate after immunoglobulin infusion. Treatment with intravenous immunoglobulin may occasionally be associated with thromboembolism, aseptic meningitis, and hemolytic anemia.[25]

Furthermore, aspirin must be used at high dosages (anti-inflammatory) of 80 to 100 mg/kg per day until the child remains afebrile for 48 hours, after which the dosage should be reduced to 3 to 5 mg/kg per day (antiplatelet aggregation dose). If aneurysms are not detected by the sixth or eighth week, aspirin administration should be discontinued. Patients with mild or moderate coronary changes should continue the aspirin at the antiplatelet aggregation dose or use clopidogrel (1 mg/kg per day), which should be maintained indefinitely.[26] However, it is worth noting that aspirin use does not reduce the frequency of aneurysms. Patients with giant or multiple aneurysms should receive an anticoagulant, such as low-molecular weight heparin or warfarin.[27]

Some factors are associated with unfavorable prognosis and should prompt earlier treatment or the initial introduction of corticosteroids in combination with immunoglobulin.

These factors include the following[28]:

- Patients younger than 12 months
- Hyponatremia

- Increased transaminases
- Neutrophilia, thrombocytopenia
- Significant increases in C-reactive protein

The first immunoglobulin infusion fails in approximately 10% to 20% of patients and the patients who persist with fever longer than 24 hours should receive a second immunoglobulin infusion. Nevertheless, 30% of the cases will not respond to retreatment. The use of corticosteroids and immunosuppressants is limited to cases with poor response to the second immunoglobulin infusion, persistent fever and systemic symptoms, or progression of coronary vasculitis.[29] The efficacy of corticosteroids in the treatment of refractory fever is explained by the suppression of cytokine production with the reduction in inflammation and endothelial expression of adhesion molecules.[30] The procoagulant activity of corticosteroids is compensated by the benefits of its anti-inflammatory activity.

A randomized clinical trial in Japan compared the efficacy of immunoglobulin alone or in combination with 2 mg/kg per day prednisolone for 15 days after the normalization of C-reactive protein levels and found that the combination treatment significantly minimized changes in the coronary arteries.[29] The authors suggested that the duration of corticosteroid administration is more important than the maximum drug concentration in suppressing inflammation and vasculitis and therefore recommended oral dosing over pulse therapy.[31] Other investigators defend the use of methylprednisolone alone in patients resistant to first immunoglobulin infusions and observed a reduction in the duration of fever as well as a reduction in cost, without differences in the incidence of aneurysms.[32]

In addition to immunoglobulin and corticosteroids, cyclophosphamide, cyclosporine, or anti-TNF-α agents can be used after the first or second immunoglobulin infusion.[33–36]

A multicenter randomized prospective trial of second immunoglobulin infusion versus infliximab in 24 children showed that both treatments were safe and well tolerated in the subjects with Kawasaki disease who were resistant to standard immunoglobulin treatment.[37] A single-dose infliximab infusion has been shown to produce better results than immunoglobulin during retreatment (after initial treatment with immunoglobulin) with respect to the speed of fever resolution and to the reduction in the duration of hospitalization. The incidence of coronary changes and adverse events were similar.[38] Another study included 20 patients refractory to immunoglobulin who were treated with infliximab 5 mg/kg initiated within 10 days of disease onset. Eighteen of 20 patients were effectively treated with regression of the dilated coronary artery to normal size in the convalescent phase.[39]

Rituximab was described as effective in one case and there are no cases reported with abatacept and tocilizumab treatment.[40]

A periodic follow-up of patients is recommended regardless of cardiovascular compromise, because these patients can develop complications during adulthood. Anticoagulation is important for disease management, especially in the case of giant aneurysms, although there is a lack of evidence-based guidelines. In some cases of advanced coronary disease, it may be necessary to perform an angioplasty or coronary artery bypass graft surgery. There are reports of use of thrombolytic agents, such as streptokinase, urokinase, tissue plasminogen activator, or abciximab, to treat myocardial infarction in children with KD as well as to reduce thrombus formation and vascular remodeling.[41,42] Statins lower cholesterol and decrease the incidence of atherosclerosis and cardiovascular disease.

Evolution and Prognosis

Although KD is an acute disease, it can progress with significant cardiac sequelae if it is not diagnosed and treated early. In males and in children younger than 1 year, prolonged fevers and prolonged inflammatory activity are known to increase the risk of aneurysm formation, which also increases with decreased hemoglobin levels, neutrophilia, hypoalbuminemia, hyponatremia, thrombocytopenia, and increased transaminase levels.[26,42] The increase in N-terminal pro-B-type natriuretic peptide (NT-pro-BNP) is associated with the presence of aneurysms and can be an important tool for predicting disease prognosis.[43]

Peak mortality occurs between 15 and 45 days after the onset of fever. At this time, coronary vasculitis can be associated with a significant increase in platelet count and a hypercoaguable state. Thrombosis of the coronary artery branch has been described. Other complications include myocarditis, macrophage activation syndrome, shock with low blood pressure, left ventricular dysfunction, mitral insufficiency, and arteriosclerosis in the long term.[44] The mortality rate in Japan is 0.08%, and nearly all deaths are related to cardiac problems.[45]

Approximately half of all aneurysms resolve within 1 to 2 years, especially small and fusiform aneurysms.[5] Approximately 20% of patients with coronary aneurysms in the acute phase will develop coronary artery stenosis. However, sudden death by heart attack can occur many years later in individuals who had aneurysm or coronary stenosis during childhood. In countries such as the United States and Japan, KD is the leading cause of heart disease acquired in childhood and is a risk factor for ischemic heart disease in adults. Many cases of myocardial infarction in young adults have been attributed to undiagnosed KD in childhood.[35,46] However, even patients without coronary changes may exhibit prolonged endothelial dysfunction and lipid profile changes.

Other complications of KD include hearing loss, which can last up to 6 months after the acute outbreak, and ophthalmic involvement with anterior uveitis, papilledema, optic neuritis, conjunctival hemorrhage, and amaurosis. Additionally, intestinal ischemia, acute abdomen, peripheral gangrene, behavioral changes and attention-deficit disorder, seizures, chorea, facial paralysis, ataxia, and cerebellar or cerebral infarctions may occur. Recurrence occurs in 4% of cases.[47]

The use of vaccines should be deferred for 11 months after receiving gamma globulin because vaccines may be ineffective during this period.

The number of patients who reach adulthood is increasing, leading to the increased participation of adult cardiologists in the management of this disease. Currently, there are no established guidelines for the evaluation and treatment of adult patients who have had KD.

Key Points

- KD is a systemic self-limiting and acute vasculitis and one of the most frequent causes of acquired heart disease.
- The diagnosis of KD is based on well-known criteria; however, diagnosis is often quite difficult because the clinical presentation may be incomplete.
- Treatment with intravenous immunoglobulin in association with aspirin early in the course of the disease shortens the duration of symptoms and decreases the frequency of coronary artery abnormalities.
- Some factors are associated with unfavorable prognosis and should prompt earlier treatment or the initial introduction of corticosteroids in combination with immunoglobulin.
- Sudden death by heart attack can occur many years later in individuals who had aneurysm or coronary stenosis during childhood.

TAKAYASU ARTERITIS

Takayasu arteritis is a chronic inflammatory vascular disease that predominantly affects large vessels, such as the aorta, its major branches, and the pulmonary artery. It is the third leading cause of primary vasculitis in children. Takayasu arteritis predominantly affects females and has many geographic and ethnic variations. There are no studies of the incidence of Takayasu arteritis in pediatric patients.

Pathogenesis

The causes of Takayasu arteritis remain unknown, but the role of genetic factors, autoimmunity, and infection in the pathogenesis of the disease are discussed. Takayasu arteritis is considered a granulomatous vasculitis mediated by T cells.

The association between the HLA genes and Takayasu arteritis has been investigated because of its importance in regulating the immune response and the disease's preference for individuals of a particular ethnicity. CD8-positive T cells are the main components of the vascular infiltrate, which reinforces the importance of HLA in the pathogenesis of this disease. These cells recognize antigens only when bound to HLA class-I molecules. Some studies suggest that HLA is important in determining Takayasu arteritis' patterns and prognosis.[48]

An association between tuberculosis and Takayasu arteritis has been suggested since the early descriptions of the disease, especially in areas of high prevalence of tuberculosis. However, the role of tuberculosis in the pathogenesis of Takayasu arteritis is not yet fully understood. A molecular mimicry of the mycobacterial 65-kDa heat-shock protein and human 65-kDa heat-shock protein has been suggested, which could cause a cross-reaction and lead to an association between the tuberculosis infection and autoimmune response.[49]

There are reports of an association of reactive T cells with mycobacterial 65-kDa heat-shock protein and its homologous human protein and the presence of serum titers of IgG antibodies for mycobacterial and human 65-kDa heat-shock protein.[50] Furthermore, the 65-kDa heat-shock protein has been detected in the middle layer and vasa vasorum in biopsies from patients with Takayasu arteritis.[51]

Some studies have shown antiaortic and antiendothelial cell antibodies in addition to B-cell infiltrates in inflamed vessels from patients with Takayasu arteritis, thus questioning the role of humoral immunity in the disease.[52,53] However, it is not clear whether humoral immunity is only an epiphenomenon or directly participates in the pathophysiology of Takayasu arteritis. Hoyer and colleagues[54] observed a greater number of antibody-secreting B cells in patients with active Takayasu arteritis.

The production of inflammatory cytokines (TNF and IL-6) and adhesion molecules in the affected region is intense and most likely participates in maintaining an altered immune response.[55] CD8-positive T cells are the main components of the vascular infiltrate. The cytotoxic activity of these cells, mediated by the release of the enzymes perforin and granzyme B, has been noted as being responsible for damaging the vascular smooth muscle cells.[56]

Clinical Presentation

The signs and symptoms with which patients with Takayasu arteritis present are caused by systemic inflammation and vascular insufficiency, leading to ischemia of the organs and limbs. Many investigators divide the clinical manifestations into an early stage, before patients have decreased pulses, and a late stage, when patients develop signs of vascular insufficiency. The early phase is characterized by nonspecific systemic signs and symptoms, and the late phase is characterized by signs and symptoms resulting from ischemia of the organs. However, this sequence in the clinical presentation occurs in a minority of patients, whereas it is rather common to see manifestations of the 2 phases simultaneously.

Systemic symptoms are observed in 60% to 70% of children with Takayasu arteritis and are characterized by fever, headache, fatigue, anorexia, weight loss, musculoskeletal symptoms (myalgia and arthralgia), night sweats, abdominal pain, and vomiting.[57] These systemic symptoms are 2 times more frequent in pediatric than adult patients.[58] In pediatric studies, headache is the most common symptom and may be present in up to 85% of the patients.[57]

Hypertension is the most common manifestation in pediatric patients with a frequency of 65% to 100% and may be the only clinical finding.[57,59] Hypertension is typically caused by renal artery stenosis with renovascular hypertension, but may be caused by the coarctation or decreased compliance of the aorta, aortic regurgitation, or baroreceptor dysfunction of the aortic and carotid sinuses.[60] In some studies, Takayasu arteritis is the most common cause of renovascular hypertension in children.[61,62]

Decreased or absent peripheral pulses are observed in more than one-half of the children, most commonly affecting a lower limb.[57] Differences in the blood pressure in limbs are also observed in more than 50% of children.[57]

The frequency of vascular bruits ranges from 29% to 58%, depending on the population studied.[57,63] Limb claudication can be observed in up to 31% of patients.[57] Dyspnea due to congestive heart failure and chest pain, as well as pericarditis, may also occur.[64]

Retinopathy is a relatively common finding in patients with Takayasu arteritis. Retinopathy may be a result of low blood flow in the carotid artery, resulting in ocular ischemia, called Takayasu retinopathy. In most cases, Takayasu retinopathy is secondary to hypertension–hypertensive retinopathy.

Neurologic manifestations, such as headache, stroke, transient ischemic attack, syncope, dizziness, amaurosis, seizures, and encephalopathy, may result from the involvement of carotid and vertebral arteries, causing cerebral ischemia, or may be secondary to hypertension.

Other findings that may be present in children with Takayasu arteritis include arthritis, skin manifestations, such as erythema nodosum and livedo reticularis, and Raynaud phenomenon.[65]

Complications are relatively common because many patients have a relapsing and progressive disease course, including valvular insufficiency, heart failure, acute myocardial infarction, stroke, renovascular hypertension, hypertensive retinopathy, amaurosis, and aneurysm rupture.

Diagnostics

There are no specific laboratory tests for Takayasu arteritis. The most common laboratory results reflect the inflammatory nature of the disease. The increased erythrocyte sedimentation rate (ESR) is the most frequent laboratory abnormality, although the ESR may not be elevated in approximately one-half of the cases. In addition, normocytic and normochromic anemia, leukocytosis, high platelet counts, and increase in other acute-phase proteins, such as C-reactive protein (CRP), alpha-1-acid glycoprotein, serum amyloid A, and fibrinogen, are also common. Some studies have reported the presence of antinuclear antibodies, rheumatoid factor, and antineutrophil cytoplasmic antibody in a small percentage of patients.[66,67] In a review study that investigated signs of Takayasu arteritis that could serve as screening tests for the diagnosis in children, an increased ESR with hypertension had a sensitivity of 65%.[68] There is evidence of increased positive results in the Mantoux tuberculin skin test in patients from certain regions. Lupi-Herrera and colleagues[66] observed a positivity rate of 81%, which was greater than that observed in the healthy population from the same region.

In recent years, the interest in evaluating the activity of Takayasu arteritis has been increasing. In clinical practice, an increased ESR is used as one of the parameters for disease activity, but the results from studies that evaluate the association of an increased ESR with disease activity are conflicting.[58,69] Both CRPs and ESRs have poor sensitivity and specificity.

Because of the difficulty of assessing the activity of Takayasu arteritis and monitoring the therapeutic response, new markers of disease activity are being investigated. Levels of serum amyloid A and C4-binding protein were significantly higher in patients with the active disease than in adult patients with the inactive phase of the disease and control group.[69] Another study observed a positive correlation of IL-6 and RANTES (regulated on activation, normal T cells expressed and secreted) with disease activity.[70] In a study on the cytokine profile in patients with Takayasu arteritis, it was observed that the levels of IL-18 were significantly reduced after treatment when the patients were in remission.[71] These studies may suggest a role of these new serologic markers in monitoring the disease.

Imaging Examinations

Imaging examinations of the aorta and its branches are fundamental for the diagnosis and monitoring of Takayasu arteritis. Digital angiography remains the gold standard for the detection of arterial injury (**Fig. 5**). However, because digital angiography is an invasive procedure, it has been replaced by other imaging methods. Magnetic resonance angiography (MRA) and computed tomography angiography (CTA) have the advantage of being noninvasive methods that evaluate the presence of edema and inflammation in the vessel walls, which are often the only changes observed in early disease. Any vascular injury may be observed, from stenosis, which is the most common, to occlusion, irregularity, dilation, aneurysm, or wall thickening.

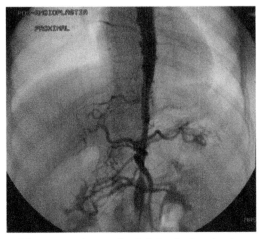

Fig. 5. Angiography with segmental stenosis of abdominal aorta above and below the level of celiac trunk.

MRA has been widely used to monitor this disease in pediatrics because it does not use radiation or nephrotoxic contrast. MRA allows the measurement of the thickened arterial wall and edema in the acute disease.[59] Doppler ultrasonography provides valuable information on the great vessels of the heart and is routinely used in most centers for monitoring lesions in the carotid artery. Doppler ultrasonography also diagnoses turbulence and increased flow rates in stenotic areas. Doppler ultrasonography has the advantage of being inexpensive and not using radiation or contrast but has the disadvantage of being operator-dependent. Additionally, it does not accurately delineate the extent of an arterial injury.

Recent studies have evaluated positron emission tomography (PET) as a promising tool for detecting the extent and intensity of inflammation in the vessel wall because it allows the visualization of lesions distribution and inflammatory activity in the aorta and its branches and the pulmonary artery.[72]

The distribution of vascular involvement in Takayasu arteritis varies according to the geographic area and the age range studied. In studies with children, the abdominal aorta and renal arteries are the arterial segments most often affected.[57,63,64] Stenosis is the most frequent type of injury in both adults and children.[73]

Angiographic classifications have been proposed over time. In recent years, the classification of the International Conference of Takayasu arteritis in Tokyo has been the most commonly used, which also includes the involvement of the pulmonary arteries or the coronary artery.[74]

Diagnosis

The delay in the diagnosis of Takayasu arteritis, particularly in pediatric patients, is due to the presence of nonspecific symptoms. A 4 times higher delay in children compared with adults has been reported.[58,73] The diagnosis of Takayasu arteritis in children is performed by the classification criteria recently proposed by the EULAR (European League Against Rheumatism)/PRES (Pediatric Rheumatology European Society)/PRINTO (Pediatric Rheumatology International Trials Organization) groups, and requires the presence of one mandatory criterion and at least one of the other criteria (**Table 1**).[75] The key to diagnosis is hypertension, vascular bruits, asymmetric blood pressure between limbs, and other ischemic symptoms associated with increased acute-phase proteins.

Table 1 Classification criteria for Takayasu arteritis	
Mandatory criteria	Abnormalities in angiography (standard, computed tomography, and magnetic resonance angiography) of the aorta, its major branches, and the pulmonary arteries (dilation/aneurysm, stenosis, occlusion and thickening of the arterial wall)
Other criteria	Reduction of the peripheral pulse and/or limb claudication
	Difference in blood pressure >10 mm Hg between limbs
	Bruits in major arteries
	Hypertension (according to age range)
	Elevation of acute-phase reactants

Data from Ozen S, Pistorio A, Lusan SM, et al. EULAR/PRINTO/PRES criteria for Henoch-Schonlein purpura, childhood polyarteritis nodosa, childhood Wegener granulomatosis and childhood Takayasu's arteritis: Ankara 2008. Part II: final classification criteria. Ann Rheum Dis 2010;69:798–806.

Imaging is necessary to confirm the diagnosis and to assess the extent of the arterial involvement. Computed tomography and magnetic resonance imaging are the most used examinations. However, these examinations are not available in all centers and are operator-dependent.

Differential Diagnosis

Some disorders that must be excluded before making a definite diagnosis of Takayasu arteritis include infectious aortitis secondary to tuberculosis, syphilis, and HIV; inherited disorders, such as Marfan syndrome, Ehlers-Danlos syndrome, coarctation of the aorta, and neurofibromatosis; and other inflammatory diseases, such as Behçet disease, KD, systemic lupus erythematosus, sarcoidosis and spondyloarthropathy, and fibromuscular dysplasia.

Treatment

There are no controlled studies of drug therapy in pediatric patients with Takayasu arteritis. The use of corticosteroids at the beginning of therapy to reduce disease activity was previously established and is one of the EULAR recommendations for the management of the disease.[76] However, the evidence is based on descriptive or case-control studies. Intravenous methylprednisolone pulse therapy or oral prednisone or prednisolone at a dose of 1 mg/kg per day is indicated and should be maintained for a month and then slowly reduced. To reduce the adverse effects of steroids, intravenous pulse therapy is preferred over oral therapy.

Despite corticosteroid therapy, Takayasu arteritis can be reactivated or remain clinically or subclinically active. In cases of extensive arterial involvement (above and below the diaphragm or involvement of pulmonary artery), cyclophosphamide is used in monthly pulse therapy (500–1000 mg/m^2). However, because of its toxicity, other therapies have been preferred.

Other immunosuppressive drugs that act as corticosteroid-sparing and maintenance therapy include azathioprine (1–2 mg/kg per day) or methotrexate (0.4–1 mg/kg per week).[77] Studies have demonstrated that methotrexate increases the remission rate, and azathioprine prevents disease progression.[75] Mycophenolate has been shown to be effective, particularly in patients who are refractory to other immunosuppressive drugs.[78]

The granulomatous nature of the histopathologic lesions led to an indication for anti-tumor necrosis factor (anti-TNF) agents in patients with disease refractory to the conventional therapy. Studies have reported success with the use of anti-TNF with remission in most patients who are refractory to other therapies, steroid-resistant, or dependent.[79,80] Currently, there is more evidence suggesting that treatment with infliximab might be more beneficial than etanercept or adalimumab.[80–82] In addition, some case reports have shown the efficacy of a humanized anti-IL-6 receptor antibody (tocilizumab) and anti-CD20 monoclonal antibody (rituximab).[54,83,84] The use of an antiplatelet dose of aspirin (50–100 mg per day) is recommended, but there is no strong evidence indicating its use. Antihypertensive drugs, such as calcium antagonists, beta-blockers, and diuretics are often used.

Surgical treatment is indicated when there is severe hypertension secondary to aortic coarctation or renal stenosis, brain and heart ischemia, ischemia of other organs and extremities, aortic regurgitation, and the possibility of aneurysm rupture.[65] It is recommended to wait for the inactive phase of the disease to perform surgery to decrease the risk of complications.

The interventional procedures most performed in Takayasu arteritis are bypass surgery, angioplasty with resection of the injured segment, endarterectomy, percutaneous transluminal angioplasty with or without stenting, valvuloplasty, and nephrectomy. However, some patients require new procedures, and deaths are rarely reported during the interventions.[85]

Evolution and Prognosis

Takayasu arteritis is a chronic disease characterized by remissions and relapses, and only 20% of patients have a monophasic course.[58]

There are no validated biomarkers to assess the response and reactivation of the disease. Clinical manifestations and markers of inflammatory activity are parameters that help monitoring the therapeutic response. Periodic imaging examinations, such as MRA and PET, can contribute to the assessment of disease activity.[72] There is little evidence that ultrasound of the carotid or subclavian vessels is useful in monitoring.

The patient is considered to be experiencing disease activity when at least 2 of the following events are present: (1) the presence of systemic manifestations that are not attributable to another condition; (2) the persistent elevation of acute-phase proteins (ESR and CRP) in the absence of infection or malignancy; (3) the presence of signs or symptoms of vascular insufficiency; and (4) vascular lesions in previously unaffected vessels diagnosed by imaging examinations.[58]

A recent study showed that the presence of more than one serious complication of the disease (retinopathy, hypertension, aortic regurgitation and aneurysm, myocardial infarction, stroke, pulmonary hypertension, and intestinal ischemia) is associated with a worse prognosis.[86]

The mortality rate has a large variability between different studies, which reflects the different populations studied, differences in clinical practice, and different follow-up times. A mortality rate of up to 35% in 5 years has been described.[87] The main causes of death are heart failure, myocardial infarction, hypertension, ruptured aneurysm, and renal failure.

Key Points

There is a delay in the diagnosis in childhood due to the lack of specific symptoms at the beginning of the disease.

Manifestations range from asymptomatic disease, findings of decreased pulses and bruits to stroke, myocardial infarction, and aneurysm rupture.

Takayasu arteritis must be ruled out in the presence of hypertension and an increased ESR.

Angiography remains the gold standard for diagnosis, although MRA and CTA have the advantage of being noninvasive methods.

Clinical manifestations and markers of inflammatory activity are parameters that are helpful to monitor the therapeutic response but disease activity is difficult to assess.

Treatment includes corticosteroids, immunosuppressive drugs, and anti-TNF agents.

SUMMARY

Childhood vasculitis is an important but still often underdiagnosed area in pediatric rheumatology with a large amount of emerging knowledge in the past years. The most common primary vasculitis is HSP, followed by KD and Takayasu arteritis. KD remains one of the most frequent causes of acquired heart disease, leading to sudden death by myocardial infarction in individuals who had aneurysm or coronary stenosis during childhood. The frequency of this complication can decrease if the treatment begins early in the course of the disease. Although well-known criteria are described, incomplete disease can exist, making the diagnosis difficult. Takayasu arteritis remains a difficult to diagnose vasculitis because of the lack of specific symptoms at the beginning of the disease. Manifestations range from asymptomatic disease, findings of decreased pulses and bruits to stroke, myocardial infarction, and aneurysm rupture. Angiography remains the gold standard for diagnosis, although other imaging examinations have the advantage of being noninvasive methods. Disease activity is difficult to assess and markers of inflammatory activity are frequently absent. Biologic agents are emerging as an alternative treatment in many cases of vasculitis that are resistant to immunosuppressive therapy.

REFERENCES

1. Ozen S, Ruperto N, Dillon MJ, et al. EULAR/PReS endorsed consensus criteria for the classification of childhood vasculitides. Ann Rheum Dis 2006;65:936–41.
2. Ball GV, Bridges SL. Pathogenesis of vasculitis. In: Ball GV, Bridges SL, editors. Vasculitis. 2nd edition. Oxford: Oxford University Press; 2008. p. 67–88.
3. Carlson JA. The histological assessment of cutaneous vasculitis. Histopathology 2010;56:3–23.
4. Zang L, Han C, Sun C, et al. Serum levels of alpha-smooth muscle actin and c-Met as biomarkers of the degree of severity of Henoch-Schonlein purpura nephritis. Transl Res 2013;161:26–36.
5. Kato H, Ichinose E, Yoshioka F, et al. Fate of coronary aneurisms in Kawasaki disease: serial coronary angiography and long-term follow-up study. Am J Cardiol 1982;49:1758–66.
6. Lau KK, Suzuki H, Novak J, et al. Pathogenesis of Henoch-Schönlein purpura nephritis. Pediatr Nephrol 2010;25:19–26.
7. Lau KK, Wyatt RJ, Moldoveanu Z, et al. Serum levels of galactose-deficient IgA in children with IgA nephropathy and Henoch-Schönlein purpura. Pediatr Nephrol 2007;22:2067–72.
8. Ozen S, Bakkaloglu A, Dusunsel R, et al. Childhood vasculitides in Turkey: a nationwide survey. Clin Rheumatol 2007;26:196–200.
9. Dillon MJ, Eleftheriou D, Brogan PA. Medium-sized-vessel vasculitis. Pediatr Nephrol 2010;25:1641–52.
10. Eleftheriou D, Dillon M, Tullus K, et al. Systemic polyarteritis nodosa in the young: a single centre experience over 32 years. Arthritis Rheum 2013;65(9): 2476–85.
11. Ozen S, Anton J, Arisoy N, et al. Juvenile polyarteritis: results of a multicenter survey of 110 children. J Pediatr 2004;145:517–22.
12. Cassidy JT, Petty RE. Vasculitis and its classification. In: Cassidy JT, Laxer RM, Petty RE, et al, editors. Textbook of pediatric rheumatology. 6th edition. Philadelphia: Saunders; 2011. p. 470–558.
13. Jennette JC, Falk RJ, Hu P, et al. Pathogenesis of antineutrophil cytoplasmic autoantibody–associated small-vessel vasculitis. Annu Rev Pathol 2013;8: 139–60.
14. Cabral DA, Uribe AG, Benseler S, et al. Classification, presentation, and initial treatment of Wegener's granulomatosis in childhood. Arthritis Rheum 2009; 60(11):3413–24.
15. Zwerina J, Eger G, Englbrecht M, et al. Churg-Strauss syndrome in childhood: a systematic review and clinical comparison with adult patients. Semin Arthritis Rheum 2008;39:108–15.
16. Hattori M, Kurayama H, Koitabashi Y. Antineutrophil cytoplasmic autoantibody–associated glomerulonephritis in children. J Am Soc Nephrol 2001;12: 1493–500.

17. Leung DY, Schlevert PM, Meissner HC. The immunopathogenesis and management of Kawasaki syndrome. Arthritis Rheum 1998;41:1538–47.
18. Yeung RS. Kawasaki disease: update on pathogenesis. Curr Opin Rheumatol 2010;22(5):551–60.
19. Pinna GS, Kafetzis DA, Tselkas OI, et al. Kawasaki disease: an overview. Curr Opin Infect Dis 2008;21(3):263–70.
20. Galeotti C, Bayry J, Kone-Paut I, et al. Kawasaki disease: aetiopathogenesis and therapeutic utility of intravenous immunoglobulin. Autoimmun Rev 2010; 9(6):441–8.
21. Hulme P. Towards evidence based emergency medicine: best BETs from the Manchester Royal Infirmary. BET 1: BCG scar changes in Kawasaki's disease. Emerg Med J 2012;29(7):598–9.
22. Soppi E, Salo E, Pelkonen P. Antibodies against neutrophil cytoplasmic components in Kawasaki disease. APMIS 1992;100:269–72.
23. Freeman AF, Shulman ST. Kawasaki disease: summary of the American Heart Association Guidelines. Am Fam Physician 2006;74(7):1141–8.
24. Guelani SJ, Sable C, Wiedermann BL, et al. Increased incidence of incomplete Kawasaki disease at a pediatric hospital after publication of 2004 American Heart Association Guidelines. Pediatr Cardiol 2012;33(7):1097–103.
25. Baba R. Effect of immunoglobulin therapy on blood viscosity and potential concerns of thromboembolism, especially in patients with acute Kawasaki disease. Recent Pat Cardiovasc Drug Discov 2008;3(2):141–4.
26. Newburger JW. Kawasaki disease: who is at risk? J Pediatr 2000;137(2):149–52.
27. Rowley AH, Shulman ST. Pathogenesis and management of Kawasaki disease. Expert Rev Anti Infect Ther 2010;8(2):197–203.
28. Seki M, Kobayashi T, Kobayashi T, et al. External validation of a risk score to predict intravenous immunoglobulin resistance in patients with Kawasaki disease. Pediatr Infect Dis J 2011;30:145–7.
29. Lang BA, Yeung RS, Oen KG, et al. Corticosteroid treatment of refractory Kawasaki disease. J Rheumatol 2006;33(4):803–9.
30. Okada Y, Shinohara M, Kobayashi T, et al. Effect of corticosteroids in addition to intravenous gamma globulin therapy on serum cytokine levels in the acute phase of Kawasaki disease in children. J Pediatr 2003;143:363–7.
31. Kobayashi T, Saji T, Takeuchi K, et al. Efficacy of immunoglobulin plus prednisolone for prevention of coronary artery abnormalities in severe Kawasaki disease (RAISE study): a randomised, open-label, blinded-endpoints trial. Lancet 2012;379:1613–20.
32. Ogata S, Bando Y, Kimura S, et al. The strategy of immune globulin resistant Kawasaki disease: a comparative study of additional immune globulin and steroid pulse therapy. J Cardiol 2009;53:15–9.
33. Luca NJ, Yeung RS. Epidemiology and management of Kawasaki disease. Drugs 2012;72(8):1029–38.
34. Wallace CA, French JW, Kahn SJ, et al. Initial intravenous gammaglobulin treatment failure in Kawasaki disease. Pediatrics 2000;105:E78.
35. Burns JC, Mason WH, Hauger SB, et al. Infliximab treatment for refractory Kawasaki syndrome. J Pediatr 2005;146:662–7.
36. Choueiter NF, Olson AK, Shen DD, et al. Prospective open-label trial of etanercept as adjunctive therapy for Kawasaki disease. J Pediatr 2010;157(6): 960–6.
37. Burns JC, Best BM, Mejias A, et al. Infliximab treatment of intravenous immunoglobulin-resistant Kawasaki disease. J Pediatr 2008;153(6):833–8.

38. Son MB, Gauvreau K, Burns JC, et al. Infliximab for intravenous immunoglobulin resistance in Kawasaki disease: a retrospective study. J Pediatr 2011;158: 644–9.
39. Mori M, Imagawa T, Hara R, et al. Efficacy and limitation of infliximab treatment for children with Kawasaki disease intractable to intravenous immunoglobulin therapy: report of an open-label case series. J Rheumatol 2012;39(4):864–7.
40. Sauvaget E, Bonello B, David M, et al. Resistant Kawasaki disease treated with anti-CD20. J Pediatr 2012;160(5):875–6.
41. Paredes N, Mondal T, Brandão LR, et al. Management of myocardial infarction in children with Kawasaki disease. Blood Coagul Fibrinolysis 2010;21(7):620–31.
42. Nakamura Y, Yashiro M, Uehara R, et al. Use of laboratory data to identify risk factors of giant coronary aneurisms due to Kawasaki disease. Pediatr Int 2004;46:33–8.
43. Kaneko K, Yoshimura K, Ohashi A, et al. Prediction of the risk of coronary arterial lesions in Kawasaki disease by brain natriuretic peptide. Pediatr Cardiol 2011; 32(8):1106–9.
44. Fukazawa R, Ogawa S. Long-term prognosis of patients with Kawasaki disease: at risk for future atherosclerosis? J Nippon Med Sch 2009;76(3):124–33.
45. Dedeoglu F, Sundel RP. Vasculitis in children. Pediatr Clin North Am 2005;52: 547–75.
46. Falcini F. Kawasaki disease. Curr Opin Rheumatol 2006;18:33–8.
47. Alves N, Magalhães C, Almeida R, et al. Prospective study of Kawasaki disease complications: review of 115 cases. Rev Assoc Med Bras 2011;57(3): 295–300.
48. Kasuya K, Hashimoto Y, Numenno F. Left ventricular dysfunction and HLA Bw52 antigen in Takayasu arteritis. Heart Vessels Suppl 1992;7:116–9.
49. Schultz DR, Arnold PI. Heat shock (stress) proteins and autoimmunity in rheumatic diseases. Semin Arthritis Rheum 1993;22(6):357–74.
50. Chauhan SK, Tripathy NK, Sinha N, et al. Cellular and humoral immune responses to mycobacterial heat shock protein-65 and its human homologue in Takayasu's arteritis. Clin Exp Immunol 2004;138:547–53.
51. Seko Y, Minota S, Kawasaki A, et al. Perforin-secreting killer cell infiltration and expression of a 65-kd heat-shock protein in aortic tissue of patients with Takayasu's arteritis. J Clin Invest 1994;93:750–8.
52. Inder SJ, Bobryshev YV, Cherian SM, et al. Immunophenotypic analysis of the aortic wall in Takayasu's arteritis: involvement of lymphocytes, dendritic cells and granulocytes in immuno-inflammatory reactions. Cardiovasc Surg 2000;8: 141–8.
53. Wang H, Ma J, Wu Q, et al. Circulating B lymphocytes producing autoantibodies to endothelial cells play a role in the pathogenesis of Takayasu arteritis. J Vasc Surg 2011;53(1):174–80.
54. Hoyer BF, Mumtaz IM, Loddenkemper K, et al. Takayasu arteritis is characterized by disturbances of B cell homeostasis and responds to B cell depletion therapy with rituximab. Ann Rheum Dis 2012;71(1):75–9.
55. Noris M. Pathogenesis of Takayasu's arteritis. J Nephrol 2001;14(6):506–13.
56. Seko Y. Takayasu arteritis: insights into immunopathology. Jpn Heart J 2000;411: 15–26.
57. Cakar N, Yalcinkaya F, Duzova A, et al. Takayasu arteritis in children. J Rheumatol 2008;35:913–9.
58. Kerr GS, Hallahan CW, Giordano J, et al. Takayasu arteritis. Ann Intern Med 1994;120:919–29.

59. Stanley P, Roebuck D, Barboza A. Takayasu's arteritis in children. Tech Vasc Interv Radiol 2003;6:158–68.
60. Jain S, Kumari S, Ganguly NK, et al. Current status of Takayasu arteritis in India. Int J Cardiol 1996;54(Suppl):S111–6.
61. Sharma BK, Sagar S, Chugh KS, et al. Spectrum of renovascular hypertension in the young in North India: A hospital based study on occurrence and clinical features. Angiology 1985;36:370–8.
62. Wiggelinkuizen J, Cremin BJ. Takayasu arteritis and renovascular hypertension in children. Pediatrics 1987;62:209–17.
63. Hahn D, Thomson PD, Kala U, et al. A review of Takayasu arteritis in children in Gauteng, South Africa. Pediatr Nephrol 1998;12:668–75.
64. Hong CY, Yung YS, Choi JY, et al. Takayasu arteritis in Korean children: clinical report of seventy cases. Heart Vessels 1992;7:91–6.
65. Gulati A, Bagga A. Large vessel vasculitis. Pediatr Nephrol 2010;25(6):1037–48.
66. Lupi-Herrera E, Sanchez-Torres G, Marcushamer J, et al. Takayasu's arteritis. Clinical study of 107 cases. Am Heart J 1977;93:94–103.
67. Arnaud L, Haroche J, Limal N, et al. Takayasu arteritis in France: a single-center retrospective study of 82 cases comparing white, North African and black patients. Medicine 2010;89(1):1–17.
68. Fieldston E, Albert D, Finkel T. Hypertension and elevated ESR as diagnostic features of Takayasu arteritis in children. J Clin Rheumatol 2003;9:156–63.
69. Ma J, Luo X, Wu Q, et al. Circulation levels of acute phase proteins patients with Takayasu arteritis. J Vasc Surg 2010;51:700–6.
70. Noris M, Daina E, Gamba S, et al. Interleukin-6 and RANTES in Takayasu arteritis: a guide for therapeutic decisions? Circulation 1999;100:55–60.
71. Park MC, Lee SW, Park YB, et al. Serum citokyne profiles and their correlations with disease activity in Takayasu's arteritis. Rheumatology 2006;45:545–8.
72. Tesuka D, Haraquchi G, Ishihara T, et al. Role of FDG PET-CT in Takayasu arteritis: sensitive detection of recurrences. JACC Cardiovasc Imaging 2012;5(4):422–9.
73. Vanoli M, Daina E, Salvarani C, et al. Takayasu's arteritis: a study of 104 Italian patients. Arthritis Rheum 2005;53:100–7.
74. Hata A, Noda M, Moriwaki R, et al. Angiographic findings of Takayasu arteritis: new classification. Int J Cardiol 1996;54(Suppl):S155–63.
75. Ozen S, Pistorio A, Lusan SM, et al. EULAR/PRINTO/PRES criteria for Henoch-Schonlein purpura, childhood polyarteritis nodosa, childhood Wegener granulomatosis and childhood Takayasu's arteritis: Ankara 2008. Part II: final classification criteria. Ann Rheum Dis 2010;69:798–806.
76. Mukhtyar C, Guillevin L, Cid MC, et al, for the European Vasculitis Study Group. EULAR recommendations for the management of large vessel vasculitis. Ann Rheum Dis 2009;68:318–23.
77. Valsakumar AK, Valappil UC, Jorapur V, et al. Role of immunosuppressive therapy on clinical, immunological and angiografic outcome in active Takayasu's arteritis. J Rheumatol 2003;30:1793–8.
78. Shinjo SK, Pereira RM, Tizziani VA, et al. Mycophenolate mofetil reduces disease activity and steroid dosage in Takayasu arteritis. Clin Rheumatol 2007;26:1871–5.
79. Filocamo G, Buoncompagni A, Viola S, et al. Treatment of Takayasu's arteritis with tumor necrosis factor antagonists. J Pediatr 2008;153:432–4.
80. Hoffman GS, Merkel PA, Brasington RD, et al. Anti-tumor necrosis factor therapy in patients with difficult to treat Takayasu arteritis. Arthritis Rheum 2004;50(7):2296–304.

81. Mekinian A, Néel A, Sibilia J, et al, Club Rhumatismes et Inflammation, French Vasculitis Study Group and Société Nationale Française de Médecine Interne. Efficacy and tolerance of infliximab in refractory Takayasu arteritis: French multicentre study. Rheumatology (Oxford) 2012;51(5):882–6.
82. Stern S, Silva GC, Reiff A, et al. Infliximab vs cyclosphosphamide in pediatric Takayasu's arteritis. Ann Rheum Dis 2012;71:433.
83. Nishimoto N, Nakahara H, Yoshio-Hoshino N, et al. Successful treatment of a patient with Takayasu's arteritis using a humanized anti-interleukin 6 receptor antibody. Arthritis Rheum 2008;58(4):1197–200.
84. Galarza C, Valencia D, Tobon GJ, et al. Should rituximab be considered as the first-choice treatment for severe autoimmune rheumatic diseases? Clin Rev Allergy Immunol 2008;34:124–8.
85. Reddy E, Robbs JV. Surgical management of Takayasu's arteritis in children and adolescents. Cardiovasc J Afr 2007;18(6):393–6.
86. Park MC, Lee SW, Park YB, et al. Clinical characteristics and outcomes of Takayasu's arteritis: analysis of 108 patients using standardized criteria for diagnosis, activity assessment and angiographic classification. Scand J Rheumatol 2005;34:284–92.
87. Morales E, Pineda C, Martínez-Lavín M. Takayasu's arteritis in children. J Rheumatol 1991;18(7):1081–4.

Developments in the Classification and Treatment of the Juvenile Idiopathic Inflammatory Myopathies

Lisa G. Rider, MD[a,b,*], James D. Katz, MD[b],
Olcay Y. Jones, MD, PhD[b,c]

KEYWORDS

- Juvenile myositis • Juvenile dermatomyositis • Juvenile polymyositis
- Overlap myositis • Myositis-specific autoantibodies • Treatment • Biologic therapies

KEY POINTS

- Juvenile dermatomyositis is the most common clinicopathologic form of the juvenile idiopathic inflammatory myopathies (IIM), but juvenile polymyositis and overlap myositis are additional distinct groups with higher morbidity and mortality rates.
- Myositis-specific and myositis-associated autoantibodies define several distinct serologic subgroups of juvenile myositis, which share many features with those of patients with adult IIM with the same autoantibodies. Of these, anti-p155/140 and anti-MJ autoantibodies are the most common in juvenile IIM.
- Based on expert consensus and a randomized controlled trial, the combination of daily prednisone with methotrexate is the initial treatment of choice for moderately active juvenile dermatomyositis. Other agents, including intravenous methylprednisolone, intravenous immunoglobulin, and cyclosporine, may be used in combination with them or may serve as alternative agents to methotrexate.
- Early evidence primarily from open-label studies and one randomized controlled trial suggest a role for additional drug and biologic therapies in treatment-refractory patients.

This research was supported in part by the Intramural Research Program of the NIH, National Institute of Environmental Health. The authors have no conflicts of interest.

[a] Environmental Autoimmunity Group, Program of Clinical Research, National Institute of Environmental Health Sciences, National Institutes of Health, CRC 4-2352, MSC 1301, 10 Center Drive, Bethesda, MD 20892-1301, USA; [b] Myositis Center, Division of Rheumatology, Department of Medicine, George Washington University, G-400, 2150 Pennsylvania Avenue Northwest, Washington, DC 20037, USA; [c] Division of Pediatric Rheumatology, Department of Pediatrics, Walter Reed National Military Medical Center, 8901 Wisconsin Avenue, America Building, 4th Floor, Bethesda, MD 20889, USA
* Corresponding author. Environmental Autoimmunity Group, Program of Clinical Research, National Institute of Environmental Health Sciences, National Institutes of Health, CRC 4-2352, MSC 1301, 10 Center Drive, Bethesda, MD 20892-1301.
E-mail address: riderl@mail.nih.gov

The juvenile idiopathic inflammatory myopathies (JIIM) are heterogeneous immune-mediated disorders characterized by chronic skeletal muscle inflammation but often include characteristic skin rashes and involvement of other organs. The diagnosis of these conditions remains based on the clinical and laboratory criteria of Bohan and Peter,[1] with acknowledged limitations that many pediatric patients with characteristic rashes do not undergo electromyography or muscle biopsy.[2] These disorders can be classified based on clinicopathologic features or on the presence of autoantibodies found almost exclusively in patients with myositis, known as the myositis autoantibodies. This subclassification of JIIM assists in understanding patients who share demographic and clinical features, laboratory abnormalities, responses to therapy, and prognoses. The authors now present an update to our understanding of the classification of juvenile myositis from work first published more than 15 years ago[3] and an update on recent advances in the treatment of JIIM, reflecting collaborative multi-center studies and the introduction of biologic therapies for these diseases.

CLINICOPATHOLOGIC CLASSIFICATION OF JIIM

The recent classification has been achieved by large registry studies that have better defined the features of the most common phenotypes and additional case series and reports that have enhanced our understanding of the spectrum of the rarer clinical phenotypes. The classification of JIIM, based on clinical and histologic features, has been recognized both in adults and children with myositis, with the finding that the same clinical subgroups exist in JIIM as adult IIM but with different relative frequencies and slight differences in manifestations and prognoses.[4,5] Although JIIM is 5-fold less common than adult IIM, in children, dermatomyositis (DM) is the most frequent of the IIMs, whereas polymyositis (PM) is relatively more frequent in adults than in children. Inclusion body myositis (IBM) and cancer-associated myositis are almost exclusively seen in adults. Since the authors' first proposal of clinicopathologic groups for JIIM,[3] several new forms of IIM have been recognized, including macrophagic myofasciitis and immune-mediated necrotizing myopathy,[6] and the spectrum of amyopathic DM has expanded to include hypomyopathic DM (**Table 1**). Infantile polymyositis is no longer recognized as a subgroup of JIIM but was found to be a muscular dystrophy (laminin alpha2 or merosin deficiency).[42]

The most common clinical phenotype of myositis in children, constituting approximately 85% of all patients with JIIM, is *juvenile DM* (JDM), which is characterized by symmetric proximal muscle weakness and the presence of characteristic rashes (ie, Gottron papules [erythematous plaques overlying the extensor joint surfaces] or heliotrope rash [a purplish or erythematous rash over the eyelids]). One of the hallmarks of JDM, vasculopathy, is evident by examining the periungual capillaries, which are often dilated, tortuous, and decreased in density because of an immune-mediated attack, which is distinct from vasculitis. Several national registry studies have expanded our understanding of the clinical spectrum of JDM as a systemic autoimmune disease.[5,7–9,43] Patients with JDM have a median age at onset of 7.5 years; in addition to the characteristic skin rashes, they have frequent malar rash, photosensitivity, linear extensor erythema, and other cutaneous findings. Their creatine kinase (CK) levels are elevated but they tend to be lower. The prognosis of JDM is variable, with a low overall mortality of 2% to 3%, and approximately 24% to 40% of patients having a monocyclic course, recovering with appropriate therapy within a 2-year period.[5,44] However, the majority (50%–60%) of patients with JDM experience a chronic illness course. Persistent periungual capillary abnormalities and active skin disease have been associated with a chronic illness course.[44,45] Patients with a

Table 1
A clinicopathologic classification of the JIIM

Clinicopathologic Phenotype	Frequency in JIIM (%)	Associations & Comments	References
DM	85	Most common form of JIIM in children with median age at onset of 7.5 y and female predominance; characterized by Gottron papules or heliotrope rash, and CD4+ T cells and dendritic cells in perivascular distribution in muscle with a type I interferon signature; approximately 50%–60% of patients have a chronic course, and 24%–40% have a monocyclic course of illness; up to 25% have skin or gastrointestinal ulcerations; calcinosis seen in 25%–40% and lipodystrophy in ∼10%, with a spectrum of other associated manifestations	5,7–11
Overlap myositis	6–12	Patients meet criteria for another autoimmune disease, most frequently systemic sclerosis, systemic lupus erythematosus, juvenile idiopathic arthritis, localized scleroderma, Sjögren syndrome, or type I diabetes; Raynaud phenomenon, interstitial lung disease, arthritis, sclerodactyly, and calcinosis are more frequent in this subgroup; mortality is high, often related to lung disease	5,8,12,13
PM	4–8	Defined by the absence of the characteristic DM rashes; pathogenesis involves CD8+ endomysial infiltration in muscle; patients tend to be older (preteen or teenage), have higher CK levels, and more severe illness onset, with frequent falling episodes as a sign of distal weakness, myalgias, more frequent cardiac involvement, and intermediate mortality	5,8,14
Amyopathic or hypomyopathic DM	1	DM skin rashes, either without muscle weakness or with subclinical muscle weakness detected only by additional testing (eg, elevated serum muscle enzymes or abnormal EMG, muscle biopsy, or MRI); approximately 25% of patients develop JDM within 3 y; calcinosis has been reported in only 4%, and cutaneous ulcerations and interstitial lung disease are very rare; none of the children have malignancy, in contrast to adults with clinically amyopathic DM whereby these associated features are common.	15–17
IBM	Rare	Characterized by slowly progressive proximal and distal weakness, low serum CK level, and rimmed vacuoles on trichrome stain of muscle biopsy, with poor responses to immunosuppressive therapy; only a few case reports in teenage boys, whereas IBM is a major clinical subgroup in adults, suggesting a degenerative pathogenesis and/or environmental triggers that are present only in older adults or that have long latency	3,18

(continued on next page)

Table 1
(continued)

Clinicopathologic Phenotype	Frequency in JIIM (%)	Associations & Comments	References
Cancer-associated myositis	<1	Malignancy in association with JIIM is so uncommon that routine screening for cancer is generally not warranted, in contrast to adults with DM and PM whereby a malignancy screen is routinely performed because of a paraneoplastic association within 2 y of myositis onset; atypical illness features, such as prominent adenopathy, hepatosplenomegaly, palpable masses, and atypical rashes, have been proposed as part of a profile of indicators that may indicate an underlying associated malignancy that has been observed in most of the 17 reported cases of cancer associated with JIIM; most common cancers in children include lymphoma, leukemia, and solid organ tumors	3,8,19–21
Focal myositis	1–2	Characterized by a subacute, often painful intramuscular swelling or mass in a single muscle group, sometimes preceded by trauma, with histologic features of myositis; most common sites of involvement are the thigh muscles, gastrocnemius, brachialis, and sternocleidomastoid; lesions often resolve spontaneously resolve, but immunosuppressive therapy or surgical resection may be beneficial in refractory cases	7,22,23
Orbital myositis	1–2	A focal myositis of the rectus muscles, which presents with ocular pain, headache, diplopia, proptosis, ocular injection, limited ocular mobility, and periorbital edema; children may have atypical presentations, including emesis, anorexia, lethargy, abdominal pain, and weight loss; inflammation of an orbital muscle must be distinguished clinically from thyroid-associated orbitopathy, but the differential diagnosis also includes rhabdomyosarcoma, lymphoproliferative disease, IgG4-related disease, or histiocytosis X; pediatric cases also differ from their adult counterparts in that they are more likely to be bilateral on presentation or associated with uveitis, disc edema, or eosinophilia; orbital myositis may be seen following an infection, such as group A streptococcus, or in the setting of other autoimmune conditions, including inflammatory bowel disease, linear scleroderma, or Kawasaki disease	7,24–27

Immune-mediated necrotizing myopathy	1	PM or DM in which the muscle biopsy demonstrates prominent muscle necrosis and little inflammation; thought to be mediated by autoantibodies, including anti-signal recognition particle or anti-3-hydroxy-3-methylglutaryl-coenzyme A reductase	6,28
Macrophagic myofasciitis	<1	An inflammatory myopathy thought to be related to aluminum-adjuvant vaccines; presents with prominent macrophagic infiltrates and aluminum detectable in the muscle; symptoms include myalgias, arthralgias, muscle weakness, chronic fatigue, and fever; in children, additional features include hypotonia, motor delay with an inability to stand or walk, and failure to thrive; typically, vaccination predates the diagnosis by 2–12 mo, and childhood-onset cases are generally in the first 5 y	29–32
Eosinophilic myositis	<1	Prominent eosinophilic infiltrates on muscle biopsy, often accompanied by peripheral eosinophilia; may be idiopathic and true polymyositis or focal in nature; may also be drug induced, related to a parasitic infection, or to an underlying hypereosinophilic syndrome; in children, it is particularly important to exclude muscular dystrophies, including calpainopathy, Becker dystrophy, and gamma sarcoglycanopathy (LGMD2 C), which have been reported to present with eosinophilic myositis	33–36
Granulomatous myositis	<1	Granulomas prominent in the muscle, which may be idiopathic or seen in association with Wegener vasculitis, sarcoidosis, or tuberculosis	37,38
Proliferative myositis	Rare	A very rare benign pseudosarcomatous lesion of skeletal muscle; may be diagnosed with fine-needle aspiration cytology, which shows hypercellular and polymorphic lesional cells and distinctive ganglion cell-like cells; most lesions resolve spontaneously within 4 mo; surgical resection is used for the remaining lesions	39,40
Graft-versus-host myositis	Rare	Polymyositis with weakness, myalgias, and elevated CK, which rarely occurs as part of graft-versus-host disease following stem cell and bone marrow transplantation); responds to prednisone and cyclosporine	41

Abbreviations: CK, creatine kinase; DM, dermatomyositis; EMG, electromyogram; Ig, immunoglobulin; MRI, magnetic resonance imaging; PM, polymyositis.

chronic illness course and poor prognosis might also have cutaneous or gastrointestinal ulcerations or, less commonly, pulmonary or gastrointestinal tract air leaks (pneumomediastinum or pneumatosis intestinalis), indicating severe vasculopathy.[46] Calcinosis occurs in 20% to 40% of patients,[5,10,43] with a lower prevalence in patients treated more aggressively who enter remission more rapidly.[47] Calcium and phosphate precipitate in the subcutaneous tissues and muscles as carbonate apatite, perhaps as a result of a loss of mineralization inhibitors.[48] The risk factors for calcinosis include delay to diagnosis, cardiac involvement, the need for additional immunosuppressive therapy, as well as a prolonged and/or severe illness course.[10] Another complication of JDM, lipodystrophy, occurs in up to 10% of patients and is characterized by progressive loss of subcutaneous fat in a localized, partial (ie, only in the extremities), or widespread distribution. Lipodystrophy has been associated with calcinosis, muscle atrophy, joint contractures, and facial rash and should be recognized early because of its association with metabolic sequelae of insulin resistance, diabetes, and hyperlipidemia, with frequencies proportionate to the degree of fat loss.[11]

Overlap myositis, in which patients meet the criteria for JIIM as well as another autoimmune disease, is the next most common clinical phenotype of JIIM, occurring in 6% to 11% of patients.[5,7] Raynaud phenomenon, interstitial lung disease, arthritis, and malar rash are more frequent illness features in this subgroup. Patients with overlap myositis are more likely to have JDM than juvenile PM (JPM), more often have myositis-associated autoantibodies, and are more often nonwhite.[5,12] Among the JIIM subgroups, overlap myositis has a relatively higher mortality rate, which is often related to lung disease.[5,13] The most common overlapping autoimmune conditions include systemic lupus erythematosus, juvenile idiopathic arthritis, systemic sclerosis, and localized scleroderma.[5] Although organ-specific autoantibodies, including those for autoimmune thyroid disease and hepatitis, type I diabetes, and celiac disease, have been observed in 2% to 15% of patients with JDM, these autoantibodies were not accompanied by overt organ-specific overlapping autoimmune diseases in one population.[49]

JPM, which is seen in about 4% to 8% of patients with JIIM, is characterized by both proximal and distal muscle weakness but lacks the characteristic rashes of JDM. The pathologic findings also differ from JDM, with frequent endomysial infiltrates in affected muscles.[5,7,8,14] Patients with JPM tend to be older, with the onset in preteen or teenage years, have higher CK levels, more myalgias, and a more severe illness onset. They often have frequent falling episodes, a sign of distal weakness; cardiac involvement occurs in approximately one-third of patients with JPM. Mortality is intermediate between JDM and overlap myositis.[5] A muscle biopsy is required for diagnosis because JPM is often misdiagnosed in patients who actually have other noninflammatory myopathies, particularly muscular dystrophies, which have more frequent myopathic features on biopsy and clinical muscle atrophy.[50] Patients with JPM also frequently have myositis-specific autoantibodies (MSAs) and myositis-associated autoantibodies (MAAs), particularly anti–aminoacyl-tRNA synthetase (anti-synthetase) and anti–signal recognition particle (SRP) autoantibodies.[5]

The other clinicopathologic phenotypes of the JIIM are uncommon (see **Table 1**). Of these, true *DM sine myositis* without evidence of muscle involvement is rare. However, *hypomyopathic DM* is occasionally observed, in which DM skin rashes are present for at least 6 months in patients who have no detectable weakness but have evidence of muscle inflammation on testing (including elevated serum muscle enzyme levels, or an abnormal electromyogram, muscle biopsy, or muscle magnetic resonance imaging [MRI]). A thorough review of 68 cases of juvenile-onset, clinically amyopathic DM, which encompasses both DM sine myositis and hypomyopathic DM, showed that

26% of the patients subsequently developed classic JDM and that this disease progression occurred up to several years later.[15,16] At the onset, only 4% of those patients had an elevated CK level; of those with a normal CK level, only a minority had an abnormal electromyogram, muscle biopsy, or MRI, suggesting that these patients can be treated symptomatically for their cutaneous disease, with close clinical monitoring for progression to muscle involvement.[15] Calcinosis was reported in only 4%, and none had ulcerations, interstitial lung disease, or malignancy,[15] which are the manifestations that are often associated with amyopathic DM in adults.[51] A case report noted cutaneous ulcerations and interstitial lung disease in a lethal case of juvenile clinically amyopathic DM.[52] The outcome of hypomyopathic DM seems to be good; for example, in 24 patients, 65% recovered spontaneously without therapy, and 5 of 10 patients treated with systemic therapy entered remission.[17]

Malignancy in association with JIIM is so uncommon that routine screening for cancer is generally not warranted. In contrast, adults with DM and PM routinely undergo malignancy screening because of an increased risk for malignancy within 2 years of myositis onset.[19] Nevertheless, a tumor may present with an autoimmune, myositis-like picture in childhood.[20] In a Brazilian registry of 189 patients with JIIM, there was an associated malignancy in 2 (1.1%) cases[8]; but in other large JIIM registry studies, coexisting cancer was not reported.[5,7,43] Atypical illness features, including prominent adenopathy, hepatosplenomegaly, palpable masses, and atypical rashes, have been proposed to be part of a profile of indicators that might indicate an underlying malignancy because at least one of those features was observed in most of the 17 reported cases of cancer in association with JIIM.[3,20,21] The most common associated cancers in children have included lymphoma, leukemia, and solid organ tumors.

Focal myositis, alternatively termed an inflammatory *pseudotumor* or *focal nodular myositis*, is characterized by an often painful intramuscular swelling or mass in a single muscle group that develops over several weeks or months, sometimes preceded by trauma. The most common sites of involvement are the thigh muscle groups, gastrocnemius, brachialis, and sternocleidomastoid; but any muscle may be affected.[22,23] This disorder must be distinguished from malignant tumors and infectious causes, including Lyme disease. Although typically an isolated phenomenon, it can be associated with other rheumatic diseases. Histologic changes include fibrosis and intramuscular inflammation, particularly infiltration of macrophages that are occasionally accompanied by prominent eosinophils and CD4+ lymphocytes. Cases with severe inflammation have elevated B cells and plasmacytoid dendritic cells.[22] Limited follow-up found spontaneous resolution in several cases, with immunosuppressive therapy or surgical resection used for refractory disease.[22] A higher CK level or erythrocyte sedimentation rate, or limb atrophy may signal an increased risk of recurrence or progression to multifocal IIM.[23]

Macrophagic myofasciitis (MMF) is an inflammatory myopathy that is thought to be related to aluminum-adjuvant vaccines. MMF often has an active lesion at the immunization site; systemic symptoms include myalgias, arthralgias, muscle weakness, chronic fatigue, and fever.[29] In children, additional features include hypotonia, motor delay with an inability to stand or walk, and failure to thrive.[30,31] Scanning electron microscopy with energy dispersive spectroscopy has been used to detect aluminum in tissue specimens.[53] Histologically, granulomas comprised of periodic acid-Schiff–positive and CD68-positive macrophages are generally seen. Typically, vaccination predates the diagnosis by 2 to 12 months but has been as long as 10 years prior.[32] MMF often occurs in individuals who have genetic susceptibility, particularly the human leukocyte antigen (HLA)-DRB1*01 allele.

Other clinicopathologic forms of JIIM are rare and are described in **Table 1**.

SEROLOGIC CLASSIFICATION OF JIIM

An alternative classification of the JIM is by the presence of myositis autoantibodies. Two classes of autoantibodies include MSAs, which are present almost exclusively in patients with myositis, and MAAs, which are present in patients with myositis and in patients with other autoimmune diseases (**Table 2**). As the recognition of myositis autoantibodies has increased recently, this has enabled the identification of a myositis autoantibody in approximately 70% of patients with JIIM.[5] These myositis autoantibodies define more homogeneous groups of patients with similar clinical features, responses to therapy, and prognoses. Of the autoantibodies studied in both children and adults, generally the same myositis autoantibodies have been seen, although some of them differ in frequency between children and adults. For example, anti-p155/140 and anti-MJ autoantibodies seem to be more prevalent in JDM than adult DM; conversely, the anti-synthetase autoantibodies, which are seen in approximately 5% of patients with JIIM, are present in 25% to 40% of patients with adult IIM.[5] There are also many similarities in the clinical and demographic features, laboratory findings, and prognoses between patients with JIIM and patients with adult IIM with the same myositis autoantibodies.[54] Myositis autoantibodies are most accurately detected by validated protein and RNA immunoprecipitation assays, with certain autoantibodies, particularly anti-p155/140 and anti-MJ, requiring additional confirmation by reverse immunoprecipitation-immunoblotting or immunodepletion methods.[55,72] A line-blot assay is almost as sensitive and specific as protein immunoprecipitation in detecting the traditional MSAs and MAAs.[73]

The most frequent MSAs in JIIM are anti-p155/140 and anti-MJ autoantibodies, and they are associated primarily with JDM.[54] Anti-p155/140 autoantibodies have reactivity to transcriptional intermediary factor 1γ and are present in 23% to 30% of patients with JIIM, particularly in those with JDM or overlap myositis with JDM. Anti-p155/140 autoantibodies are associated with extensive photosensitive skin rashes, including the characteristic rashes of JDM, malar rash, V-sign and shawl-sign rashes, and linear extensor erythema, as well as periungual capillary changes, skin ulceration, and generalized lipodystrophy.[11,54,55] Patients with JIIM with anti-p155/140 autoantibodies frequently have a chronic illness course.[54] In patients with adult IIM, but not in patients with JIIM, anti-p155/140 autoantibodies are frequently associated with cancer-associated myositis.[56] Anti-MJ autoantibodies are present in 20% to 25% of patients with JIIM and are seen primarily in patients with JDM who have frequent muscle cramps, dysphonia, joint contractures, and a monocyclic disease course.[54,57,58] Patients with this autoantibody group have more severe illness, with one report finding a higher frequency of calcinosis,[57] another report detailing frequent muscle atrophy,[58] and a third report showing more frequent hospitalizations and increased frequency of gastrointestinal ulceration.[54]

Of the traditional MSAs, anti-synthetase autoantibodies, which are present in less than 5% of patients with JIIM overall, are less frequent in JIIM than adult IIM. They are more often seen in patients with JPM or juvenile overlap myositis, with a frequency of 9% and 13%, respectively.[54] Anti-Jo-1 autoantibodies are the most common of the anti-synthetase autoantibodies. As in adults, children with these autoantibodies also have frequent interstitial lung disease, arthritis, Raynaud phenomenon, fevers, and mechanic's hands.[54] Among the MSA phenotypes, this group also has the highest mortality rate, caused by interstitial lung disease.[13,54] Anti-SRP autoantibodies are seen primarily in African American girls with severe JPM who have proximal and distal muscle weakness, frequent falling episodes, Raynaud phenomenon, very high CK levels, wheelchair use, and a chronic illness course.[28,54] Cardiac disease is also likely associated with these autoantibodies; similar to patients with adult IIM with anti-SRP autoantibodies, their disease is refractory to many therapies.[28] Myonecrosis, consistent with an immune-mediated necrotizing myopathy, is characteristic of the muscle pathology.[28]

Other MSAs and MAAs are described in **Table 2**. Anti-Mi-2 is a traditional MSA that is associated with JDM and its cutaneous features. Anti-CADM-140, which is associated with rapidly progressive interstitial lung disease, cutaneous ulcerations, and mucinous papules, and anti–small ubiquitin like modifier activating enzyme autoantibodies have been described in patients with JIIM only in case reports.[59,60,63] Anti-200/100, an MSA that targets 3-hydroxy-3-methyl-glutaryl–CoA reductase, is associated with an immune-mediated necrotizing myopathy that resembles PM in adult patients and is more frequent in patients who have taken statins; it has not yet been described in patients with JIIM.[6]

MAAs, including anti-U1RNP, anti-Ro, anti-PM-Scl, and anti-Ku autoantibodies, are present in up to 15% of patients with JIIM overall but are more frequent in patients with overlap myositis.[5,12] Relatively little is known about their associated clinical features in JIIM, and the limited clinical correlative information is based primarily on adult IIM cohorts.[66–71] Individuals who have no identified MSAs or MAAs currently compose approximately 28% of patients. Although disease in this subgroup seems to be mild, it is likely comprised of several currently unrecognized autoantibody phenotypes. The strength of the clinical associations and prognostic information from the MSAs suggest that serologic data are likely valuable in guiding therapy.

TREATMENT APPROACHES FOR JDM

The development of new therapies for JIIM has been historically hampered not only by the rarity of these conditions but also by a lack of common outcome measures and controlled clinical trials and by vastly different approaches to therapy by geographic region and specialty. Important advances in the past decade should help provide a foundation for the development of new therapies for JIIM. Two large international clinical research consortia, the International Myositis Assessment and Clinical Studies Group (IMACS) and the Pediatric Rheumatology International Trials Organization (PRINTO), have developed and preliminarily validated core set measures of myositis disease activity and damage as well as preliminary definitions of improvement to be used as end points for therapeutic trials.[74–76] These measures, including the assessment of muscle strength and physical function by manual muscle testing, the Childhood Myositis Assessment Scale, the Child Health Assessment Questionnaire, and extramuscular activity and global activity assessments, were readily adopted for use in clinical studies and trials, which resulted in standardized outcome assessment and an improved ability to monitor responses to therapies. Ancillary measures to assess cutaneous disease activity, physical disability, and quality of life have also been developed.[74] The first large randomized controlled trials of treatments for JDM have recently been conducted, including the first use of targeted biologic therapies.[77,78] The Childhood Arthritis and Rheumatology Research Alliance (CARRA) has developed consensus guidelines for the treatment of moderately active patients and for corticosteroid dose reduction,[79,80] which help greatly to standardize the care of patients.

The following discussion of therapy emphasizes 3 aspects of the current state of treatment of JDM, including new aspects of the initial treatment; drug and biologic therapies for refractory patients (**Table 3**); and the treatment of cutaneous disease, calcinosis, and rehabilitation. Most of the therapeutic experience in the JIIM is related to studies and trials in JDM. Although these therapies are applicable to other forms of

Table 2
A serologic classification of the JIIM

Serologic Group	Frequency (%)	Clinical Subgroup Association in JIIM	Comments	References
MSA				
Anti-p155/140 (TIF1-γ)	23–30	JDM and JDM with overlap myositis	Associated with extensive photosensitive skin rashes, including the characteristic rashes of JDM, malar rash, V-sign and shawl-sign rashes, and linear extensor erythema, as well as periungual capillary changes, skin ulceration, and generalized lipodystrophy; patients frequently have a chronic illness course; not associated with cancer-associated myositis, which differs from patients with adult IIM with this autoantibody	5,11,54–56
Anti-MJ (NXP-2)	20–25	Primarily JDM	Frequent muscle cramps, dysphonia, joint contractures, and a monocyclic illness course; this autoantibody group seems to have more severe illness, with some reports of increased calcinosis, frequent muscle atrophy, more frequent hospitalizations and gastrointestinal ulceration	5,54,57,58
Anti-aminoacyl-tRNA synthetases (Jo1 & non-Jo1 synthetases)	2–4	JDM, JPM, & overlap myositis	More common in JPM (9%) and patients with juvenile overlap myositis (8%–13%); frequent ILD, arthritis, Raynaud phenomenon, fevers, and mechanic's hands, similar to adults with these autoantibodies; among the MSA phenotypes, this group has the highest mortality caused by ILD	5,12,13,54
Anti-SRP	1	JPM	More common in JPM (18%); seen primarily in African American girls with JPM who have severe to profound proximal and distal muscle weakness, frequent falling episodes, Raynaud phenomenon, very high CK levels, wheelchair use, and a chronic illness course; cardiac disease is also likely associated, and these patients are refractory to several therapies, similar to patients with adult IIM with anti-SRP autoantibodies	5,28,54
Anti-Mi-2 (NuRD)	2–13	JDM & overlap myositis	JDM with classic cutaneous findings of Gottron papules, heliotrope rash, and malar rash; predominantly seen in Hispanic patients; mild disease, but children have higher CK levels than adults with this autoantibody	5,49,54,58

Autoantibody	Disease	Frequency	Description	References
Anti-CADM-140 (MDA-5)	JDM	Unknown	Associated with DM and clinically amyopathic DM in adults who frequently have rapidly progressive ILD, cutaneous ulceration, and palmar papules, with a high fatality rate; 7 patients with JDM or amyopathic JDM and ILD have been reported with this autoantibody; to date, most reports are from Japan, and mortality has been high	59–62
Anti-SAE	JDM	0.2	Associated with DM cutaneous manifestations, which predate development of muscle symptoms, an absence of constitutional manifestations, and low frequency of ILD	5,63–65
MAA				
Anti-U1-RNP	JDM, JPM, & overlap myositis	5–10	More common in JPM (12%) and overlap myositis (20%–27%); associated with arthritis, Raynaud phenomenon, and sclerodactyly	5,12,58,66,67
Anti-Ro	JDM, JPM, & overlap myositis	2–6	More common in overlap myositis (8%–15%); little known about the associated clinical features; associated with impaired lung function in 1 report; in adults, patients respond well to prednisone alone; may be seen in association with anti-Jo1 autoantibodies	5,12,67,68
Anti-PM-Scl	JDM, JPM, & overlap myositis	1–4	More common in JPM (6%) and overlap myositis (10%–25%); based on adult cohorts, this autoantibody is associated with Raynaud phenomenon, arthritis, ILD, and esophageal dysmotility; most frequent in Caucasian patients with an HLA DRB1*0301 immunogenetic association	5,12,69,70
Anti-Ku	JDM, JPM, & overlap myositis	0.2	More common in overlap myositis (2%); based on adult cohorts, frequently associated manifestations include arthralgia, Raynaud phenomenon, myalgias, dysphagia, and less commonly, ILD; patients respond well to corticosteroids alone, except those with lung disease	49,71
Other MAAs: anti-U2-, U3- or U5-RNP; anti-La; anti-Sm; anti-Th	JDM, JPM, & overlap myositis	<1	Each autoantibody is present more frequently in overlap myositis (1%–10%); little known, primarily associated with overlap myositis	5,12
Myositis autoantibody negative	JDM, JPM, & overlap myositis	28–57	Relatively mild disease in this subgroup; this group is likely heterogeneous, with several different unrecognized autoantibody groups contained within	5,12

Abbreviations: ILD, interstitial lung disease; JDM, juvenile dermatomyositis; JPM, juvenile polymyositis; MAA, myositis-associated autoantibodies; MDA-5, melanoma differentiation-associated gene 5; MSA, myositis-specific autoantibodies; NuRD, nucleosome remodeling deacetylase complex; SAE, small ubiquitinlike modifier activating enzyme; SRP, signal recognition particle; TIF1-γ, transcriptional intermediary factor 1γ.

Table 3
Medications used to treat JDM[a]

Medication	Recommended Regimen	Support & Comments	References
Primary therapy[b]			
Prednisone	Dosage starting at 2 mg/kg/d po; maximum 60 mg/d gradually tapered by 2- to 4-wk intervals, with a minimum recommended duration of 10–12 mo	Daily prednisone considered the mainstay of treatment of JDM and other JIIM, throughout the illness course, and has led to dramatic improvements in mortality (now less than 2% for JDM) and functional disability	3,79,80
IVMP	30 mg/kg/d IV; maximum 1 g, 3 d in a row at diagnosis, then optional once weekly	Used as an adjunct therapy with daily corticosteroids during the initial treatment of moderate to severe JDM; provides better absorption of corticosteroid, aiding in rapid improvement of disease activity; also valuable for acute or life-threatening manifestations, such as severe dysphagia, interstitial lung disease, myocarditis; may be used later in the illness course for flares or persistent activity	3,79,81,82
Methotrexate	1 mg/kg or 15 mg/m² once weekly SQ; max 40 mg weekly	Most commonly used adjunct therapy with steroids, used as first-line therapy for moderate to severe disease; efficacy in combination with steroids is superior to prednisone alone, including a shorter time to inactive disease; methotrexate used in conjunction with steroids from time of diagnosis results in fewer cataracts, less weight gain, and less reduction in growth velocity, and a lower cumulative dose of prednisone	78,79,83
IVIG	2 g/kg IV; max 70 g, every 2 wk × 3, then monthly	Adjunct therapy for moderate to severe disease; usually combined with steroids and methotrexate; used both as an agent for initial treatment of moderately severe disease and for refractory cases; rapid onset of action and lack of immunosuppression are potential benefits; may be helpful in patients with acute, potentially life-threatening manifestations (dysphagia, marked weakness, ulceration), and for treatment of skin disease and calcinosis	3,79,84
Cyclosporine	2.5–7.5 mg/kg/d po divided bid (max 150 mg bid) to maintain trough blood level ≤300 ng/mL	Preferred agent in European centers compared with other continents; used for initial treatment but more so for refractory patients; efficacy in combination with steroids is superior to prednisone alone, including a shorter time to inactive disease; however, side effects are greater than with methotrexate	3,78

Therapies for refractory disease[c]

Mycophenolate mofetil	20–40 mg/kg/d po divided bid or 800–1350 mg/m²/d	Used to treat severe or refractory disease, with improvements in muscle strength and skin activity and reduction in corticosteroid dose	82,85
Tacrolimus	Initial dosage of 0.04–0.08 mg/kg/d po divided bid (max 2–3 mg bid), with gradual increase to 0.1–0.25 mg/kg/d divided bid (max 3–6 mg bid) to maintain trough level of 5–10 ng/mL	Used for severe or treatment-refractory disease, particularly with severe weakness, interstitial lung disease, or with anti-synthetase or anti-SRP autoantibodies	86,87
Cyclophosphamide	500–1000 mg/m²/mo IV	Used for life-threatening disease activity, severe dysphagia, interstitial lung disease, gastrointestinal or cutaneous ulcerations or other forms of vasculitis, or in patients with severe disease activity that is treatment refractory; improvements in muscle strength and function, skin, extramuscular activity, and calcinosis reported	88,89
Rituximab	575 mg/m² or 750 mg/m² (max 1 g) per dose for 2 weekly infusions	Used for refractory patients who failed to improve on other DMARDs; approximately 80% of treatment-refractory patients have improved in a randomized controlled trial and in open-label studies; onset of improvement lags for about 3 mo after infusion; efficacy more toward muscle rather than skin disease activity; helpful in patients with myositis autoantibodies	77,90–93
Anti-TNFα (infliximab, etanercept)	Infliximab: 3–6 mg/kg IV at weeks 0, 2, 6 and then every 4 wk	Infliximab has best success for JDM in open-label study and small case series of treatment-refractory patients; reported improvement in muscle strength and physical function, muscle enzyme levels, skin rashes, and global activity in >70% of treatment-refractory patients; calcinosis improved in 46%; mixed experience in adult DM/PM, and some reports of disease worsening with anti-TNFα therapy, which may be related to induction of the interferon signature	94,95

Abbreviations: DMARD, disease-modifying anti-rheumatic drug; IV, intravenous; IVIG, intravenous immunoglobulin; IVMP, intravenous methylprednisolone; max, maximum; SQ, subcutaneous; TNFα, tumor necrosis factor α.

[a] Experience with additional agents with more limited supporting data, as well as the treatment of cutaneous disease, calcinosis, and rehabilitation, is discussed in the text.

[b] Per the Childhood Arthritis and Rheumatology Research Alliance treatment consensus for moderately severe disease, dietary modifications and dietary consultation if possible (to minimize prednisone weight gain), photoprotective measures, and folic acid are adjunctive primary therapies. Calcium and vitamin D supplementation and referral to physical therapy and/or occupational therapy are also recommended.[79]

[c] Combinations of several primary therapies and therapies for refractory disease may also be used.

JIIM, the sequence and use of these medications differs slightly among the clinical and serologic phenotypes; therapy for other JIIM phenotypes is often best directed from adult IIM studies.[96]

The goals of therapy include the elimination of active disease (which may result from inflammation [including type I interferons and proinflammatory cytokines], from vasculopathy, or from myogenic factors, such as endoplasmic reticulum stress responses[97]) and the prevention of disease damage to muscle and other organ systems in order to reduce morbidity while minimizing the side effects of medication.[43,98] Aggressive initial treatment of JDM disease activity is thought to be essential in preventing the development of calcinosis. This idea is based on observations that, among patients who have received long-term high-dose corticosteroids, including intravenous pulse methylprednisolone (IVMP) therapy, or who were treated with multiple immunosuppressive therapies, fewer developed calcinosis and most of them more readily entered remission.[47,81] Complete and rapid treatment of underlying inflammation is thought to be essential not only to fully restore muscle function but also to prevent damage, including scarring and atrophy in the muscle and skin; to shorten the illness course; and to reduce or prevent calcinosis.[44,45] Cutaneous activity, including panniculitis, is a risk factor for the development of calcinosis and lipodystrophy[11] and, thus, requires attention in therapy. New biomarkers of disease activity, which include the evaluation of the vasculopathy and immune activation,[99] and the use of MRI can aide in the assessment of occult active disease and muscle damage.

Initial Therapy

Current practice among pediatric rheumatologists for the treatment of JDM has been summarized in several recent publications.[9,100,101] Daily oral corticosteroid therapy is universally used in the care of these patients. Stringer and colleagues[100] surveyed more than 160 North American pediatric rheumatologists and found that corticosteroid doses vary based on disease severity; nonetheless, an initial dose of prednisone at 2 mg/kg/d was preferred by more than half of the respondents, and dosages tend to remain higher in severe cases. The use of IVMP is common, particularly for moderate and severe cases, with a trend to deliver 3 to 5 daily doses of 30 mg/kg initially, followed by intermittent subsequent doses, particularly for severe disease. Almost 90% of respondents favored the use of corticosteroids in combination with a disease-modifying antirheumatic drug (DMARD), most commonly methotrexate. Hydroxychloroquine is used mostly for mild disease and cases with predominantly cutaneous manifestations, and cyclophosphamide was preferred for ulcerative cases (45%) or for interstitial lung disease (ILD). Intravenous immunoglobulin (IVIG) was used to treat severe or refractory cases or those with predominant skin disease. A large PRINTO study of 145 patients with recent-onset JDM and 130 patients experiencing a disease flare[101] found that patients in North and South America more frequently received intravenous pulse corticosteroids at the beginning of illness compared with patients in Europe (59%–74% vs 19%–38%). The use of methotrexate was similar throughout these regions, but cyclosporine and IVIG were favored in Europe for patients experiencing illness flares (16%–40%). Guseinova and colleagues[9] conducted one of the largest retrospective reviews on treatment practice, involving 490 patients with JIIM receiving care at 27 pediatric rheumatology centers in Europe and South America from 1980 to 2004. They found that methotrexate and IVMP were used in approximately 50% of patients, antimalarials in 32%, cyclosporine in 25%, and IVIG in 17%. Although treatment with high-dose IVMP, in combination with a DMARD, such as cyclosporine, cyclophosphamide, or azathioprine, was common in European centers, methotrexate and antimalarial medications were preferred by South American providers.

Recently, CARRA developed consensus protocols to optimize the initial therapy of patients with moderately severe JDM.[79,80] Three consensus treatment protocols have been proposed; given the risks of poorer outcomes for untreated or longstanding disease, as discussed earlier, as well as the adverse effects of high-dose, long-term corticosteroid use,[83] all 3 options propose combinations of therapies from the time of diagnosis. The use of steroids (2 mg/kg/d) and methotrexate (15 mg/m^2 or 1 mg/kg per dose) is common to all 3 treatment arms, with 2 other arms adding IVMP (30 mg/kg, maximum of 1 g, 3 days in a row and then optional once weekly) or IVMP with IVIG (2 g/kg every 2 weeks × 3, then monthly). The early use of IVMP and other parenteral therapies is done in part to overcome the poor absorption of oral corticosteroids because of the underlying vasculopathy[82] and to diminish disease activity more rapidly so as to potentially improve outcomes.[44,45,47,81] Early introduction of corticosteroid-sparing medications, such as methotrexate, may also decrease the frequency of corticosteroid toxicity, including excessive weight gain, decreased growth velocity, and cataracts.[83] CARRA is currently conducting prospective studies of these 3 treatment protocols. This treatment consensus represents an important advance, by considering steroid-sparing agents as part of the initial therapy of JDM and including multiple agents simultaneously as part of the initial therapy for some patients with high levels of disease activity or serious illness manifestations. A follow-up consensus report from the CARRA pediatric rheumatologists determined that patients with clinical improvement may undergo corticosteroid dose reduction every 2 weeks, or monthly for lower steroid doses, such that steroids would be discontinued by 10 to 12 months after diagnosis. Importantly, the criteria for reducing corticosteroid therapy include improvement or normalization of muscle strength, muscle enzymes, skin rashes, and other disease manifestations, emphasizing that all aspects of disease activity must be completely treated before therapy is further reduced or discontinued.[80]

A recent large, multicenter, randomized controlled trial by PRINTO of 139 patients with newly diagnosed JDM demonstrated a trend toward greater response to therapy at 6 months when prednisone and methotrexate (74%) were used compared with prednisone and cyclosporine (67%) or prednisone alone (52%).[78] The time to inactive disease was significantly shorter and the time to major therapeutic changes was significantly longer in the combination groups (prednisone with cyclosporine or methotrexate) compared with prednisone alone. The number of adverse events was highest in the group treated with cyclosporine (51%) compared with methotrexate (28%) or prednisone alone (21%). This first large randomized controlled trial for the initial treatment of JDM suggests that combination of prednisone with methotrexate or cyclosporine is more effective than prednisone alone, but the safety profile favors the use of methotrexate over cyclosporine.

Treatment of Refractory Disease

The use of other therapies to treat refractory disease is appropriate in patients with unacceptable medication toxicity and in patients with severe disease activity, with certain severe illness manifestations (such as interstitial lung disease and cutaneous or gastrointestinal ulcerations), or with a poor prognosis (such as the presence of anti-synthetase or anti-SRP autoantibodies). The use of IVIG to treat JDM was initially inspired by a double-blind placebo-controlled trial in adult DM[102] and small case series or anecdotal reports in JDM.[3] Lam and colleagues[84] published a retrospective review of their experience using monthly IVIG infusions in 30 patients with JDM who failed initial therapy compared with 48 patients who did not go on to receive IVIG.

The comparison of treatment outcomes was confounded for the IVIG group, which consisted of patients with more severe disease activity and included 2 subgroups of patients, namely, steroid-resistant patients (who failed to respond to 6 weeks of initial therapy with corticosteroids often with methotrexate or who had severe disease with dysphagia and marked weakness that required initial treatment with IVIG) and steroid-dependent patients (who improved with the initial 6 weeks of treatment but flared after subsequent dose reduction of corticosteroids). The IVIG group, particularly the steroid-resistant subgroup, achieved lower disease activity 30 days to 4 years after treatment compared with the corticosteroid-only group, based on analyses that used bias-reduction methods. Although IVIG infusions were generally tolerated well and most patients remained on IVIG for more than 2 years, IVIG preparations containing a high level of immunoglobulin A were more frequently associated with fever, malaise, nausea, and vomiting.[103] IVIG may also be used in the initial treatment of patients with JDM with moderately severe disease, as discussed earlier,[79] including patients with severe weakness or dysphagia, ulcerative disease, or calcinosis.[3]

Mycophenolate mofetil is one of the few medications that have been studied formally in children with JDM, albeit in a small retrospective case series involving 50 children. That study demonstrated the efficacy of 12 months of therapy in refractory patients who had an average disease duration of 3.6 years. Skin and muscle activity steadily improved in most patients, based on a significant reduction in their Disease Activity Scores. Those patients who responded to mycophenolate mofetil also tolerated steroid dose reduction, with a mean decrease of 0.2 mg/kg/d. The most common adverse event was minor infection (upper respiratory, sinusitis, and otitis media), with a similar rate of infection in the first 6 months of therapy as in the months before the initiation of mycophenolate mofetil. Dagher and colleagues[85] reported similar observations in 8 children with refractory JDM who received mycophenolate mofetil (800–1350 mg/m^2/d) along with oral corticosteroids. There was improvement in Childhood Myositis Assessment Scale scores and manual muscle testing scores, as well as a decrease in the daily steroid dose by an average of 18%. Rashes resolved in 2 patients, and calcinosis improved in 1 patient. Mycophenolate mofetil was tolerated well, except in one case with transient neutropenia.

Other treatments have been reported to be beneficial for specific types of patients. Oral tacrolimus, which has been beneficial in patients with adult DM/PM with refractory disease, particularly in patients with interstitial lung disease and anti-synthetase or anti-SRP autoantibodies,[86] has been reported to be beneficial for a few patients with refractory JDM, particularly those with cutaneous disease, enabling them to reduce their corticosteroid dose.[87] Intravenous pulse cyclophosphamide therapy (0.5–1.0 g/m^2 monthly for 6–14 dosages) was used in 12 patients with cutaneous or gastrointestinal ulceration or other signs of vasculitis, interstitial lung disease, and/or extremely refractory disease.[88] Although 2 patients died, the remaining 10 patients who received a full course of therapy had significant improvement in muscle strength and function, skin and extramuscular disease activity, and serum levels of lactate dehydrogenase. Clinical improvement continued or was maintained for 6 months to 7 years after discontinuation of cyclophosphamide. The primary adverse events were reversible lymphopenia, infection with *Herpes zoster*, and alopecia. In London, at the Great Ormond Street Hospital, similar success was preliminarily reported in a larger series of 56 patients for whom cyclophosphamide pulse therapy was used.[89] In addition, calcinosis improved in 9 of 14 patients (64%).

The use of adrenocorticotropic hormone (ACTH) gel administered subcutaneously (80 IU once or twice weekly) in 5 adult treatment-refractory DM patients, including one adult with JDM, resulted in moderately improved muscle strength, physical function, and skin rashes and decreased pain over 12 weeks.[104] ACTH gel is the only medication approved by the Food and Drug Administration for the treatment of myositis. Although additional studies in adults will clarify its safety and effectiveness, ACTH gel could be used in selected treatment-refractory patients who are having trouble with absorption of oral corticosteroids because of vasculopathy,[82] in patients who are noncompliant with oral medications, and as a bridge medication for a brief period.

Biologic Therapies

Several open-label studies, case reports, and small trials have been recently completed that provide initial insights into the role of biologic therapies to treat refractory JDM.

Rituximab depletes CD20+ B cells, which are elevated in the peripheral blood and muscle of patients with active disease, and might also diminish the production of myositis autoantibodies. Rituximab demonstrated early promise in open-label trials and case reports, with more than 70% of treatment-refractory patients improving clinically.[90] In an early report, 3 of 4 patients with treatment-refractory JDM entered remission after rituximab administration for up to 12 to 14 months.[91] A review of rituximab use in 12 patients with treatment-refractory JDM (most received rituximab weekly at a dose of 375 mg/m^2 for 4 weeks) found that 9 patients (75%) had improved muscle or cutaneous disease activity, and 5 (42%) achieved remission for up to 20 months.[105] However, an open-label trial of rituximab in 8 adult patients with refractory DM showed that 3 patients improved their muscle strength at week 24, but there was no benefit for DM skin disease.[92]

A large, multicenter, randomized controlled trial has now been completed in which 48 patients with JDM, 76 with adult DM, and 76 with adult PM were randomized to receive rituximab (575 mg/m^2 or 750 mg/m^2 per dose for 2 weekly infusions or placebo at weeks 0 and 1 followed by placebo, or placebo followed by rituximab at weeks 8 and 9), using a randomized placebo-phase design.[93] Although 83% of these treatment-refractory patients responded to rituximab and could significantly decrease the corticosteroid dose after rituximab therapy, there was no difference in the time to response in the two treatment arms, the primary trial end point. However, the study was not designed to have adequate power to detect a significant difference between treatment arms within the JDM cohort.[93] For JDM, the time to response was a median of 12 weeks, compared with 20 weeks overall. It is unclear from this trial whether rituximab is effective in myositis or whether there was a failure of trial design, including too short a placebo period to detect a difference in the clinical response of the early rituximab group versus placebo and/or a failure of the preliminarily validated outcome measures.[106] Patients with JDM, with anti-synthetase or anti-Mi-2 autoantibodies, and those with a lower disease damage score seem to have a more rapid response to rituximab.[77] Safety concerns with rituximab include infusion reactions (many of which respond to adequate premedication regimens), infections, and, rarely, progressive multifocal leukoencephalopathy.[93,107] Accordingly, the authors do not recommend routine re-administration of rituximab at scheduled times after completion of one course of rituximab but rather when there is evidence of worsening disease activity following B cell return. Whether rituximab will prove useful in the treatment of early disease or whether other B cell–depleting agents may be helpful in the IIM remains to be determined.

The biologic rationales for the use of anti–tumor necrosis factor (TNFα) in the therapy for JDM are that elevated levels of TNFα are present in the muscle and peripheral blood of patients with active disease[97,99] and that a proinflammatory TNFα promoter polymorphism is associated with the development of calcinosis and ulcerations.[108] Reports suggest mixed benefit and some worsening in patients receiving anti-TNFα therapies. Perhaps the greatest benefit observed was with the use of infliximab in open-label studies of patients with treatment-refractory JDM. One case series of 5 patients with refractory JDM given infliximab reported improvement in muscle strength and other core set activity measures as well as in calcinosis.[94] A larger study of 30 patients with JDM treated with infliximab found improvement in muscle strength and physical function, muscle enzyme levels, skin rashes, and physician global disease activity in more than 70% of treatment-refractory patients.[95] Calcinosis improved in 46%. Improvements were not as dramatic or frequent using other anti-TNFα agents, including etanercept and adalimumab.[95]

A randomized controlled trial of infliximab in 11 patients with refractory adult PM and 1 with DM had mixed success; approximately 25% had improved muscle strength and function during the randomized portion of the trial,[109] and 7 of 12 patients (58%) met the criteria for the IMACS preliminary definition of improvement. Other reports of infliximab to treat adult patients with refractory DM and PM also show mild benefit,[110] but several open-label trials later reported disease progression or worsening with infliximab therapy in patients with refractory adult DM and PM.[111] In one trial of infliximab in 9 adult patients with refractory DM, PM, or IBM, 3 improved by the IMACS definition of improvement, 4 were unchanged, and 2 worsened; no patient improved in muscle strength by manual muscle testing. Muscle edema on MRI worsened in 5 patients, and proinflammatory cytokines and type I interferon activity increased after treatment.[112]

An open-label trial of etanercept in 10 patients with refractory JDM reported mild improvement in overall disease activity by the Disease Activity Score but no improvement in muscle strength, function, or skin activity.[113] In contrast, in a randomized placebo-controlled trial of etanercept in adult DM, 11 etanercept-treated patients had a longer time to disease flare and greater ability to lower prednisone dose compared with 5 patients receiving placebo.[114] Although core set measures of disease activity, including physician global activity, muscle strength, and physical function, improved during the 52-week trial, there was no difference between etanercept-treated patients and those in the placebo group. Reports of the development or exacerbation of adult DM after the use of etanercept or adalimumab for the treatment of arthritis suggest further caution in the use of anti-TNFα therapies in the treatment of JIIM.[115]

The evidence for using other biologic therapies to treat JDM is even sparser, consisting of single open-label trials in patients with adult IIM or case reports in patients with treatment-refractory JIIM. For example, an open-label trial of anakinra in 15 patients with refractory adult DM, PM, and IBM showed clinical response in 7 patients, which correlated best with those who had higher extramuscular activity, muscle macrophages, and interleukin (IL)-1α expression.[116] There are no reports to date of IL-1 blockade in JDM.

In an early phase IB randomized, placebo controlled, dose-ranging study of the anti-interferon α monoclonal antibody sifalimumab in adult DM and PM, the type I interferon gene signature and interferon-inducible proteins were suppressed in the peripheral blood by 53% to 66% from 28 to 98 days after administration and in the muscle by 47% at day 98. Patients with a greater degree of improvement in manual muscle testing scores showed greater inhibition of the interferon gene signature.[117]

A single patient with severe refractory JDM gained improvement in muscle strength, function, and skin activity, including cutaneous ulcerations, after administration of abatacept.[118] A beneficial effect of tocilizumab was reported in 2 adult patients with refractory PM who had improved CK levels and muscle edema on MRI.[119]

Alemtuzumab (CAMPATH 1H) at an immunoablative dose was used to treat a single patient with severe refractory JPM.[120] Clinical improvement began 6 months after the infusion and continued to 12 months; 2 courses were required for sustained remission, with achievement of normal strength and function, normal enzyme levels, and ability to taper off all immunosuppressive medication. A nonablative regimen of alemtuzumab was examined in an open-label trial of 13 patients with IBM in which strength improved by a mean of 11% after 6 months of therapy, and 8 patients (62%) had moderate improvement in their daily life functional activities, which compared favorably with the prior decline in strength and function before the initiation of treatment. Endomysial inflammation, including expression of CD3+ T lymphocytes and stressor molecules in the muscle, was reduced following therapy.[121]

Cell-based therapy has been reserved for treatment-resistant and life-threatening IIM. Three patients with severe treatment-refractory JDM who failed to respond to several conventional therapies improved dramatically after autologous stem cell transplantation.[122,123] Two of these patients with JDM who were wheelchair bound and had severe, extensive disease activity entered sustained remission after an immunoablative conditioning regimen of fludarabine, cyclophosphamide, and anti–thymocyte globulin, and engraftment of a CD3/CD19-depleted graft. These patients had near normalization of strength and function and discontinued other medications; one patient also had dissolution of extensive calcinosis.[123]

Treatment of Skin Disease and Rehabilitation

Evidence of a role for UV radiation in the cause of DM and other systemic autoimmune diseases is mounting. A direct relationship was found between UV radiation exposure, based on UV surface exposure at the patients' residence location, and the proportion of patients with DM versus PM, as well as the proportion of patients with DM-associated MSAs, including anti-p155/140 and anti-Mi-2 autoantibodies.[124] UV radiation may lead to local inflammation in the skin and alter the expression of auto-antigens.[125,126] Daily application of sunscreens protecting against both UV-A and UV-B light with an sun protection factor of at least 30 and reapplication after 2 hours in the sun is recommended for patients with JDM, based on expert consensus.[127,128] The use of other photoprotective measures, such as sun avoidance, photoprotective clothing, wide-brimmed hats, and the use of laminated glass in car windows may also be helpful.[129]

Many therapeutic agents used to treat muscle disease are also effective for treating cutaneous disease. Specific use of topical corticosteroids or topical immunomodulators (tacrolimus, pimecrolimus) can be helpful for limited rashes when disease activity is confined to the skin and not amenable to systemic therapy or for more severe rashes, including scalp involvement.[127] Antihistamines and moisturizers are helpful for treating associated pruritus, given the presence of dermal mast cells in the skin of patients with JDM.[130] Hydroxychloroquine, which inhibits Toll-like receptor activation, has anecdotally been helpful as an adjunctive agent, and has been shown to improve cutaneous and renal disease activity and prevent disease damage in lupus.[131] Cutaneous ulcerations have anecdotally been reported to improve with IVIG, cyclophosphamide, abatacept, and with the surgical use of artificial skin and wound debridement protocols.[118,132]

Therapeutic approaches for the treatment of calcinosis, which are based on small open-label case series and reports, include aggressive antiinflammatory therapy for the underlying JDM disease activity, such as treatment with IVIG, IVMP pulses, mycophenolate mofetil, cyclophosphamide, infliximab, abatacept, and others, with reports of improvement in calcinosis lesions in more than half of patients.[85,94] Medications that alter the metabolism of calcium or phosphorous, such as calcium channel blockers, aluminum hydroxide, and probenecid, have had mixed success.[133,134] In 8 patients with JDM, bisphosphonates, particularly pamidronate, which inhibit the conversion of calcium phosphate into crystalline hydroxyapatite and the nucleation of hydroxyapatite, as well as inhibit macrophage function, were reported to improve calcinosis lesions and arrest progression.[133,134] Sodium thiosulfate, a calcium chelator and vasodilator that has been used to treat calciphylaxis, was reported to improve severe calcinosis in a few patients when applied topically and administered intravenously.[118] Surgical resection, extracorporeal shock wave lithotripsy, and carbon dioxide laser therapy may improve associated pain and functional disability for severe lesions.[133,134]

Aerobic fitness is a significant health challenge to patients with JIIM. Studies have documented decreased aerobic capacity related to disease activity, muscle damage, and duration of active disease.[135] However, evidence is slowly accruing that exercise training for patients with JIIM is safe and beneficial. A single isometric strengthening exercise session did not increase muscle inflammation in children with active or inactive JDM, as assessed by serum muscle enzymes and MRI.[136] However, longer-term interventions are needed. Several studies in adult IIM have found that isometric and isotonic strengthening, range of motion, and aerobic exercise of 6 to 24 weeks' duration were safe in patients with inactive or chronic active disease, without inducing muscle inflammation. Most of these 16 primarily uncontrolled studies also documented improvement in strength, muscle endurance, physical function, and quality of life.[137] A single open-label pilot trial in 10 patients with mild, chronic JDM examined the effects of supervised, twice-weekly aerobic and resistance exercise training.[138] Deleterious effects on muscle enzymes were not observed. On the other hand, muscle strength and function, aerobic conditioning, bone mass, muscle mass, global disease activity, and health-related quality of life all improved after 12 weeks of exercise training.

SUMMARY

The JIIM are heterogeneous diseases defined by clinicopathologic groups and myositis autoantibody phenotypes, which segregate patients sharing similar demographic and clinical features, laboratory abnormalities, and prognoses into more homogeneous subsets. These phenotypes are similar in children and adults within the same subgroup. Treatments have advanced to include more aggressive approaches in the initial treatment of JDM, typically consisting of daily oral prednisone and methotrexate, often in conjunction with another medication. Thus far, several open-label studies and a few randomized trials support the use of several drugs and biologic agents for patients with treatment-refractory disease, severe illness manifestations, and poor prognoses. Attention to the therapy for skin disease, including photoprotective measures, and rehabilitation are also important. Recognition of the heterogeneity of juvenile myositis will lead to tailored, individualized therapies aimed at optimizing each patient's outcome. In addition, the use of validated core set outcome measures has laid a foundation for needed randomized trials and quality clinical studies that should better inform future therapies.

ACKNOWLEDGMENTS

The authors thank Drs Adriana Almeida de Jesus and Hanna Kim for the critical reading of the article, Dr Frederick Miller for his support of this research on natural history and therapy for juvenile myositis, and the CureJM Foundation for their support of the George Washington University Myositis Clinic. The authors also thank the patients and physicians who have participated in the Childhood Myositis Heterogeneity Study and the George Washington University Myositis Clinic for helping to better define the classification of the juvenile idiopathic inflammatory myopathies.

REFERENCES

1. Bohan A, Peter JB. Polymyositis and dermatomyositis. Parts 1 and 2. N Engl J Med 1975;292:344–7, 3403–7.
2. Brown VE, Pilkington CA, Feldman BM, et al. An international consensus survey of the diagnostic criteria for juvenile dermatomyositis (JDM). Rheumatology (Oxford) 2006;45:990–3.
3. Rider LG, Miller FW. Classification and treatment of the juvenile idiopathic inflammatory myopathies. Rheum Dis Clin North Am 1997;23:619–55.
4. Rider LG, Miller FW. Deciphering the clinical presentations, pathogenesis, and treatment of the idiopathic inflammatory myopathies. JAMA 2011;305:183–90.
5. Shah M, Targoff IN, Rice MM, et al. The clinical phenotypes of the juvenile idiopathic inflammatory myopathies. Medicine 2013;92:25–41.
6. Mohassel P, Mammen AL. Statin-associated autoimmune myopathy and anti-HMGCR autoantibodies: a review. Muscle Nerve 2013. [Epub ahead of print]. http://dx.doi.org/10.1002/mus.23854.
7. McCann LJ, Juggins AD, Maillard SM, et al. The juvenile dermatomyositis national registry and repository (UK and Ireland)–clinical characteristics of children recruited within the first 5 yr. Rheumatology (Oxford) 2006;45:1255–60.
8. Sato JO, Sallum AM, Ferriani VP, et al. A Brazilian registry of juvenile dermatomyositis: onset features and classification of 189 cases. Clin Exp Rheumatol 2009;27:1031–8.
9. Guseinova D, Consolaro A, Trail L, et al. Comparison of clinical features and drug therapies among European and Latin American patients with juvenile dermatomyositis. Clin Exp Rheumatol 2011;29:117–24.
10. Sallum AM, Pivato FC, Doria-Filho U, et al. Risk factors associated with calcinosis of juvenile dermatomyositis. J Pediatr (Rio J) 2008;84:68–74.
11. Bingham A, Mamyrova G, Rother KI, et al. Predictors of acquired lipodystrophy in juvenile-onset dermatomyositis and a gradient of severity. Medicine (Baltimore) 2008;87:70–86.
12. Wedderburn LR, McHugh NJ, Chinoy H, et al. HLA class II haplotype and autoantibody associations in children with juvenile dermatomyositis and juvenile dermatomyositis-scleroderma overlap. Rheumatology (Oxford) 2007;46:1786–91.
13. Huber AM, Mamyrova G, Lee JA, et al. Illness features associated with an increased risk of mortality in children with juvenile idiopathic inflammatory myopathies. Arthritis Rheum 2012;64(Suppl 10):S127–8.
14. Lorenzoni PJ, Scola RH, Kay CS, et al. Idiopathic inflammatory myopathies in childhood: a brief review of 27 cases. Pediatr Neurol 2011;45:17–22.
15. Gerami P, Walling HW, Lewis J, et al. A systematic review of juvenile-onset clinically amyopathic dermatomyositis. Br J Dermatol 2007;157:637–44.
16. Mukamel M, Brik R. Amyopathic dermatomyositis in children: a diagnostic and therapeutic dilemma. J Clin Rheumatol 2001;7:191–3.
17. Plamondon S, Dent PB. Juvenile amyopathic dermatomyositis: results of a case finding descriptive survey. J Rheumatol 2000;27:2031–4.
18. Dimachkie MM, Barohn RJ. Inclusion body myositis. Curr Neurol Neurosci Rep 2013;13:321.

19. Limaye V, Luke C, Tucker G, et al. The incidence and associations of malignancy in a large cohort of patients with biopsy-determined idiopathic inflammatory myositis. Rheumatol Int 2013;33:965–71.

20. Ibarra M, Chou P, Pachman LM. Ovarian teratoma mimicking features of juvenile dermatomyositis in a child. Pediatrics 2011;128:e1293–6.

21. Morris P, Dare J. Juvenile dermatomyositis as a paraneoplastic phenomenon: an update. J Pediatr Hematol Oncol 2010;32:189–91.

22. Auerbach A, Fanburg-Smith JC, Wang G, et al. Focal myositis: a clinicopathologic study of 115 cases of an intramuscular mass-like reactive process. Am J Surg Pathol 2009;33:1016–24.

23. Smith AG, Urbanits S, Blaivas M, et al. Clinical and pathologic features of focal myositis. Muscle Nerve 2000;23:1569–75.

24. Fraser CL, Skalicky SE, Gurbaxani A, et al. Ocular myositis. Curr Allergy Asthma Rep 2013;13:315–21.

25. Costa RM, Dumitrascu OM, Gordon LK. Orbital myositis: diagnosis and management. Curr Allergy Asthma Rep 2009;9:316–23.

26. Wallace ZS, Khosroshahi A, Jakobiec FA, et al. IgG4-related systemic disease as a cause of "idiopathic" orbital inflammation, including orbital myositis, and trigeminal nerve involvement. Surv Ophthalmol 2012;57:26–33.

27. Kondolot M, Unal E, Poyrazoglu G, et al. Orbital myositis associated with focal active colitis in a teenage girl. Childs Nerv Syst 2012;28:641–3.

28. Rouster-Stevens KA, Pachman LM. Autoantibody to signal recognition particle in African American girls with juvenile polymyositis. J Rheumatol 2008;35: 927–9.

29. Israeli E, Agmon-Levin N, Blank M, et al. Macrophagic myofasciitis a vaccine (alum) autoimmune-related disease. Clin Rev Allergy Immunol 2011;41: 163–8.

30. Gruis KL, Teener JW, Blaivas M. Pediatric macrophagic myofasciitis associated with motor delay. Clin Neuropathol 2006;25:172–9.

31. Rivas E, Gomez-Arnaiz M, Ricoy JR, et al. Macrophagic myofasciitis in childhood: a controversial entity. Pediatr Neurol 2005;33:350–6.

32. Lach B, Cupler EJ. Macrophagic myofasciitis in children is a localized reaction to vaccination. J Child Neurol 2008;23:614–9.

33. Pickering MC, Walport MJ. Eosinophilic myopathic syndromes. Curr Opin Rheumatol 1998;10:504–10.

34. Dourmishev LA, Dourmishev AL. Activity of certain drugs in inducing of inflammatory myopathies with cutaneous manifestations. Expert Opin Drug Saf 2008; 7:421–33.

35. Brown RH Jr, Amato A. Calpainopathy and eosinophilic myositis. Ann Neurol 2006;59:875–7.

36. Baumeister SK, Todorovic S, Milic-Rasic V, et al. Eosinophilic myositis as presenting symptom in gamma-sarcoglycanopathy. Neuromuscul Disord 2009;19: 167–71.

37. Hewer E, Goebel HH. Myopathology of non-infectious inflammatory myopathies - the current status. Pathol Res Pract 2008;204:609–23.

38. Le RK, Streichenberger N, Vial C, et al. Granulomatous myositis: a clinical study of thirteen cases. Muscle Nerve 2007;35:171–7.

39. Wong NL, Di F. Pseudosarcomatous fasciitis and myositis: diagnosis by fine-needle aspiration cytology. Am J Clin Pathol 2009;132:857–65.

40. Talbert RJ, Laor T, Yin H. Proliferative myositis: expanding the differential diagnosis of a soft tissue mass in infancy. Skeletal Radiol 2011;40:1623–7.

41. Stevens AM, Sullivan KM, Nelson JL. Polymyositis as a manifestation of chronic graft-versus-host disease. Rheumatology (Oxford) 2003;42:34–9.
42. Pegoraro E, Mancias P, Swerdlow SH, et al. Congenital muscular dystrophy with primary laminin alpha2 (merosin) deficiency presenting as inflammatory myopathy. Ann Neurol 1996;40:782–91.
43. Ravelli A, Trail L, Ferrari C, et al. Long-term outcome and prognostic factors of juvenile dermatomyositis: a multinational, multicenter study of 490 patients. Arthritis Care Res (Hoboken) 2010;62:63–72.
44. Stringer E, Singh-Grewal D, Feldman BM. Predicting the course of juvenile dermatomyositis: significance of early clinical and laboratory features. Arthritis Rheum 2008;58:3585–92.
45. Christen-Zaech S, Seshadri R, Sundberg J, et al. Persistent association of nail fold capillaroscopy changes and skin involvement over thirty-six months with duration of untreated disease in patients with juvenile dermatomyositis. Arthritis Rheum 2008;58:571–6.
46. Miles L, Bove KE, Lovell D, et al. Predictability of the clinical course of juvenile dermatomyositis based on initial muscle biopsy: a retrospective study of 72 patients. Arthritis Rheum 2007;57:1183–91.
47. Kim S, El-Hallak M, Dedeoglu F, et al. Complete and sustained remission of juvenile dermatomyositis resulting from aggressive treatment. Arthritis Rheum 2009;60:1825–30.
48. Eidelman N, Boyde A, Bushby AJ, et al. Microstructure and mineral composition of dystrophic calcification associated with the idiopathic inflammatory myopathies. Arthritis Res Ther 2009;11:R159.
49. Aikawa NE, Jesus AA, Liphaus BL, et al. Organ-specific autoantibodies and autoimmune diseases in juvenile systemic lupus erythematosus and juvenile dermatomyositis patients. Clin Exp Rheumatol 2012;30:126–31.
50. Mamyrova G, Katz JD, Jones RV, et al. Clinical and Laboratory Features Distinguishing Juvenile Polymyositis and Muscular Dystrophy. Arthritis Care and Reseach 2013, in press.
51. Gerami P, Schope JM, McDonald L, et al. A systematic review of adult-onset clinically amyopathic dermatomyositis (dermatomyositis sine myositis): a missing link within the spectrum of the idiopathic inflammatory myopathies. J Am Acad Dermatol 2006;54:597–613.
52. Abe Y, Koyasu Y, Watanabe S, et al. Juvenile amyopathic dermatomyositis complicated by progressive interstitial pneumonia. Pediatr Int 2010;52:149–53.
53. Kalil RK, Monteiro A Jr, Lima MI, et al. Macrophagic myofasciitis in childhood: the role of scanning electron microscopy/energy-dispersive spectroscopy for diagnosis. Ultrastruct Pathol 2007;31:45–50.
54. Rider LG, Shah M, Mamyrova G, et al. The myositis autoantibody phenotypes of the juvenile idiopathic inflammatory myopathies. Medicine 2013;92(4):223–43.
55. Gunawardena H, Wedderburn LR, North J, et al. Clinical associations of autoantibodies to a p155/140 kDa doublet protein in juvenile dermatomyositis. Rheumatology (Oxford) 2008;47:324–8.
56. Trallero-Araguas E, Rodrigo-Pendas JA, Selva-O'Callaghan A, et al. Usefulness of anti-p155 autoantibody for diagnosing cancer-associated dermatomyositis: a systematic review and meta-analysis. Arthritis Rheum 2012;64:523–32.
57. Gunawardena H, Wedderburn LR, Chinoy H, et al. Autoantibodies to a 140-kd protein in juvenile dermatomyositis are associated with calcinosis. Arthritis Rheum 2009;60:1807–14.

58. Espada G, Maldonado Cocco JA, Fertig N, et al. Clinical and serologic characterization of an Argentine pediatric myositis cohort: identification of a novel autoantibody (anti-MJ) to a 142-kDa protein. J Rheumatol 2009;36:2547–51.
59. Kobayashi I, Okura Y, Yamada M, et al. Anti-melanoma differentiation-associated gene 5 antibody is a diagnostic and predictive marker for interstitial lung diseases associated with juvenile dermatomyositis. J Pediatr 2011;158:675–7.
60. Sakurai N, Nagai K, Tsutsumi H, et al. Anti-CADM-140 antibody-positive juvenile dermatomyositis with rapidly progressive interstitial lung disease and cardiac involvement. J Rheumatol 2011;38:963–4.
61. Koga T, Fujikawa K, Horai Y, et al. The diagnostic utility of anti-melanoma differentiation-associated gene 5 antibody testing for predicting the prognosis of Japanese patients with DM. Rheumatology (Oxford) 2012;51:1278–84.
62. Cao H, Pan M, Kang Y, et al. Clinical manifestations of dermatomyositis and clinically amyopathic dermatomyositis patients with positive expression of anti-melanoma differentiation-associated gene 5 antibody. Arthritis Care Res (Hoboken) 2012;64:1602–10.
63. Fujimoto M, Hamaguchi Y, Kaji K, et al. Myositis-specific anti-155/140 autoantibodies target transcription intermediary factor 1 family proteins. Arthritis Rheum 2012;64:513–22.
64. Fujimoto M, Matsushita T, Hamaguchi Y, et al. Autoantibodies to small ubiquitin-like modifier activating enzymes in Japanese patients with dermatomyositis: comparison with a UK Caucasian cohort. Ann Rheum Dis 2013;72:151–3.
65. Tarricone E, Ghirardello A, Rampudda M, et al. Anti-SAE antibodies in autoimmune myositis: identification by unlabelled protein immunoprecipitation in an Italian patient cohort. J Immunol Methods 2012;384:128–34.
66. Vancsa A, Gergely L, Ponyi A, et al. Myositis-specific and myositis-associated antibodies in overlap myositis in comparison to primary dermatopolymyositis: relevance for clinical classification: retrospective study of 169 patients. Joint Bone Spine 2010;77:125–30.
67. Koenig M, Fritzler MJ, Targoff IN, et al. Heterogeneity of autoantibodies in 100 patients with autoimmune myositis: insights into clinical features and outcomes. Arthritis Res Ther 2007;9:R78.
68. Marie I, Hatron PY, Dominique S, et al. Short-term and long-term outcome of anti-Jo1-positive patients with anti-Ro52 antibody. Semin Arthritis Rheum 2012;41:890–9.
69. Mahler M, Raijmakers R. Novel aspects of autoantibodies to the PM/Scl complex: clinical, genetic and diagnostic insights. Autoimmun Rev 2007;6:432–7.
70. Marie I, Lahaxe L, Benveniste O, et al. Long-term outcome of patients with polymyositis/dermatomyositis and anti-PM-Scl antibody. Br J Dermatol 2010;162:337–44.
71. Rigolet A, Musset L, Dubourg O, et al. Inflammatory myopathies with anti-Ku antibodies: a prognosis dependent on associated lung disease. Medicine (Baltimore) 2012;91:95–102.
72. Targoff IN, Mamyrova G, Trieu EP, et al. A novel autoantibody to a 155-kd protein is associated with dermatomyositis. Arthritis Rheum 2006;54:3682–9.
73. Ghirardello A, Rampudda M, Ekholm L, et al. Diagnostic performance and validation of autoantibody testing in myositis by a commercial line blot assay. Rheumatology (Oxford) 2010;49:2370–4.
74. Rider LG, Werth VP, Huber AM, et al. Measures of adult and juvenile dermatomyositis, polymyositis, and inclusion body myositis: Physician and Patient/Parent Global Activity, Manual Muscle Testing (MMT), Health Assessment Questionnaire

(HAQ)/Childhood Health Assessment Questionnaire (C-HAQ), Childhood Myositis Assessment Scale (CMAS), Myositis Disease Activity Assessment Tool (MDAAT), Disease Activity Score (DAS), Short Form 36 (SF-36), Child Health Questionnaire (CHQ), physician global damage, Myositis Damage Index (MDI), Quantitative Muscle Testing (QMT), Myositis Functional Index-2 (FI-2), Myositis Activities Profile (MAP), Inclusion Body Myositis Functional Rating Scale (IBMFRS), Cutaneous Dermatomyositis Disease Area and Severity Index (CDASI), Cutaneous Assessment Tool (CAT), Dermatomyositis Skin Severity Index (DSSI), Skindex, and Dermatology Life Quality Index (DLQI). Arthritis Care Res (Hoboken) 2011;63(Suppl 11):S118–57.

75. Rider LG, Giannini EH, Brunner HI, et al. International consensus on preliminary definitions of improvement in adult and juvenile myositis. Arthritis Rheum 2004; 50:2281–90.

76. Ruperto N, Pistorio A, Ravelli A, et al. The Paediatric Rheumatology International Trials Organisation provisional criteria for the evaluation of response to therapy in juvenile dermatomyositis. Arthritis Care Res (Hoboken) 2010;62: 1533–41.

77. Oddis CV, Reed AM, Aggarwal R, et al. Rituximab in the treatment of refractory adult and juvenile dermatomyositis and adult polymyositis: a randomized, placebo-phase trial. Arthritis Rheum 2013;65:314–24.

78. Ruperto N, Pistorio A, Oliveira S, et al. A randomized trial in new onset juvenile dermatomyositis: prednisone versus prednisone plus cyclosporine versus prednisone plus methotrexate. Arthritis Rheum 2012;64(Suppl 10):S1042–3.

79. Huber AM, Giannini EH, Bowyer SL, et al. Protocols for the initial treatment of moderately severe juvenile dermatomyositis: results of a Children's Arthritis and Rheumatology Research Alliance Consensus Conference. Arthritis Care Res (Hoboken) 2010;62:219–25.

80. Huber AM, Robinson AB, Reed AM, et al. Consensus treatments for moderate juvenile dermatomyositis: beyond the first two months. Results of the second Childhood Arthritis and Rheumatology Research Alliance Consensus Conference. Arthritis Care Res (Hoboken) 2012;64:546–53.

81. Seshadri R, Feldman BM, Ilowite N, et al. The role of aggressive corticosteroid therapy in patients with juvenile dermatomyositis: a propensity score analysis. Arthritis Rheum 2008;59:989–95.

82. Rouster-Stevens KA, Gursahaney A, Ngai KL, et al. Pharmacokinetic study of oral prednisolone compared with intravenous methylprednisolone in patients with juvenile dermatomyositis. Arthritis Rheum 2008;59:222–6.

83. Ramanan AV, Campbell-Webster N, Ota S, et al. The effectiveness of treating juvenile dermatomyositis with methotrexate and aggressively tapered corticosteroids. Arthritis Rheum 2005;52:3570–8.

84. Lam CG, Manlhiot C, Pullenayegum EM, et al. Efficacy of intravenous Ig therapy in juvenile dermatomyositis. Ann Rheum Dis 2011;70:2089–94.

85. Dagher R, Desjonqueres M, Duquesne A, et al. Mycophenolate mofetil in juvenile dermatomyositis: a case series. Rheumatol Int 2012;32:711–6.

86. Wilkes MR, Sereika SM, Fertig N, et al. Treatment of antisynthetase-associated interstitial lung disease with tacrolimus. Arthritis Rheum 2005;52:2439–46.

87. Hassan J, van der Net JJ, van Royen-Kerkhof A. Treatment of refractory juvenile dermatomyositis with tacrolimus. Clin Rheumatol 2008;27:1469–71.

88. Riley P, Maillard SM, Wedderburn LR, et al. Intravenous cyclophosphamide pulse therapy in juvenile dermatomyositis. A review of efficacy and safety. Rheumatology (Oxford) 2004;43:491–6.

89. Moraitis E, Arnold K, Pilkington C. Effectiveness of intravenous cyclophospha-mide in severe or refractory juvenile dermatomyositis - a national cohort study UK and Ireland [abstract]. Arthritis Rheum 2012;64(Suppl 10):S130–1.

90. Aggarwal R, Oddis CV, Bandos A, et al. Effect of B cell depletion therapy with rituximab on myositis associated autoantibody levels in idiopathic inflammatory myopathy. Arthritis Rheum 2012;64(Suppl 10):S325.

91. Rios FR, Callejas Rubio JL, Sanchez CD, et al. Rituximab in the treatment of dermatomyositis and other inflammatory myopathies. A report of 4 cases and review of the literature. Clin Exp Rheumatol 2009;27:1009–16.

92. Cooper MA, Willingham DL, Brown DE, et al. Rituximab for the treatment of juvenile dermatomyositis: a report of four pediatric patients. Arthritis Rheum 2007;56:3107–11.

93. Chung L, Genovese MC, Fiorentino DF. A pilot trial of rituximab in the treatment of patients with dermatomyositis. Arch Dermatol 2007;143:763–7.

94. Riley P, McCann LJ, Maillard SM, et al. Effectiveness of infliximab in the treat-ment of refractory juvenile dermatomyositis with calcinosis. Rheumatology (Oxford) 2008;47:877–80.

95. Boulter EL, Beard L, Ryder C, et al. Juvenile Dermatomyositis Research Group. Effectiveness of anti-tumor necrosis factor- agents in the treatment of refractory juvenile dermatomyositis. Arthritis Rheum 2011;63(Suppl 10):S795.

96. Aggarwal R, Oddis CV. Therapeutic advances in myositis. Curr Opin Rheumatol 2012;24:635–41.

97. Nagaraju K, Lundberg IE. Polymyositis and dermatomyositis: pathophysiology. Rheum Dis Clin North Am 2011;37:159–71, v.

98. Rider LG, Lachenbruch PA, Monroe JB, et al. Damage extent and predictors in adult and juvenile dermatomyositis and polymyositis as determined with the myositis damage index. Arthritis Rheum 2009;60:3425–35.

99. Robinson AB, Reed AM. Clinical features, pathogenesis and treatment of juve-nile and adult dermatomyositis. Nat Rev Rheumatol 2011;7:664–75.

100. Stringer E, Bohnsack J, Bowyer SL, et al. Treatment approaches to juvenile der-matomyositis (JDM) across North America: the Childhood Arthritis and Rheuma-tology Research Alliance (CARRA) JDM Treatment Survey. J Rheumatol 2010; 37:1953–61.

101. Hasija R, Pistorio A, Ravelli A, et al. Therapeutic approaches in the treatment of juvenile dermatomyositis in patients with recent-onset disease and in those experiencing disease flare: an international multicenter PRINTO study. Arthritis Rheum 2011;63:3142–52.

102. Dalakas MC, Illa I, Dambrosia JM, et al. A controlled trial of high-does intrave-nous immune globulin infusions as treatment for dermatomyositis. N Engl J Med 1993;329:1993–2000.

103. Manlhiot C, Tyrrell PN, Liang L, et al. Safety of intravenous immunoglobulin in the treatment of juvenile dermatomyositis: adverse reactions are associated with immunoglobulin A content. Pediatrics 2008;121:e626–30.

104. Levine T. Treating refractory dermatomyositis or polymyositis with adrenocortico-tropic hormone gel: a retrospective case series. Drug Des Devel Ther 2012;6: 133–9.

105. Chiu YE, Co DO. Juvenile dermatomyositis: immunopathogenesis, role of myositis-specific autoantibodies, and review of rituximab use. Pediatr Dermatol 2011;28:357–67.

106. de Visser M. The efficacy of rituximab in refractory myositis: the jury is still out. Arthritis Rheum 2013;65:303–6.

107. Molloy ES, Calabrese LH. Progressive multifocal leukoencephalopathy associated with immunosuppressive therapy in rheumatic diseases: evolving role of biologic therapies. Arthritis Rheum 2012;64:3043–51.
108. Mamyrova G, O'Hanlon TP, Sillers L, et al. Cytokine gene polymorphisms as risk and severity factors for juvenile dermatomyositis. Arthritis Rheum 2008;58: 3941–50.
109. Coyle K, Pokrovnichka A, French K, et al. A randomized, double-blind, placebo-controlled trial of infliximab in patients with polymyositis and dermatomyositis. Arthritis Rheum 2008;58(Suppl 9):S923–4.
110. Hengstman GJ, van den Hoogen FH, Barrera P, et al. Successful treatment of dermatomyositis and polymyositis with anti-tumor-necrosis-factor-alpha: preliminary observations. Eur Neurol 2003;50:10–5.
111. Hengstman GJ, De Bleecker JL, Feist E, et al. Open-label trial of anti-TNF-alpha in dermato- and polymyositis treated concomitantly with methotrexate. Eur Neurol 2008;59:159–63.
112. Dastmalchi M, Grundtman C, Alexanderson H, et al. A high incidence of disease flares in an open pilot study of infliximab in patients with refractory inflammatory myopathies. Ann Rheum Dis 2008;67:1670–7.
113. Miller ML, Smith RL, Abbott KA, et al. Use of etanercept in chronic juvenile dermatomyositis (JDM). Arthritis Rheum 2002;46(Suppl 9):S306.
114. Muscle Study Group. A randomized, pilot trial of etanercept in dermatomyositis. Ann Neurol 2011;70:427–36.
115. Klein R, Rosenbach M, Kim EJ, et al. Tumor necrosis factor inhibitor-associated dermatomyositis. Arch Dermatol 2010;146:780–4.
116. Zong M, Dorph C, Dastmalchi M, et al. Anakinra treatment in patients with refractory inflammatory myopathies and possible predictive response biomarkers: a mechanistic study with 12 months follow-up. Ann Rheum Dis 2013. [Epub ahead of print].
117. Higgs BW, Zhu W, Morehouse C, et al. A phase 1b clinical trial evaluating sifalimumab, an anti-IFN-alpha monoclonal antibody, shows target neutralisation of a type I IFN signature in blood of dermatomyositis and polymyositis patients. Ann Rheum Dis 2013. [Epub ahead of print].
118. Arabshahi B, Silverman RA, Jones OY, et al. Abatacept and sodium thiosulfate for treatment of recalcitrant juvenile dermatomyositis complicated by ulceration and calcinosis. J Pediatr 2012;160:520–2.
119. Narazaki M, Hagihara K, Shima Y, et al. Therapeutic effect of tocilizumab on two patients with polymyositis. Rheumatology (Oxford) 2011;50:1344–6.
120. Reiff A, Shaham B, Weinberg KI, et al. Anti-CD52 antibody-mediated immune ablation with autologous immune recovery for the treatment of refractory juvenile polymyositis. J Clin Immunol 2011;31:615–22.
121. Dalakas MC, Rakocevic G, Schmidt J, et al. Effect of Alemtuzumab (CAMPATH 1-H) in patients with inclusion-body myositis. Brain 2009;132: 1536–44.
122. Wu FQ, Luan Z, Lai JM, et al. Treatment of refractory rheumatism among preschool children with autologous peripheral blood hematopoietic stem cell transplantation. Zhonghua Er Ke Za Zhi 2007;45:809–13.
123. Holzer U, van Royen-Kerkhof A, van der Torre P, et al. Successful autologous stem cell transplantation in two patients with juvenile dermatomyositis. Scand J Rheumatol 2010;39:88–92.
124. Shah M, Targoff IN, Rice MM, et al. Childhood Myositis Heterogeneity Collaborative Study Group. Brief report: ultraviolet radiation exposure is associated with

clinical and autoantibody phenotypes in juvenile myositis. Arthritis Rheum 2013; 65(7):1934–41.

125. Widel M. Bystander effect induced by UV radiation; why should we be interested? Postepy Hig Med Dosw (Online) 2012;66:828–37.

126. Kripke ML. Reflections on the field of photoimmunology. J Invest Dermatol 2013; 133:27–30.

127. Walling HW, Gerami P, Sontheimer RD. Juvenile-onset clinically amyopathic dermatomyositis: an overview of recent progress in diagnosis and management. Paediatr Drugs 2010;12:23–34.

128. Sambandan DR, Ratner D. Sunscreens: an overview and update. J Am Acad Dermatol 2011;64:748–58.

129. Wang SQ, Balagula Y, Osterwalder U. Photoprotection: a review of the current and future technologies. Dermatol Ther 2010;23:31–47.

130. Shrestha S, Wershil B, Sarwark JF, et al. Lesional and nonlesional skin from patients with untreated juvenile dermatomyositis displays increased numbers of mast cells and mature plasmacytoid dendritic cells. Arthritis Rheum 2010; 62:2813–22.

131. Olsen NJ, Schleich MA, Karp DR. Multifaceted effects of hydroxychloroquine in human disease. Semin Arthritis Rheum 2013. http://dx.doi.org/10.1016/j.semarthrit.2013.01.001. pii:S0049–0172(13)00006-1. [Epub ahead of print].

132. Matsuda H, Goto M, Fujiwara S. Successful treatment of intractable ulceration associated with dermatomyositis by debridement and the skin implantation of an artificial dermis sheet. J Dermatol 2011;38:1027–30.

133. Chander S, Gordon P. Soft tissue and subcutaneous calcification in connective tissue diseases. Curr Opin Rheumatol 2012;24:158–64.

134. Gutierrez A Jr, Wetter DA. Calcinosis cutis in autoimmune connective tissue diseases. Dermatol Ther 2012;25:195–206.

135. Mathiesen PR, Orngreen MC, Vissing J, et al. Aerobic fitness after JDM–a long-term follow-up study. Rheumatology (Oxford) 2013;52:287–95.

136. Maillard SM, Jones R, Owens CM, et al. Quantitative assessments of the effects of a single exercise session on muscles in juvenile dermatomyositis. Arthritis Rheum 2005;53:558–64.

137. Alexanderson H, Lundberg IE. Exercise as a therapeutic modality in patients with idiopathic inflammatory myopathies. Curr Opin Rheumatol 2012;24:201–7.

138. Omori CH, Silva CA, Sallum AM, et al. Exercise training in juvenile dermatomyositis. Arthritis Care Res (Hoboken) 2012;64:1186–94.

New Developments in Juvenile Systemic and Localized Scleroderma

Ivan Foeldvari, MD

KEYWORDS

- Juvenile localized scleroderma • Juvenile systemic sclerosis
- Doppler ultrasonography • Biomarkers

KEY POINTS

- The main organ, and that which is always involved in juvenile localized scleroderma (jLS) and juvenile systemic sclerosis (jSS), is the skin.
- The Modified Rodnan Skin Score was developed to assess the skin involvement in adult patients with systemic sclerosis, and is a primary outcome measure in therapeutic trials. It is a simple bedside examination to measure skin thickening (not tethering) in 17 anatomic areas and score it from 0 to 3.
- Ultrasonography combined with Doppler is nowadays a readily available and noninvasive imaging modality that has great potential to aid monitoring of localized scleroderma disease activity and, eventually, jSS, because it allows for the evaluation of both superficial and deep soft tissues.

INTRODUCTION

Juvenile localized scleroderma (jLS) and juvenile systemic sclerosis (jSS) are both orphan diseases, with jLS around 10 times more frequent than jSS. According a more recent cross-sectional national survey from the United Kingdom and Ireland, the incidence rate per million children per year is 3.4 (95% confidence interval [CI] 2.7–4.1) for jLS, including an incidence rate of 2.5 (95% CI 1.8–3.1) for linear scleroderma, and 0.27 (95% CI 0.1–0.5) for jSS.[1] According the German National Pediatric Rheumatology Registry (Kerndokumentation), in 2011 19 of 14 million children in Germany had documented jSS, which would give a prevalence of 1.36 per million children in Germany (Dr Kirsten Minden, Deutsche Rheumaforschungszentrum, 2013, personal communication).

Hamburger Zentrum für Kinder- und Jugendrheumatologie, Dehnhaide 120, Hamburg 22081, Germany
E-mail address: Sprechstunde@kinderrheumatologie.de

Rheum Dis Clin N Am 39 (2013) 905–920
http://dx.doi.org/10.1016/j.rdc.2013.05.003   rheumatic.theclinics.com
0889-857X/13/$ – see front matter © 2013 Elsevier Inc. All rights reserved.

It still takes some time to be diagnosed with the systemic and localized forms of juvenile scleroderma. According the cross-sectional survey conducted around 2003/2004 by Martini and colleagues,[2] the median time to be diagnosed with jSS was 1 year (range 0.2–18.8 years). The time gap between the appearance of symptoms and diagnosis is becoming significantly shorter; according to a current assessment in the United Kingdom this is 7 months for jSS (range 0–50 months),[3] but the range is still impressively wide. The time to be diagnosed with jLS is longer, with a median delay from onset of symptoms to being seen in a secondary care center varying from 13.1 months (range 6.9–36.5)[4] to 15 months (range 1–103).[3] In a recent study from Switzerland, the mean disease duration until diagnosis was 11.1 months (range 1.8–79) and the mean time to initiation of therapy was after disease duration of 16.6 months (range 1.8–113.4).[5]

This review focuses on the new classifications of jSS and jLS, and on the developments and adaptations of the outcome measures for certain organ involvements whereby progress has been made regarding pediatric patients.

CLASSIFICATION CRITERIA OF JUVENILE SYSTEMIC SCLEROSIS

For a long time there were no specific classification criteria for jSS.[6] As jSS differs in the course of development of organ involvement from adult systemic sclerosis, the pediatric rheumatologic community, in its capacity as the juvenile scleroderma working group of the Pediatric Rheumatology European Society (PRES), initiated a multidisciplinary project using the Delphi method, with the participation of adult rheumatologists and pediatric and adult dermatologists, which ultimately established new proposed classification criteria (**Box 1**). This new classification is accepted by PRES, the European League Against Rheumatism (EULAR), and the American College of Rheumatology.[7]

This classification should enable an earlier diagnosis of patients. The first publications to apply these criteria are appearing.[8] This new system has one major criterion, namely proximal skin sclerosis/induration of the skin, and several minor criteria (see **Box 1**). The patient has to fulfill 1 major and at least 2 minor criteria (see **Box 1**). Each criterion was defined in the publication and represents an organ-specific presentation of juvenile scleroderma. This classification system has to be prospectively validated in a larger pediatric cohort. One of the validation projects is the Juvenile Scleroderma Inception Cohort Project (www.juvenile-scleroderma.com), in which patients with less than 18 months' disease duration after the first non-Raynaud symptom are included and prospectively followed with a standardized assessment.

CLASSIFICATION OF JUVENILE LOCALIZED SCLERODERMA

Localized scleroderma is a distinct entity from systemic sclerosis, and as yet there is no accepted uniform terminology. Dermatologists like to use the word "morphea" and rheumatologists and pediatric rheumatologists the term "localized scleroderma." In the framework of the PRES Scleroderma Working Group a preliminary proposed classification of jLS was suggested,[9,10] but this is not as widely accepted as the new classification of jSS. In **Table 1** this preliminary proposed classification, which consists of 5 types with some subgroups, is summarized. The classification criteria have not yet been prospectively tested.

OUTCOME MEASURES

A major problem in the care of children with jLS and jSS lies in assessing the activity of the disease, especially in the skin, and vascular involvement. Not even in adults are all

Box 1
Classification criteria for juvenile systemic sclerosis

Major Criterion (Required)

Proximal skin sclerosis/induration of the skin

Minor Criteria (At Least 2 Required)

Cutaneous

    Sclerodactyly

Peripheral vascular

    Raynaud phenomenon

    Nailfold capillary abnormalities

    Digital tip ulcers

Gastrointestinal

    Dysphagia

    Gastroesophageal reflux

Cardiac

    Arrhythmias

    Heart failure

Renal

    Renal crisis

    New-onset arterial hypertension

Respiratory

    Pulmonary fibrosis (high-resolution computed tomography/radiography)

    Decreased diffusing capacity of carbon monoxide

    Pulmonary arterial hypertension

Neurologic

    Neuropathy

    Carpal tunnel syndrome

Musculoskeletal

    Tendon friction rubs

    Arthritis

    Myositis

Serologic

    Antinuclear antibodies

    Systemic sclerosis–selective autoantibodies (anticentromere, anti–topoisomerase I [Scl-70], antifibrillarin, anti-PMScl, antifibrillin, or anti–RNA polymerase I or III)

Data from Zulian F, Woo P, Athreya BH, et al. The Pediatric Rheumatology European Society/ American College of Rheumatology/European League against Rheumatism provisional classification criteria for juvenile systemic sclerosis. Arthritis Rheum 2007;57(2):203–12.

Table 1
Preliminary proposed classification for juvenile localized scleroderma

Main Group	Subtype/Definition
1. Circumscribed morphea	A, Superficial B, Deep

2. Linear scleroderma	A, Trunk/limbs
	B, Head
	    c, En coup de sabre
	    cc, Parry-Romberg or progressive hemifacial atrophy

3. Generalized morphea	Four or more plaques (>3 cm) and involves at least 2 of 7 anatomic sites
4. Pansclerotic morphea	Circumferential involvement of the limbs, affecting all tissue layers including the bone
5. Mixed morphea	Combination of 2 or more previous types

Data from Laxer RM, Zulian F. Localized scleroderma. Curr Opin Rheumatol 2006;18(6):606–13.

organ-involvement assessments validated according to the OMERACT criteria.[11,12] A good outcome measure should be relevant to the goal of treatment, easy to administer, and easy to score. It should be reliable and valid and at the same time sensitive to change.

ASSESSMENT OF SKIN INVOLVEMENT

The main organ, and that which is always involved in jLS and jSS, is the skin. The extent of skin involvement can be palpated with the fingers of the physician and assessed using the Modified Rodnan Skin Score (MRSS). The skin, especially the subcutaneous components, changes during the maturation of the child, therefore the "normal skin score" changes with age.[13]

Modified Rodnan Skin Score

The MRSS was developed to assess skin involvement in adult patients with systemic sclerosis, and is a primary outcome measure in therapeutic trials. It is a simple bedside examination to measure skin thickening (not tethering) in 17 anatomic areas and award a score from 0 to 3. The MRSS has large intraobserver variability and has never been validated in children. Foeldvari and Wierk[14] applied it in 217 consecutive healthy children to establish norm values. Surprisingly, healthy children had a mean MRSS of 13.92, which is significantly elevated. It was suggested that the MRSS should be adjusted according to the age and Tanner stage of the child. The prospective assessment of the MRSS in a larger jSS patient population is pending. It is routinely applied in the Localized Scleroderma Cutaneous Assessment Tool.[15]

Durometer

The durometer is a hand-held device that assesses hardness of the skin, expressed in arbitrary units from 0 to 100 in linear distribution. The measurement can be conducted in seconds. In patients with systemic sclerosis a correlation between durometer and MRSS assessments has been found.[16,17] It has a lower intraobserver variability than the MRSS,[18] and has been used in patients with localized[19,20] and systemic scleroderma[21] to assess the treatment effect. Merkel and colleagues[21] established norm values for anatomic areas similar to those used in the MRSS. The durometer assessment showed good intraobserver correlation (0.82–0.92), and the baseline durometer values showed a good correlation with the MRSS values ($r = 0.7$). Foeldvari and colleagues (unpublished data, 2013) conducted a study to establish norm values for the durometer in children whereby values less than 30 appeared normal and were equivalent to an MRSS score of 0. The durometer cannot be used in all anatomic areas, especially if a bony surface is directly under the skin, such as the dorsal site of the fingers. Otherwise a durometer is a reliable device to access skin thickening more objectively.

Ultrasonography with Doppler to Assess Skin Involvement

Ultrasonography combined with Doppler is nowadays a readily available and noninvasive imaging modality that has great potential to aid monitoring of localized scleroderma disease activity and eventually jSS, because it allows for the evaluation of both superficial and deep soft tissues. Li and colleagues[22] established a protocol to evaluate Doppler ultrasonography in jLS for the assessment of activity. The lesions were assessed by clinicians, and features such as erythema, warmth, violaceous color, new lesion, expansion of lesion, and induration were considered to indicate active disease. The Ultrasound Disease Activity (U-DA) was assessed by a radiologist, comparing the site of the lesion with the control healthy site. The U-DA is a composite score of the echogenicity and vascularity of dermis, hypodermis, and deep tissue. Hypovascularity or hypoechogenicity had a score of -1 compared with the healthy site. No difference from the control site was scored as 0. Increased vascularity was scored 1 to 3, and increased echogenicity was scored depending on the tissue layer: dermis $+1$, hypodermis 1 to 3, and deep tissue 1 to 2. The U-DA was significantly different between active and inactive skin lesions ($P = .0010$) with significant differences found for the parameters total echogenicity, hypodermis echogenicity, and deep tissue layer vascularity ($P = .0014$, $P = .0023$, and $P = .0374$, respectively). No significant differences were found for tissue layer thickness or the Tissue Thickness Score. The U-DA promises to be a useful tool in the identification of localized scleroderma activity. Ultrasonography is not universally applicable, because it cannot be used over a bony surface situated directly under the lesion, such as on the scalp, near the eyes, or on the shin. The findings of Li and colleagues were confirmed in a further color Doppler study by Wortsman and colleagues,[23] in which the most accurate sonographic signs of lesion activity were increased subcutaneous tissue echogenicity and increased blood flow, with sensitivity and specificity both of 100%. In this study the sonographic findings correlated with histologic findings. Further prospective studies are needed to validate this Doppler ultrasonography scoring system.

Thermography and Laser Color Doppler

Thermography is not a widely available method for the assessment of activity of skin lesions, being time consuming and expensive. Infrared thermography (IRT) is of value for the assessment of the inflammatory changes associated with jLS.[24] Patients need to acclimatize to a standardized room temperature at least for 15 minutes. IRT measures skin temperature as a surrogate measure of blood flow. It is a sensitive technique but can show false-positive results in "older/dystrophic" inactive lesions. In these "burned" lesions the heat conduction is increased and therefore the lesion appears "hot" despite clinical inactivity. Martini and colleagues[25] found that the sensitivity of thermography was 92% and specificity 68%. Full concordance between the 2 clinicians involved was observed in 91% of lesions, with a κ coefficient of 0.82, implying very high reproducibility of this technique.

If IRT is combined with other measurements of activity, it becomes more sensitive. Howell and colleagues[24] combined it with laser Doppler measurement, which assesses the blood flow/vascularity of the lesion by digital photographic techniques to provide a record of the temperature, blood flow, and appearance of each localized scleroderma lesion. These investigators developed norm values for thermography and laser Doppler measurements for certain anatomic areas such as forehead, cheek, abdomen, back, arm, and leg. Of note, a temperature difference of 1°C occurred in contralateral sites in healthy individuals. Zulian and colleagues[26] used thermography measurements as one of the outcome measures in the first controlled trial of jLS with methotrexate.

Weibel and colleagues[27] conducted a study with laser Doppler and thermography to assess the activity of jLS lesions. Seventy-five active lesions (34%) and 147 inactive lesions (66%) were identified clinically. The median relative increase in blood flow measured by laser Doppler flowmetry was +89% (range −69% to +449%) for clinically active lesions and +11% (range −46% to +302%) for clinically inactive lesions ($P<.001$). Thermography showed a median difference in temperature of +0.5°C (range −0.1°C to +4.1°C) and +0.3°C (range −1.9°C to +2.7°C) for clinically active lesions and clinically inactive lesions, respectively ($P = .024$). Using a cutoff level of 39% to indicate increase in blood flow, a sensitivity of 80% and specificity of 77% to detect clinically active lesions were observed. For thermography, no useful cutoff level was identified. Howell and colleagues[24] showed that a +1°C difference can also occur in healthy skin. The correlation between differences in blood flow and differences in temperature was small, but significant ($r^2 = 0.120$, $P<.001$). In daily practice, thermography seems fairly time consuming, with extensive personnel and cost. Laser Doppler is sensitive in assessing blood flow and vascularity and thus the activity of the lesion, but it is not readily available and, hence, not an ideal tool to assess activity.

Optical Coherence Tomography

A recent publication describes the newly applied method of optical coherence tomography (OCT), in a pilot study in 21 systemic sclerosis patients and 22 healthy controls, as "virtual skin biopsy by optical coherence tomography: the first quantitative imaging biomarker for scleroderma."[28] OCT is a powerful imaging technology providing high-contrast images with 4-μm resolution, comparable with microscopy ("virtual biopsy"). OCT uses a low-intensity infrared laser beam and is capable of producing high-contrast images of skin up to 2 mm deep with resolutions of 4 to 10 μm. Both features make it an ideal tool to explore the most superficial layers of the skin. Visualizing the superficial structures of the skin, it can assess the early fibrotic changes (eg, capillary rarefaction and perivascular infiltration) that are foremost represented in the superficial dermis. Indeed, recent work has shown a pivotal interaction between keratinocytes and superficial dermis in early skin fibrosis in systemic sclerosis.[29] Comparisons of OCT images with skin histology indicated a progressive loss of visualization of the dermal-epidermal junction associated with dermal fibrosis. Furthermore, skin affected by systemic sclerosis showed a consistent decrease of optical density (OD) in the papillary dermis, progressively worse in patients with a worse MRSS ($P<.0001$). In addition, clinically unaffected skin was also distinguishable from healthy skin for its specific pattern of OD decrease in the reticular dermis ($P<.001$). The technique showed an excellent intraobserver and interobserver reliability (intraclass correlation coefficient >0.8). This tool has not yet been not tested in pediatric jLS or jSS patients, but its use seems intriguing because it is not invasive, the interpreter does not need any special training as with ultrasonography, and it is not time consuming (<10 seconds for each site examination).

Composite Index to Assess Localized Scleroderma Skin Damage and Physician Global Assessment of Disease Damage

The composite index was developed because even nowadays, as already described, there is no simple, feasible, or reliable tool to assess activity of jLS. Ultrasonography, thermography, laser Doppler, and OCT all require availability of specific equipment and sometimes special training to use and interpret the results. Arkachaisri and colleagues[15] established the first composite index to assess disease activity in jLS. The Localized Scleroderma Skin Severity Index (LoSSI) (**Table 2**) consists of the assessment in 18 anatomic areas of the surface area (SA), erythema (ER), skin thickness (ST), and new lesion/extension of the localized scleroderma lesions. Interrater reliability was excellent for ER (intraclass correlation coefficient [ICC] 0.71), ST (ICC 0.70), LoSSI (ICC 0.80), and Physician Global Assessment (PhysGA-A) (ICC 0.90), but poor for SA (ICC 0.35); thus, LoSSI was modified to mLoSSI. In mLoSSI the SA of the lesion is excluded, because it had low interrater reliability and was not sensitive to change. Examiners' experience did not affect the scores, but training and practice improved reliability. Intrarater reliability was excellent for ER, ST, and LoSSI (Spearman $\rho = 0.71–0.89$) and moderate for SA. The PhysGA-A was based on 4 clinical criteria (appearance of new lesion, extension of existing lesion, erythema, and skin thickening) and 2 laboratory variables (erythrocyte sedimentation rate and C-reactive protein). mLoSSI correlated moderately with PhysGA-A and the Patient Global Assessment of Disease Severity (PtGA-S). Both mLoSSI and PhysGA-A were sensitive to change following therapy. To deal with the age-specific skin thickness,[13] each involved skin area was compared with the contralateral healthy area from the same person. The LoSSI and PhysGA-A appeared to be easy to use in a busy clinic. In the next step the same group established the Localized Scleroderma Skin Damage Index (LoSDI) (see **Table 2**) and the Physician Global Assessment of Disease Damage (PGA-D).[30] Although jLS is not a life-threatening disease, regardless of subtype, it almost always results in chronic and/or irreversible changes in the skin or underlying tissue. Therefore the assessment of damage is important. Damage was defined as irreversible/persistent changes (>6 months) caused by previous active disease/complications of therapy. LoSDI was calculated by summing 3 scores for cutaneous features of damage (dermal atrophy [DAT], subcutaneous atrophy [SAT], and dyspigmentation [DP]) measured at 18 anatomic sites. LoSDI and its domains DAT, SAT, DP, and PGA-D demonstrated excellent interrater and intrarater reliability (reliability coefficients 0.86–0.99 and 0.74–0.96, respectively). PGA-D and PtGA-S were also validated. At each visit patients were instructed to consider the past month for their answers.

For PGA-D, raters assessed global disease damage (using clinical variables with high content validity) on a 100-mm visual analog scale with the anchors being 0 (no damage) and 100 (severe damage). For PtGA-S, anchors were 0 (not severe) and 100 (very severe). PtGA-S was completed by patients older than 8 years, or otherwise by the accompanying parent blinded to the physician ratings. LoSDI correlated moderately with PhysGA-A and poorly with PtGA-S. A prospective assessment on this activity and damage score is being conducted by the LOCUS group. From the results of this prospective study we will be able to discern to what extent the damage index is static, and whether a regression of the damage will occur over time. It is hoped that this score will enable us to more easily conduct future clinical therapeutic trials.

Histologic Criteria for Assessment of Activity of Localized Skin Lesions

Histopathologic changes (skin biopsy) accurately reflect stages of localized skin disease but are limited by sampling bias, and repeated biopsies are inconvenient and

Table 2
Localized Scleroderma Skin Severity Index (LoSSI)

Localized Scleroderma Cutaneous Assessment Tool

	mLoSSI Localized Scleroderma Skin **Activity** Index			LoSDI Localized Scleroderma Skin **Damage** Index		
Site	New/ enlarge (within 1 mo) 0 = none 3 = N/E	Erythema 0 = none 1 = pink 2 = red 3 = dark red/ violaceous	Skin Thickness 0 = none 1 = mild 2 = moderate 3 = marked	Dermal Atrophy 0 = none 1 = shiny 2 = visible vessel 3 = obvious 'cliffdrop'	Subcutaneous Atrophy 0 = none 1 = flat 2 = concave 3 = marked atrophy	Dyspigmentation (hypo/hyperpig) 0 = none 1 = mild 2 = moderate 3 = marked
Scalp/ face						
Neck						
Chest						
Abdomen						
Upper back						
Lower back						
RT arm						
forearm						
hand						
thigh						
leg						
foot						
LT arm						
forearm						
hand						
thigh						
leg						
foot						

<u>Total Score:</u>   mLoSSI (Activity) _____   LoSDI (Damage) _____

PLEASE MARK WITH A STRAIGHT LINE:

Physician Global Assessment of Disease <u>Activity</u>

———

0   100
Inactive   Markedly active

Physician Global Assessment of Disease <u>Damage</u>

———

0   100
No damage   Markedly damage

Comment:

From Arkachaisri T, Vilaiyuk S, Torok KS, et al. Development and initial validation of the localized scleroderma skin damage index and physician global assessment of disease damage: a proof-of-concept study. Rheumatology (Oxf) 2010;49(2):373–81; with permission.

not well accepted by patients. Therefore this method is not routinely applied and should not be applied for assessment of activity, although, interestingly, in one dermatologic study[23] the ultrasonographic findings correlated with the histologic findings:

1. Active lesion
   a. Inflammatory cellular infiltrates (lymphocytes, histiocytes, plasma cells, or a combination of these)
   b. Collagen deposition
2. Inactive lesion
   a. Increased collagen deposits without inflammatory infiltrates
3. Atrophic lesion
   a. Decreased thickness of all cutaneous layers with disappearance of skin appendages
   b. Collagen deposits arranged into actual bundles (sclerosis)

"White" Uveitis in Localized Scleroderma

"White" uveitis, whereby no redness of the eye and no pain occurs, is a known phenomenon to pediatric rheumatologists who are following patients with juvenile idiopathic arthritis. This type of uveitis occurs in around 3.2% to 8.3% of patients with jLS.[31,32] Twenty-four (16 female and 8 male) of 750 patients (3.2%) revealed a significant ocular involvement.[31] Sixteen patients (66.7%) had scleroderma en coup de sabre of the face, 5 (20.8%) had the linear subtype, 2 (8.3%) had generalized morphea, and 1 (4.2%) had plaque morphea. Of the 24 patients with eye involvement, 10 (41.7%) reported adnexa (eyelids and eyelashes) abnormalities, 7 (29.2%) anterior segment inflammation (5 anterior uveitis, 2 episcleritis), and 3 central nervous system–related abnormalities. Four patients presented with singular findings such as paralytic strabismus,[1] pseudopapilledema,[1] and refractive errors.[2]

Consequently the Juvenile Scleroderma Working Group of PRES suggested at the last consensus meeting in Hamburg (2011) a screening schedule for these patients (Foeldvati and colleagues, 2013, unpublished data). In the absence of clear evidence, the group recommended screening every 6 months for uveitis with slit-lamp examination for the first 4 years of the disease if the lesion involves the scalp or the face, and screening every 12 months if the lesions do not involve the scalp or face. A prospective observational trial is planned by the working group to assess the validity of these suggestions.

Temporomandibular Joint Involvement in jLS

The involvement of the temporomandibular joint (TMJ) is another underrecognized extracutaneous characteristic of jLS. At present there are no data on the occurrence of this involvement, so the Juvenile Scleroderma Working Group of PRES suggested at the last consensus meeting in Hamburg (2011) a screening schedule for such patients (Foeldvati and colleagues, unpublished data). In the absence of clear evidence it is advised to screen clinically for signs of TMJ involvement, tenderness of the joint, crepitus at mouth opening, lateral protrusion of the mandible at mouth opening, or a history of TMJ involvement (eg, morning stiffness, pain at chewing) every 6 months if the patients have lesions on the face or scalp. For this extracutaneous part of the disease, a prospective observational trial is planned to assess the validity of this suggestion.

Assessment of Vascular Involvement in jSS

Vascular involvement is the most common organ involvement after skin involvement in jSS, but not in jLS. The degree of vascular involvement correlates with internal organ involvement.

Capillaroscopy

Capillaroscopy is a noninvasive examination that can take 5 to 10 minutes, which can be annoying for some younger children. Capillaroscopy can be conducted routinely with a dermatoscope or in more detail with a capillary microscope. Some studies have examined the capillaroscopy pattern of healthy children. Herrick and colleagues[33] evaluated 110 healthy children and found in this cross-sectional study that there was a significant trend for arterial and venous dimensions to increase with age, which was not present for apical and loop diameters. Results did not differ between males and females. Terreri and colleagues[34] assessed 329 healthy individuals with a mean age of 8.2 years with a stereomicroscope at 16× magnification, addressing the following parameters: capillary morphology, capillary enlargement, devascularization, microhemorrhage, and subpapillary venous plexus visibility (PVS). Atypical capillary morphology was observed in 118 of the studied cases (36%), mainly bizarre capillaries in 90 (27%), meandering capillaries in 32 (10%), and bushy capillaries in 20 (6%). The enlarged capillary phenomenon was uncommon, being observed in 30 cases (9%). The number of capillaries per millimeter varied from 5 to 9. Deletion areas were detected in only 7 individuals (2%). The subpapillary venous plexus was not visualized in 13 (4%) cases.

Younger children presented higher PVS scores and fewer capillaries per millimeter in comparison with older children. PVS scores were lower in males and in nonwhite children. Other variables were not associated with sex or ethnicity.

Dolezalova and colleagues[35] compared 17 healthy children with 26 children with various connective tissue diseases (CTD), using a color digital video camera attached to a stereomicroscope for the capillaroscopy. Six parameters of each image were measured: linear capillary density, capillary width, capillary tortuosity, avascular areas, capillary disarrangement, and the number of abnormal vessels. Capillary density and width was found to be age related, younger children having fewer (for all children: 6.9 [0.9] capillaries/mm) and wider (for all children: 3.1 [2.2–9.4] mm) capillaries than older children. Healthy children partly had tortuous, bizarrely shaped capillaries, with median tortuosity index of 29%.[5–49] The CTD group had lower linear density (4.9 [1.7] capillaries/mm) and increased capillary width (10.7 [7.3] mm), and had more than 2 abnormal capillaries in at least 2 nailfolds. Avascularity was a specific finding for CTD.

Looking at these data, there is still a need to prospectively establish normal values for each age group using a standardized method and nomenclature. Age-specific norm values that are able differentiate which capillary changes are clearly suggestive of an evolving autoimmune disease are needed. Sulli and colleagues[36] classified a clear capillary pattern in adult patients with systemic scleroderma systemic scleroderma, consisting of: (1) enlarged capillary: an increase in capillary diameter (homogeneous or irregular) of greater than 20 mm; (2) giant capillary: homogeneously enlarged loops with a diameter greater than 50 mm; (3) microhemorrhage: dark mass due to hemosiderin deposit; (4) loss of capillaries: reduction of the capillary number below normal range (the normal range was adopted from the literature: average of 9 capillaries per linear millimeter, counted at distal row of the nailfold); (5) disorganization of the microvascular array: irregular capillary distribution and orientation, together with shape heterogeneity of the loops; (6) capillary ramifications: branching, bushy or coiled capillaries, often originating from a single normal-sized capillary suggestive of scleroderma. These changes in scleroderma pattern, defined in the capillaroscopy of adults, partially overlap with the findings in healthy children.

Infrared Thermography

There is growing evidence that infrared thermography can be used to more objectively assess the microvascular changes in Raynaud phenomenon.[37] Thermographic parameters showing agreement with clinical end points in therapeutic trials included baseline hand/finger absolute temperature and parameters derived following local cold challenge, including longitudinal thermal gradients and percent rewarming. More studies are needed to standardize this assessment tool.

Assessment of Physical Fitness/Cardiopulmonary Function

The 6-minute walk test (6MWT) is the accepted and validated indicator of cardiopulmonary function. It is the one of the primary end points approved by the Food and Drug Administration in prospective clinical trials for adult patients with pulmonary hypertension there are guidelines regarding the conduction of the 6MWT,[38] although establishing norm values for pediatric patients is ongoing. It is known that peak oxygen consumption is reached around the age of 14 years, and increases between age 8 and 16 years by about 80% in girls and 150% in boys. Exercise capacity is influenced by cardiorespiratory fitness, improved motor skills, and movement efficiency. Li and colleagues[39] established height-specific and age-specific standards for Chinese patients, which unfortunately differ significantly from values in a similar study in the United Kingdom population.[40] The 6MWT seems to correlate with age, height, and weight of the patients. A study by Foeldvari and colleagues (EULAR 2013, only published as abstract) found norm values in German schoolchildren similar to those in the United Kingdom group. These established norm values will help to assess the cardiopulmonary function/stamina of pediatric patients, and to enable trials for the treatment of pulmonary hypertension in children. Unfortunately, patients with systemic sclerosis can have restriction of the 6MWT without any cardiopulmonary problems because of the joint, muscle, or vascular involvement of the disease.[41]

BIOMARKERS

Serum KL-6 is a high molecular weight, mucin-like glycoprotein, strongly expressed on type II pneumocytes. Serum KL-6 was measured in 6 jSS patients with interstitial lung disease (ILD) (defined with high-resolution computed tomography)[42] 6 jSS patients without ILD, and 20 healthy age-matched controls. KL-6 expression was significantly higher in patients with ILD. Patients without ILD and healthy controls had similar values. It would be interesting to assess serum KL-6 as a possible surrogate measure of grade in interstitial fibrosis and, thus, reduce the number of HRCT assessments of the lung and decrease radiation exposure. It has been shown in adults with systemic sclerosis and ILD that KL-6 correlates with the changes in diffusion capacity.

Pronatriuretic Hormone

The prognostic value of B-type natriuretic peptide (BNP) in children with pulmonary arterial hypertension (PAH) was assessed by Lammers and colleagues.[43] BNP was measured in 50 children with PAH aged 8.4 ± 5.1 years, all receiving pronatriuretic hormone–specific therapies. Mean BNP value was 143.5 ± 236.2 pg/mL (range <5–1250). BNP correlated with Functional Class II, III, and IV (50.8 ± 61.3, 196.9 ± 291.2, and 280.0 ± 276.5, respectively; $P = .01$), and with echocardiographic assessment of right ventricular function ($P<.01$), hypertrophy ($P<.01$), and dilatation ($P<.01$) In idiopathic PAH, BNP correlated with pulmonary arterial pressure and, on inhaled nitric oxide, also with vascular resistance. Data on jSS-associated PAH is lacking but would be worthwhile to collect prospectively, to learn whether it behaves similarly to idiopathic PAH.

PROGRESS IN TREATMENT
Localized Scleroderma

The first double-blind controlled trial showing the efficacy of methotrexate in the treatment of localized scleroderma was published in 2011.[26] Methotrexate was chosen as treatment for the active arm, which is the first choice of therapy, based on previous retrospective evaluations of treated patients and on clinical experience summarized in a current survey by the Childhood Arthritis and Rheumatology Research Alliance (CARRA) group.[44] The main issue remains which lesions should be treated with methotrexate. There is still considerable ongoing debate between pediatric rheumatologists and dermatologists regarding this issue. The pediatric rheumatologists believe that cosmetically potentially disfiguring lesions, lesions crossing joints, or lesions near joints should be treated with methotrexate to prevent contractures and limb-length discrepancies. This idea was reinforced in the framework of the consensus meeting, conducted in Hamburg 2011, of participating pediatric rheumatologists and dermatologists (Foeldvari and colleagues, 2013, personal communication, proceedings in preparation). Zulian and colleagues presented positive data on a small number of patients using methotrexate as first-choice therapy, in combination with glucocorticoids as bridging therapy, until methotrexate showed a therapeutic effect. The trial design compared methotrexate over 12 months plus glucocorticoids for the first 3 months, with glucocorticoids in the control arm for the first 3 months without any accompanying therapy. The methotrexate dose (15 mg/m^2 body surface area/week) used was the standard dose applied in pediatric rheumatology. Perhaps because of the relatively low number of patients, no significant change could be demonstrated between the 2 arms regarding several outcome parameters. The accompanying editorial points out the problems of the study in detail.[45]

In a small pilot study including 10 patients, the efficacy of mycophenolate was shown, all patients being methotrexate resistant.[46] In 6 patients, mycophenolate was taken in addition to methotrexate. No published data exist as yet on theoretically promising biologics such as tocilizumab, rituximab, or imatinib.

Systemic Sclerosis

There are no published controlled studies on jSS. Most of the treatment is based on the adult experience. The EULAR recently published guidelines for the treatment of systemic sclerosis,[47] which summarize the data from 2008, and updated guidelines are expected soon. At present the results of the controlled tocilizumab study are expected; preliminary results from 2 treated patients showed a significant softening of the skin.[48] Results of autologous bone marrow transplantation are intriguing, based on data from phase I and phase II studies.[49,50] The final results of the phase III trials are pending.[51] The Autologous Stem Cell Transplantation International Scleroderma (ASTIS) trial, a phase III trial, has reached completion and shows promising results in cases where the patients underwent transplantation before the disease was too far advanced. This trial enrolled more than 150 patients between 2001 and 2009, and randomized patients to autologous bone marrow transplantation or intravenous pulse cyclophosphamide treatment. As of May 1, 2012, significantly more deaths have occurred in the conventional treatment group. Half of the deaths in the stem cell transplantation group occurred early and were deemed treatment-related according to an independent data-monitoring committee. In the conventional treatment group, by contrast, none of the deaths were deemed to be treatment related; but more deaths occurred later and most were related to progressive disease (Farge and colleagues, EULAR 2012 abstract). The Scleroderma: Cyclophosphamide or Transplantation (SCOT) trial is still ongoing, and results are expected in approximately 2 years. All trials apply a different conditioning regimen: 2 are nonmyeloablative (ASTIS and American Scleroderma Stem Cell vs Immune Suppression [ASSIST]) and 1 myeloablative (SCOT), and patients younger than 18 years were excluded. Only the ASSIST trial is a treatment-failure trial that allows a crossover after treatment failure.

SUMMARY

Progress has been made in the assessment of activity of jLS and in some aspects of jSS. The currently ongoing juvenile scleroderma inception cohort for jSS (www. juvenile-scleroderma.com) will help us understand useful measures for the prospective assessment of jSS. The LOCUS group and the Juvenile Scleroderma Working Group of PRES are currently assessing project outcomes of jLS. The Juvenile Scleroderma Working Group of the PRES has already held two consensus conferences, one regarding the diagnosis and care of children with jLS and another on patients with Raynaud phenomenon (both proceedings in preparation). The CARRA group has proposed therapeutic pathways for the treatment of jLS.

REFERENCES

1. Herrick AL, Ennis H, Bhushan M, et al. Incidence of childhood linear scleroderma and systemic sclerosis in the UK and Ireland. Arthritis Care Res (Hoboken) 2010;62(2):213–8.
2. Martini G, Foeldvari I, Russo R, et al. Systemic sclerosis in childhood: clinical and immunologic features of 153 patients in an international database. Arthritis Rheum 2006;54(12):3971–8.
3. Hawley DP, Baildam EM, Amin TS, et al. Access to care for children and young people diagnosed with localized scleroderma or juvenile SSc in the UK. Rheumatology (Oxford) 2012;51(7):1235–9.
4. Herrick AL, Ennis H, Bhushan M, et al. Clinical features of childhood localized scleroderma in an incidence cohort. Rheumatology (Oxford) 2011;50(10): 1865–8.
5. Weibel L, Laguda B, Atherton D, et al. Misdiagnosis and delay in referral of children with localized scleroderma. Br J Dermatol 2011;165(6):1308–13.
6. Preliminary criteria for the classification of systemic sclerosis (scleroderma). Subcommittee for scleroderma criteria of the American Rheumatism Association Diagnostic and Therapeutic Criteria Committee. Arthritis Rheum 1980;23:581.
7. Zulian F, Woo P, Athreya BH, et al. The Pediatric Rheumatology European Society/American College of Rheumatology/European League against Rheumatism provisional classification criteria for juvenile systemic sclerosis. Arthritis Rheum 2007;57(2):203–12.
8. Russo R, Katsicas MM. Clinical characteristics of children with juvenile systemic sclerosis: follow up of 23 patients in a single tertiary center. Pediatr Rheumatol Online J 2007;5:6.
9. Laxer RM, Zulian F. Localized scleroderma. Curr Opin Rheumatol 2006;18(6): 606–13.
10. Zulian F. Systemic sclerosis and localized scleroderma in childhood. Rheum Dis Clin North Am 2008;34(1):239–55, ix.

11. Tugwell P, Boers M, Brooks P, et al. OMERACT: an international initiative to improve outcome measurement in rheumatology. Trials 2007;8:38.

12. Chung L, Denton CP, Distler O, et al. Clinical trial design in scleroderma: where are we and where do we go next? Clin Exp Rheumatol 2012;30(2 Suppl 71): S97–102.

13. de Rigal J, Escoffier E, Pharm M, et al. Assessment of aging of the human skin by in vivo ultrasound imaging. J Invest Dermatol 1989;93:621–5.

14. Foeldvari I, Wierk A. Healthy children have a significantly increased skin score assessed with the modified Rodnan skin score. Rheumatology 2006;45:76–8.

15. Arkachaisri T, Vilaiyuk S, Li S, et al. The localized scleroderma skin severity index and physician global assessment of disease activity: a work in progress toward development of localized scleroderma outcome measures. J Rheumatol 2009;36(12):2819–29.

16. Falanga V, Bucalo B. Use of a durometer to assess skin hardness. J Am Acad Dermatol 1993;29(1):47–51.

17. Aghassi D, Monoson T, Braverman I. Reproducible measurements to quantify cutaneous involvement in scleroderma. Arch Dermatol 1995;131(10):1160–6.

18. Kissin EY, Schiller AM, Gelbard RB, et al. Durometry for the assessment of skin disease in systemic sclerosis. Arthritis Rheum 2006;55(4):603–9.

19. Kroft EB, Groeneveld TJ, Seyger MM, et al. Efficacy of topical tacrolimus 0.1% in active plaque morphea: randomized, double-blind, emollient-controlled pilot study. Am J Clin Dermatol 2009;10(3):181–7.

20. Kroft EB, van de Kerkhof PC, Gerritsen MJ, et al. Period of remission after treatment with UVA-1 in sclerodermic skin diseases. J Eur Acad Dermatol Venereol 2008;22(7):839–44.

21. Merkel PA, Silliman NP, Denton CP, et al. Validity, reliability, and feasibility of durometer measurements of scleroderma skin disease in a multicenter treatment trial. Arthritis Rheum 2008;59(5):699–705.

22. Li SC, Liebling MS, Haines KA, et al. Initial evaluation of an ultrasound measure for assessing the activity of skin lesions in juvenile localized scleroderma. Arthritis Care Res (Hoboken) 2011;63(5):735–42.

23. Wortsman X, Wortsman J, Sazunic I, et al. Activity assessment in morphea using color Doppler ultrasound. J Am Acad Dermatol 2011;65(5):942–8.

24. Howell KJ, Lavorato A, Visentin MT, et al. Validation of a protocol for the assessment of skin temperature and blood flow in childhood localised scleroderma. Skin Res Technol 2009;15(3):346–56.

25. Martini G, Murray KJ, Howell KJ, et al. Juvenile-onset localized scleroderma activity detection by infrared thermography. Rheumatology (Oxford) 2002; 41(10):1178–82.

26. Zulian F, Martini G, Vallongo C, et al. Methotrexate treatment in juvenile localized scleroderma: a randomized, double-blind, placebo-controlled trial. Arthritis Rheum 2011;63(7):1998–2006.

27. Weibel L, Howell KJ, Visentin MT, et al. Laser Doppler flowmetry for assessing localized scleroderma in children. Arthritis Rheum 2007;56(10):3489–95.

28. Abignano G, Aydin SZ, Castillo-Gallego C, et al. Virtual skin biopsy by optical coherence tomography: the first quantitative imaging biomarker for scleroderma. Ann Rheum Dis 2013. [Epub ahead of print].

29. Chung L, Chen H, Khanna D, et al. Dyspnea assessment and pulmonary hypertension in patients with systemic sclerosis: utility of the University of California, San Diego, Shortness of Breath Questionnaire. Arthritis Care Res (Hoboken) 2013;65(3):454–63.

30. Arkachaisri T, Vilaiyuk S, Torok KS, et al. Development and initial validation of the localized scleroderma skin damage index and physician global assessment of disease damage: a proof-of-concept study. Rheumatology (Oxford) 2010;49(2): 373–81.

31. Zulian F, Vallongo C, Woo P, et al. Localized scleroderma in childhood is not just a skin disease. Arthritis Rheum 2005;52(9):2873–81.

32. Zannin ME, Martini G, Athreya BH, et al. Ocular involvement in children with localised scleroderma: a multi-centre study. Br J Ophthalmol 2007;91(10):1311–4.

33. Herrick ML, Moore T, Hollis S, et al. The influence of age on nailfold capillary dimension in childhood. J Rheumatol 2000;27:797–800.

34. Terreri MT, Andrade LE, Puccinelli ML, et al. Nail fold capillaroscopy: normal findings in children and adolescents. Semin Arthritis Rheum 1999;29(1):36–42.

35. Dolezalova P, Young SP, Bacon PA, et al. Nailfold capillary microscopy in healthy children and in childhood rheumatic diseases: a prospective single blind observational study. Ann Rheum Dis 2003;62:444–9.

36. Sulli A, Pizzorni C, Smith V, et al. Timing of transition between capillaroscopic patterns in systemic sclerosis. Arthritis Rheum 2012;64(3):821–5.

37. Pauling JD, Shipley JA, Harris ND, et al. Use of infrared thermography as an endpoint in therapeutic trials of Raynaud's phenomenon and systemic sclerosis. Clin Exp Rheumatol 2012;30(2 Suppl 71):S103–15.

38. Society AT. ATS statement: guidelines for the six-minute walk test. Am J Respir Crit Care Med 2002;166(1):111–7.

39. Li AM, Yin J, Au JT, et al. Standard reference for the six-minute-walk test in healthy children aged 7 to 16 years. Am J Respir Crit Care Med 2007;176(2): 174–80.

40. Lammers AE, Hislop AA, Flynn Y, et al. The 6-minute walk test: normal values for children of 4-11 years of age. Arch Dis Child 2008;93(6):464–8.

41. Garin MC, Highland KB, Silver RM, et al. Limitations to the 6-minute walk test in interstitial lung disease and pulmonary hypertension in scleroderma. J Rheumatol 2009;36(2):330–6.

42. Vesely R, Vargova V, Ravelli A, et al. Serum level of KL-6 as a marker of interstitial lung disease in patients with juvenile systemic scleroderma. J Rheumatol 2004;31:795–800.

43. Lammers AE, Hislop AA, Haworth SG. Prognostic value of B-type natriuretic peptide in children with pulmonary hypertension. Int J Cardiol 2009;135(1):21–6.

44. Li SC, Feldman BM, Higgins GC, et al. Treatment of pediatric localized scleroderma: results of a survey of North American pediatric rheumatologists. J Rheumatol 2010;37(1):175–81.

45. Foeldvari I. Methotrexate in juvenile localized scleroderma: adding to the evidence. Arthritis Rheum 2011;63(7):1779–81.

46. Martini G, Ramanan AV, Falcini F, et al. Successful treatment of severe or methotrexate-resistant juvenile localized scleroderma with mycophenolate mofetil. Rheumatology (Oxford) 2009;48(11):1410–3.

47. Kowal-Bielecka O, Landewe R, Avouac J, et al. EULAR recommendations for the treatment of systemic sclerosis: a report from the EULAR Scleroderma Trials and Research group (EUSTAR). Ann Rheum Dis 2009;68(5):620–8.

48. Shima Y, Kuwahara Y, Murota H, et al. The skin of patients with systemic sclerosis softened during the treatment with anti-IL-6 receptor antibody tocilizumab. Rheumatology (Oxford) 2010;49:2408–12.

49. Milanetti F, Bucha J, Testori A, et al. Autologous hematopoietic stem cell transplantation for systemic sclerosis. Curr Stem Cell Res Ther 2011;6(1):16–28.

50. Burt RK, Shah SJ, Dill K, et al. Autologous non-myeloablative haemopoietic stem-cell transplantation compared with pulse cyclophosphamide once per month for systemic sclerosis (ASSIST): an open-label, randomised phase 2 trial. Lancet 2011;378(9790):498–506.
51. Naraghi K, van Laar JM. Update on stem cell transplantation for systemic sclerosis: recent trial results. Curr Rheumatol Rep 2013;15(5):326.

Outcomes Research in Childhood Autoimmune Diseases

Esi Morgan DeWitt, MD, MSCE[a,b,*]

KEYWORDS

- Outcomes research • Patient outcome assessment • Registries
- Quality improvement • Rheumatology • Pediatrics • Health services research

KEY POINTS

- Outcomes research is the study of the impact of treatments, health care, or quality improvement interventions on patient-relevant end points such as disease control, function, or quality of life.
- Longitudinal registries require high-quality data for patient outcomes studies to be valid. Information technology may facilitate use of electronic medical record data.
- Reliable and routine assessment of health status using standardized outcome measures allows for objective, comparable measurement of the impact of different interventions on outcomes.
- Patient-reported measures add unique information to other clinical end points to assess response to therapy, describe preferences, assess impact on quality of life, and track long-term outcomes.
- Outcomes research has its most impact on optimizing patient outcomes when research findings on best practices are rapidly translated into delivery of health care.

INTRODUCTION

Outcomes research, also known as patient-centered outcomes research or comparative effectiveness research (CER), is oriented toward studies of health care practices such as specific medications, behavioral interventions, care delivery systems, and

Disclosures: The author has no financial or commercial interests to disclose. Dr Morgan DeWitt is Chair of the Pediatric Rheumatology Care and Outcomes Improvement Network. She is also a principal investigator in the Patient Reported Outcomes Measurement Information System (PROMIS) network.
The author receives funding from NIH Grant number U01AR0757940 (PI Morgan DeWitt) and from AHRQ (Agency for Healthcare Research and Quality) grant number U19HS021114 (PI Lannon).
[a] Department of Pediatrics, College of Medicine, University of Cincinnati, 3333 Burnet Avenue, Cincinnati, OH 45229, USA; [b] Division of Rheumatology, Cincinnati Children's Hospital Medical Center, 3333 Burnet Avenue, MLC 4010, Cincinnati, OH 45229, USA
* James M. Anderson Center for Health Systems Excellence, Cincinnati Children's Hospital Medical Center, 3333 Burnet Avenue, MLC 4010, Cincinnati, OH 45229.
E-mail address: esi.morgan_dewitt@cchmc.org

0889-857X/13/$ – see front matter © 2013 Elsevier Inc. All rights reserved.
rheumatic.theclinics.com

their impact on best outcomes for individual patients.[1,2] For this research to make a difference, there must be investment in activities to disseminate this knowledge, to implement the findings into practice, and to measure and improve quality of care delivered.[3]

Although this is not a new field of study, there has been increased emphasis and enthusiasm for this line of research as a result of changes in federal legislation and recent substantial funding for CER. The American Recovery and Reinvestment Act of 2009 allocated $1.1 billion to fund CER between the Agency for Healthcare Research and Quality, the Department of Health and Human Services, and the National Institutes of Health (NIH). In 2010, the Patient Protection and Affordable Care Act served to establish the Patient-Centered Outcomes Research Institute (PCORI), a not-for-profit, independent organization funded through the Patient-Centered Outcomes Research Trust Fund (PCORTF) with income from the Treasury and from a fee to Medicare, private insurers, or self-insurance plans. It is estimated that PCORI will receive $3.5 billion up to September 30, 2019.[4,5]

The spirit and distinguishing characteristics of this research are evident in the definition of CER used by the Federal Coordinating Council for Comparative Effectiveness Research:

> CER is the conduct and synthesis of systematic research comparing different interventions and strategies to prevent, diagnose, treat and monitor health conditions. The purpose of this research is to inform patients, providers, and decision-makers, responding to their expressed needs, about which interventions are most effective for which patients under specific circumstances. To provide this information, comparative effectiveness research must assess a comprehensive array of health-related outcomes for diverse patient populations. Defined interventions compared may include medications, procedures, medical and assistive devices and technologies, behavioral change strategies, and delivery system interventions. This research necessitates the development, expansion, and use of a variety of data sources and methods to assess comparative effectiveness.[6]

The emphasis is for delivery of high-quality topics of relevance and importance to patients and families that allows them to make informed decisions about their health care. A central aspect of that evidence is the analysis of the impact of a particular intervention (ie, as defined earlier) on patient-relevant outcomes. These outcomes may include patient-reported outcomes (PROs) of symptoms or function, side effects, economic impact, or impact on social or societal participation. CER thus necessitates high-quality registries for longitudinal patient follow-up and outcome measures that have proved to be valid and responsive to change. Another distinguishing feature is the recognition that there are multiple stakeholders who require this information to make informed health care decisions, including not only clinicians, researchers, and patients but also policy makers and insurers.[2]

Once information has been generated from outcomes research on which interventions or treatments are most effective, it needs to be efficiently distributed in such a way that it can identify in which setting the intervention will be most beneficial. There is a significant time lag in translation of research evidence into clinical practice.[1] Furthermore, there are widespread disparities in care received in which people who might benefit from a treatment do not receive it.[7] The CER definition places emphasis on the mission "to inform." The quality of delivered care may be monitored and evaluated in part on whether or not patients who would benefit from a given treatment receive it.[8]

REGISTRIES IN PEDIATRIC RHEUMATOLOGY

Longitudinal registries with high-quality data are essential to the validity of patient outcomes studies. Clinic-based data sets, in contrast to administrative data sets such as medical insurance claims, allow for collection of information on disease severity such as clinician measures of disease activity and PRO measures.

There is a growing number of national and international registries in pediatric rheumatology, of which only a few examples are described here. The organizing principles, format, frequency of visits, measures collected, disease populations, funding sources, and other features vary across the registries (**Table 1**). This variation renders aggregation of the data or replication of study findings challenging.

PharmaChild is a network of registries from multiple European Union (EU) countries for the purpose of pharmacovigilance regarding treatments of juvenile idiopathic arthritis (JIA). PharmaChild is funded by the EU and pharmaceutical companies and organized by the Pediatric Rheumatology International Trials Organization.[9] In North America, the Pediatric Rheumatology Collaborative Study Group has maintained post-marketing surveillance registries after completion of randomized controlled trials for JIA treatments.[10]

The example of national, population-based databases shows comparative effectiveness studies under favorable circumstances. Such registries confer advantages such as reduction in bias, full ascertainment of the population avoids selection bias, and ensuring representativeness of the sample. A national registry minimizes censoring and loss to follow-up. Equally important is the standardization of outcomes assessment for patients across different clinic sites.

Studies from Germany, such as the German Etanercept Registry, have described long-term safety and efficacy of etanercept in JIA. Another recent German registry[11] examined the clinical experience with oral versus subcutaneous administration of methotrexate on disease control, as well as adverse effects of treatment. The investigators found no advantage of using subcutaneously injected methotrexate over orally administered methotrexate, despite practitioner debates to the contrary. Is this a question of interest to the patient? A study by Mulligan and colleagues[12] showed the importance of addressing this question as far as implications for health-related quality of life (HRQOL) of patients and caregivers. In the study, methotrexate use in general was described as having a negative impact on HRQOL, but administration in the form of injections was identified as a significant independent predictor of distress.

The Dutch National Biologics Register provides another example of a registry providing longitudinal follow-up of etanercept-treated patients used to address a question likely of general interest to the public, payers, and policy makers: do the treatment benefits of etanercept justify the high cost of the biological medication? The study entailed an economic evaluation comparing estimates of costs and usefulness in the 12 months preceding the medication use and 27 months after initiation. The Health Utility Index Mark 3 was given to most sites that participated (7 of 9), in order to calculate quality-adjusted life years, in addition to routine collection of clinical variables and PROs. It was concluded that the medication was cost-effective.[13] In the United States, it is stipulated that CER focuses on effectiveness of treatments rather than results to be used in policy decisions to minimize costs.

In the United States, the Childhood Arthritis and Rheumatology Research Alliance (CARRA) registry represents 59 pediatric rheumatology centers and more than 6000 patients with JIA (see **Table 1**). The CARRA registry also collects information on multiple childhood rheumatic diseases, including systemic lupus erythematosus, juvenile dermatomyositis, linear scleroderma, vasculitis, and fibromyalgia. One of the purposes of

Table 1
Pediatric rheumatology disease registries in North America

Registry	Purpose	Population	Data Collected	Frequency of Data Collection	Funding	Contact
ARChiVe	Research	Vasculitis	Clinical, laboratory tests, imaging	Onset, and up to 2 mo after diagnosis	Foundations	Email: pedvas@cw.bc.ca
CAPRI–ReACCh Out	Research	JIA	Clinical, PRO, laboratory tests, medications	Every 6–12 mo	Arthritis Society, CIHR, various	Web: http://www.icaare.ca/
CARRA	Research, pharmaco-vigilance	JIA SLE MCTD JDM LS SS Vasculitis Sarcoid JPFS	Clinical, PRO, laboratory tests, medications	Every 6 mo	NIH, Arthritis Foundation, various	Web: https:// carranetwork.org
PR-COIN	Quality improvement, research	JIA	Clinical, PRO, laboratory tests, medications	Continuous	Arthritis Foundation, AHRQ CERT, various	Web: http://pr-coin.org Email: PR-COIN@cchmc.org

Abbreviations: AHRQ CERTS, Agency for Healthcare Research and Quality Center for Education and Research of Therapeutics; ARChiVe, A Registry for Children with Vasculitis e-entry; CAPRI, Canadian Alliance of Pediatric Rheumatology Investigators; CARRA, Childhood Arthritis and Rheumatology Research Alliance; CIHR, Canadian Institutes for Health Research; JDM, juvenile dermatomyositis; JIA, juvenile idiopathic arthritis; JPFS, juvenile primary fibromyalgia syndrome; LS, linear scleroderma; MCTD, mixed connective tissue disease; NIH, National Institutes of Health; PR-COIN, Pediatric Rheumatology Care and Outcomes Improvement Network; PRO, patient reported outcomes; REACCH OUT, Research on Arthritis in Canadian Children Emphasizing Outcomes; SLE, systemic lupus erythematosus; SS, systemic sclerosis.
Data from Refs.[18,47–49]

the registry is to identify patients eligible for clinical trials, to conduct CER and long-term safety studies. Cross-sectional studies have characterized a descriptive epidemiology of the study population, including disease and demographic characteristics and pre-scribing patterns in the United States.[14,15] Longitudinal follow-up is planned and under way. The CARRA registry overlies an informatics framework based on the Informatics for Integrating Biology and the Bedside and NIH-funded National Center for Biomedical Computing.[16] It is a scalable, federated system whereby individual centers have owner-ship of their own data and can contribute data to network studies with permission.[17]

The ARChiVe (A Registry for Childhood Vasculitis), based in Canada, is a registry targeting children with ANCA (antineutrophil cytoplasmic antibody)-associated vascu-litis, established in cooperation with the CARRA network.[18]

Comparative effectiveness in observational databases creates significant chal-lenges to the validity of findings. Principal among these challenges are bias, of which there are several types, and confounding.[19] For example, confounding by indication occurs when both the study outcome of interest and the treatment selected are related to the severity of disease. A choice of treatment that is believed to be the strongest may thus go to the sickest patients, who are most refractory to treat, and the potential benefit of the treatment of the disease may be underestimated. There are statistical analytical techniques that minimize these challenges, such as use of propensity scores or instrumental variables, but these may not be able to sufficiently overcome the problem and risk of flawed conclusions.

Variation in how patients are treated in clinical practice also poses additional diffi-culty to analysis and interpretation of observational data. According to clinical prac-tice, geography, and other considerations, there is wide variability in the care that patients receive.[20] There is inconsistency in the way providers may approach patients that makes it difficult to analyze clinical data. For instance, there may be differences across providers in treatment selection, medication dosing, follow-up intervals, whether clinical variables and outcomes measures are assessed and if so which mea-sures are used, missing data, all which introduce significant noise into the database. In the face of such unwarranted variability, even sophisticated statistical techniques are unlikely to detect whether an intervention is effective.

A way to try to minimize variability as well as bias is the use of treatment guidelines, which if followed drive standardization. For example, guidelines may provide specified treatment options and dosing, approach to intensification or taper of medication reg-imens, standard visit intervals, and assessment schedules that specify clinical labora-tory and PRO measures. There are examples of treatment guidelines by various professional organizations, including consensus treatment plans generated by CARRA for systemic arthritis, juvenile dermatomyositis, localized scleroderma, lupus nephritis[21,22,23,24] and polyarticular JIA (Ringold S, Weiss PF, Colbert RA, et al. Child-hood Arthritis and Rheumatology Research Alliance Consensus Treatment Plans for New Onset Polyarticular Juvenile Idiopathic Arthritis. Submitted for publication).

NETWORKS FOR IMPROVEMENT AND RESEARCH

The Pediatric Rheumatology Care and Outcomes Improvement Network (PR-COIN) is an international quality improvement (QI) network that aims to improve the outcomes for children with JIA.[25] Learning networks are practice-based clinical networks that use data to conduct research, including CER, and use proven QI methods and tools to improve process of care delivery and child health outcomes. Such networks func-tion as collaborations among clinicians with patients and families, along with re-searchers and communities.[26] PR-COIN is a growing network, which was launched in 2011, and now includes 10 active PR-COIN sites and more than 1000 enrolled patients, with close to 4000 encounters.

The network sites of PR-COIN use a shared registry platform for longitudinal data collection, the Rheumatology Clinical Registry of the American College of Rheumatology (ACR).[27] Data are collected at point of care on process measures of care and outcome measures. Process measures of care and target goals are based on published proposed process measures of care for JIA.[28] For instance, data are recorded to determine whether children with JIA receive uveitis screening according to published guidelines in order to reduce risk of unrecognized inflammatory eye disease and avert development of vision loss. Other process measures track medication safety monitoring, and whether clinical outcome and PROs are assessed reliably. Outcome measures are based on clinical outcomes prioritized by stakeholders and reflect the proportion of patients with (1) inactive disease, (2) optimal physical function, and (3) no or mild pain.

Data are used in a timely manner to inform on improvement activities. Registry data are used to generate statistical process control charts, funnel charts, and other graphical presentations of site performance on measures over time. An individual site's performance is compared against other sites' performance and network aggregate benchmarks on a monthly basis. This prompt feedback on performance is used to direct subsequent QI activities and learning. For example, if a site is not meeting targets for uveitis screening, 90-day goals are set and teams design and carry out small tests of change with plan-do-study-act cycles. Sites then adapt, adopt, or abandon the test interventions depending on whether they result in an improvement.[29]

In the current system of health care delivery for JIA, (1) site performance at baseline leaves an uncomfortably high number of patients with active disease, physical disability, and more than mild pain, and (2) there is variation in performance across centers. However, as a network, with sharing of learning and QI activities, there has been initial improvement in performance on process measures of care. Interventions and change in concepts for improving care are based on the improving chronic illness care model,[30] using the model for improvement for reliability of implementation.

The ideal state for the PR-COIN registry is to meet the goal of data in once, with repurposing of data. One site has piloted upload of data from the electronic health record into the registry database, effectively being able to reuse the data, starting with entry once for clinical care. Subsequently, the same data are being used for QI and research purposes. Reuse of data becomes an essential strategy for such networks, because it reduces costs of participation in the registry, by eliminating double data entry. This gain in efficiency allows for enrollment of a larger proportion of a clinic population into the registry, enabling spread of interventions (such as the concept of previsit planning) to more patients, generating a more representative sample of patients, thereby reducing bias and increasing validity of findings and also giving a more accurate picture of the health status of the clinic population and quality of care delivered.[26]

Learning networks aspire to the model of a learning health care system, as described by the Institute of Medicine. Information technology may facilitate use of electronic medical record data as infrastructure for research and support integration of health care, health care improvement, outcomes research, and innovation. Communities of patients, clinicians, and researchers engage in generating and addressing research questions of interest to guide decision making and QI activities.[26]

CLINICAL OUTCOMES ASSESSMENT

In outcomes research, consistent, reliable, and routine assessment of health status using standard outcomes measures is important for objective measurement of disease progression over time. In QI, clinical outcomes assessment can feature either a process measure of care (eg, are complete joint counts being performed? Is physician global assessment recorded?) or measures to evaluate quality of care with respect to health outcomes.

For clinical trials, use of the ACR JIA Core Set of Variables is a means of describing treatment responses in terms of percentage of improvement. The core set variables include: (1) physician global assessment of disease activity; (2) parent/patient assessment of overall well-being; (3) functional ability; (4) number of joints with active arthritis; (5) number of joints with limited range of motion; and (6) erythrocyte sedimentation rate (ESR) or C-reactive protein (CRP) (eg,, 30% improvement as defined in terms of changes to core set variables, 30% or more improvement from baseline in 3 of any variables in the core set, with no more than 1 variable worsening by more than 30%). When a patient achieves 30% improvement, they are classified in the proportion of responders to an intervention meeting a JIA ACR 30 response. Fifty percent improvement corresponds to JIA ACR 50, and so forth, for 70% response, 90% response, and 100% response.[31] There are also criteria defining flare of disease in terms of the core set variables.[32]

Although the ACR JIA Core Set is an established measure of change over time used in randomized clinical trials, and in longitudinal outcomes studies, it is not typically used in routine clinical practice, because it is not a continuous measure of current health status, but rather a measure of change, and it is not straightforward to calculate. Furthermore, not all components needed to calculate the measure are collected at each routine clinic visit.

An easy-to-use and continuous measure of disease activity for JIA has not been established. However, a promising new disease activity score is the Juvenile Arthritis Disease Activity Score (JADAS), for which a validation study in a clinical practice setting has recently been published.[33] It is a composite disease activity score comprising 4 variables: (1) active joint count, (2) physician global assessment, (3) parent/patient global assessment of well-being, and (4) ESR. There are various versions depending on the number of joints assessed, with the numeric modifier indicating the total joint count (eg, JADAS-71, JADAS-27, JADAS-10).[34]

In recognition that requiring an ESR to determine a JADAS scale score is problematic in patient situations in which blood draws are not being performed concurrent with a visit, or do not seem indicated based on a patient's having excellent clinical status, an alternative version, the JADAS-3, has been studied. The JADAS-3 omits the ESR from calculations and is well correlated with the full JADAS. The JADAS-3 alternative reduces a missing data problem in evaluating this measure routinely to track patient clinical status.

There is a dichotomous measure of JIA disease activity: the ACR provisional criteria for defining clinical inactive disease.[35] There are 6 components to this measure, all of which must be as noted for a patient to be considered in clinical inactive disease: (1) no joints with active arthritis, (2) no fever, rash, serositis, splenomegaly, or generalized lymphadenopathy (ie, features of systemic arthritis) attributable to JIA, (3) no active uveitis (per Standardization of Uveitis Nomenclature Working Group), (4) ESR or CRP level within normal limits established by performing laboratory tests, unless known to be increased as a result of another cause (eg, concurrent illness), (5) physician global assessment at best possible value on scale, (6) duration morning stiffness less than or up to 15 minutes. As noted in the example with the JADAS, the requirement of inclusion of the ESR laboratory value may result in a missing data point in a clinical setting. This measure is clinician based, and aside from the morning stiffness value, does not consider patient report.

As part of the PR-COIN learning network, sites are encouraged to collect all variables that are included in the ACR Criteria for inactive disease at each clinic visit (laboratory tests every 3 months), although quality measures are less stringent in terms of frequency of assessment. Given the speed with which new treatments for JIA take effect, interim changes may not be observed to characterize the trajectory of the disease course and timing of medication effect if assessments are collected only at 6-month intervals. Now that a validated continuous measure of disease activity in the form of JADAS-3 is available, it offers a value by which to track patient status at a single point in time, in addition to the ability to monitor progress over time. This measure may prove useful in a clinical setting, and also as part of CER analyses.

PRO ASSESSMENT

PROs add information that is complementary to other clinical parameters such as physical examination findings and laboratory tests to assess response to therapy, monitor disease control, and track long-term outcomes. PROs are self-reports from patients that can capture a broad array of the patient experience, including health symptoms (pain, fatigue), functioning, mental health, HRQOL, participation in activities, and self-efficacy.[36] Other topics such as satisfaction with care, treatment goals, and preferences can also be elicited by patient self-reporting. Assessing PROs helps to examine patient-centered outcomes and provision of care that is responsive to patient needs that may not otherwise be identified in a clinical setting.

In selecting a PRO for a clinical study, or for clinical care, there are several factors to consider. These factors include the psychometric theory underlying development, whether it is based on classic test theory or modern item-response theory (IRT). The content covered by the measure, whether validity studies were performed, and measurement properties such as sensitivity at high and low ends of the scale, and whether it is responsive to change, need to be reviewed. There are some practical considerations such as whether a scale is publicly available or has licensing fees, ease of administration including the mode (paper and pencil, computer, hand-held electronic device, automated telephone surveys, or interview), respondent burden, ease of scoring, and interpretability of results. In pediatrics, another consideration is whether the scale is developmentally appropriate, and whether there is a companion proxy-administered version of the measure for young children unable to self-report (<8 years old).

There are a multitude of PRO instruments to choose from in pediatric rheumatology. There are generic and cross-cutting measures intended to be used across diseases, and then there are disease-specific scales. An important concept is that of a health domain. A domain represents a one-dimensional health attribute, such as fatigue or anxiety. Domain-specific instruments can be generic and suitable for use across diseases, because such health attributes are not specific to a given disease, although a given disease may have a characteristic profile of the attribute.[36] Disease-specific PRO instruments lose the flexibility of being used across studies and conditions. A consequence of numerous PRO measurement options is that if the same instruments are not used uniformly across studies or clinical populations, it results in the inability to compare results of interventions or treatments across different studies or to perform meta-analyses of treatment effectiveness.

Development of PRO instruments has shifted from classic test theory to an IRT approach. PRO instruments, or tests, are designed to measure an underlying health construct or attribute. Tests developed with classic test theory include a range of items to enable use for patients at high and low ends of the construct being measured.

All items must be administered for the test to be scored. In order to administer items that cover the entire range of a trait without high respondent burden, there is a trade-off between efficiency and precision. Such tests may be subject to floor and ceiling effects and not sensitive to change.

For tests developed using IRT, each item is calibrated on the trait along a measurement continuum. IRT models characterize the probability of the respondent's level on the construct based on the response option chosen for a calibrated item. Some advantages are that item banks can be created for each heath attribute, which can be large to allow for precision coverage at different levels of the attribute, yet any 1 respondent needs to be given only a subset of items relevant to their level on the trait. For instance, a person who endorses ability to run a mile does not need to answer a question about whether they can walk on flat ground. Advantages are shorter instruments with fewer items (efficiency, less respondent burden), more precision of measurement, and increased ability to detect change. Tests can be administered as static short forms, off-the-shelf or customized for a target level of a trait, or as computerized adaptive tests. The NIH Patient Reported Outcomes Measurement Information System (PROMIS) cooperative network was created in 2004 to support a publicly available assessment system of PROs created with state-of-the-art measurement science, including IRT (http://www.nihpromis.org).[37]

There are several instruments for PRO assessment in pediatric rheumatology. The reader is encouraged to review measure validation studies before selection of a PRO measure, because such detail is beyond the scope of this review. Generic measures of HRQOL tested in pediatric rheumatic disease samples, and as reviewed by Hullmann and colleagues,[38] include the DISABKIDS, Pediatric Quality of Life Inventory (PedsQL) 4.0 Generic Core Scales, and Quality of My Life Questionnaire, all of which are claimed to be useful in clinical and research settings. The Child Health Questionnaire is lengthy for clinical use but perhaps more useful in a research setting. Examples of JIA disease-specific measures of quality of life reviewed by Carle and colleagues[39] include the PedsQL Rheumatology Module 3.0, which was evaluated as useful in clinical and research settings. The Juvenile Arthritis Quality of Life Questionnaire and Pediatric Rheumatology Quality of Life Scale may be most useful in clinical settings.

Physical function PRO measures studied in JIA include the Child Health Assessment Questionnaire (CHAQ),[40] Juvenile Arthritis Functionality Scale (JAFS),[41] and Activities Scale for Kids (ASK). The CHAQ is well known to have a strong ceiling effect, which may limit its usefulness in detecting differences at low levels of disability (or high function); nonetheless, it is used widely in clinical and research settings. ASK has been used in research settings more for primary orthopedic disorders.[42]

PROMIS offers IRT-based measures to assess a variety of health domains that have been tested in children with JIA (http://www.nihpromis.org). These health domains include measures of mobility, upper extremity function, fatigue, pain interference, anxiety, and depressive symptoms. Qualitative analysis show good content validity[43] and construct validity and responsiveness studies are under way.[44]

As PROs are developed that offer efficient, precise estimates of patient self-reported health end points with less respondent burden and time demand, it increases the feasibility of incorporating PROs into routine clinical care. PROs can be administered electronically and incorporated directly into the electronic health record. There are examples of health systems that are already using such systems to guide medical decision making.[45,46] Electronic health record vendors, including Epic (Epic Systems Corporation, Verona, WI, USA), are integrating such PRO packages into their software. The routine assessment of PROs in clinical care has potential to influence the focus of care at patient visits and improve disease management, particularly if a system is used whereby PRO scales are automatically scored and results presented to the clinician in an interpretable and actionable way. Routine collection of PROs in clinical care will increase the ability to use data from clinical encounters to monitor patient status longitudinally and conduct CER of treatments and interventions in a clinical setting.

FUTURE CONSIDERATIONS/SUMMARY

Patient-centered outcomes research is motivated to inform about the best health care decisions according to a particular patient's circumstances and preferences. By understanding the impact of treatments, health care or QI interventions on patient-relevant end points such as disease control, function, or quality of life, the appropriate treatment can be selected for a patient that will optimize their outcome. Longitudinal registries with high-quality data are essential to patient outcomes studies, and advances in information technology are anticipated to allow use of data from clinical encounters to be repurposed for outcomes research. Reliable and routine assessment of health status using standardized outcomes measures allows for objective, comparable measurement of impact of different interventions on outcomes. PRO assessment in a clinical setting, when entered into the electronic record, will enable PROs to be part of the calculus on impact on patients of interventions being evaluated in CER. Rapid translation of research on best practices into clinical care, as facilitated by QI learning networks, leads to timely and meaningful improvement in patient outcomes.

REFERENCES

1. Dougherty D, Conway PH. The "3T's" road map to transform US health care: the "how" of high-quality care. JAMA 2008;299(19):2319–21.
2. Clancy CM. Commentary: precision science and patient-centered care. Acad Med 2011;86:667–70.
3. Conway PH, Clancy C. Comparative-effectiveness research–implications of the Federal Coordinating Council's report. N Engl J Med 2009;361(4):328–30.
4. Selby JV, Beal AC, Frank L. The Patient-Centered Outcomes Research Institute (PCORI) national priorities for research and initial research agenda. JAMA 2012;307(15):1583–4.
5. Patient Centered Outcomes Research Institute. How We're Funded. Available at: http://www.pcori.org/about-us/how-were-funded/. Accessed June 3, 2013.
6. Tunis SR, Benner J, McClellan M. Comparative effectiveness research: policy context, methods development and research infrastructure. Stat Med 2010; 29(19):1963–76.
7. Flores G. Technical report–racial and ethnic disparities in the health and health care of children. Pediatrics 2010;125(4):e979–1020.
8. Chin MH, Alexander-Young M, Burnet DL, et al. Health care quality-improvement approaches to reducing child health disparities. Pediatrics 2009;124(Suppl 3): S224–36.
9. Wulffraat NM, Swart JF. An international registry for biologics used in children with Juvenile Idiopathic Arthritis: a challenging collaboration between paediatric rheumatologists and pharmaceutical industry. Ann Paediatr Rheumatol 2012;1: 106–11.
10. Ruperto N, Martini A. Networking in paediatrics: the example of the Paediatric Rheumatology International Trials Organisation (PRINTO). Arch Dis Child 2011; 96(6):596–601.
11. Klein A, Kaul I, Foeldvari I, et al. Efficacy and safety of oral and parenteral methotrexate therapy in children with juvenile idiopathic arthritis: an observational

study with patients from the German Methotrexate Registry. Arthritis Care Res (Hoboken) 2012;64(9):1349–56.

12. Mulligan K, Kassoumeri L, Etheridge A, et al. Mothers' reports of the difficulties that their children experience in taking methotrexate for juvenile idiopathic arthritis and how these impact on quality of life. Pediatr Rheumatol Online J 2013;11(1):23.

13. Prince FH, de Bekker-Grob EW, Twilt M, et al. An analysis of the costs and treatment success of etanercept in juvenile idiopathic arthritis: results from the Dutch Arthritis and Biologicals in Children register. Rheumatology (Oxford) 2011;50(6):1131–6.

14. Ringold S, Beukelman T, Nigrovic PA, et al. Race, ethnicity, and disease outcomes in juvenile idiopathic arthritis: a cross-sectional analysis of the Childhood Arthritis and Rheumatology Research Alliance (CARRA) Registry. J Rheumatol 2013;40(6):936–42.

15. Beukelman T, Ringold S, Davis TE, et al. Disease-modifying antirheumatic drug use in the treatment of juvenile idiopathic arthritis: a cross-sectional analysis of the CARRA Registry. J Rheumatol 2012;39(9):1867–74.

16. i2b2: Informatics for Integrating Biology and the Bedside. A National Center for Biomedical Computing. Available at: https://www.i2b2.org. Accessed June 17, 2013.

17. Natter MD, Quan J, Ortiz DM, et al. An i2b2-based, generalizable, open source, self-scaling chronic disease registry. J Am Med Inform Assoc 2013;20(1):172–9.

18. Cabral DA, Uribe AG, Benseler S, et al. Classification, presentation, and initial treatment of Wegener's granulomatosis in childhood. Arthritis Rheum 2009; 60(11):3413–24.

19. Bernatsky S, Lix L, O'Donnell S, et al. Consensus statements for the use of administrative health data in rheumatic disease research and surveillance. J Rheumatol 2013;40(1):66–73.

20. Mangione-Smith R, DeCristofaro AH, Setodji CM, et al. The quality of ambulatory care delivered to children in the United States. N Engl J Med 2007;357(15): 1515–23.

21. DeWitt EM, Kimura Y, Beukelman T, et al. Consensus treatment plans for new-onset systemic juvenile idiopathic arthritis. Arthritis Care Res (Hoboken) 2012; 64(7):1001–10.

22. Huber AM, Robinson AB, Reed AM, et al. Consensus treatments for moderate juvenile dermatomyositis: beyond the first two months. Results of the second Childhood Arthritis and Rheumatology Research Alliance consensus conference. Arthritis Care Res (Hoboken) 2012;64(4):546–53.

23. Li SC, Torok KS, Pope E, et al. Development of consensus treatment plans for juvenile localized scleroderma: a roadmap toward comparative effectiveness studies in juvenile localized scleroderma. Arthritis Care Res (Hoboken) 2012; 64(8):1175–85.

24. Mina R, von Scheven E, Ardoin SP, et al. Consensus treatment plans for induction therapy of newly diagnosed proliferative lupus nephritis in juvenile systemic lupus erythematosus. Arthritis Care Res (Hoboken) 2012;64(3):375–83.

25. Pediatric Rheumatology Care and Outcomes Improvement Network. Available at: http://pr-coin.org. Accessed June 17, 2013.

26. Clancy CM, Margolis PA, Miller M. Collaborative networks for both improvement and research. Pediatrics 2013;131(Suppl 4):S210–4.

27. American College of Rheumatology. Rheumatology clinical registry. Available at: http://www.rheumatology.org/Practice/Clinical/Rcr/Rheumatology_Clinical_Registry/. Accessed June 17, 2013.

28. Lovell DJ, Passo MH, Beukelman T, et al. Measuring process of arthritis care: a proposed set of quality measures for the process of care in juvenile idiopathic arthritis. Arthritis Care Res (Hoboken) 2011;63(1):10–6.
29. Langley G, Moen R, Nolan K, et al. The improvement guide: a practical approach to enhancing organizational performance. 2nd edition. San Francisco (CA): Jossey-Bass; 2009.
30. Coleman K, Austin BT, Brach C. Evidence on the chronic care model in the new millennium. Health Aff (Millwood) 2009;28(1):75–85.
31. Giannini EH, Ruperto N, Ravelli A, et al. Preliminary definition of improvement in juvenile arthritis. Arthritis Rheum 1997;40(7):1202–9.
32. Brunner HI, Lovell DJ, Finck BK, et al. Preliminary definition of disease flare in juvenile rheumatoid arthritis. J Rheumatol 2002;29(5):1058–64.
33. McErlane F, Beresford MW, Baildam EM, et al. Validity of a three-variable Juvenile Arthritis Disease Activity Score in children with new-onset juvenile idiopathic arthritis. Ann Rheum Dis 2012. [Epub ahead of print].
34. Consolaro A, Ruperto N, Bazso A, et al. Development and validation of a composite disease activity score for juvenile idiopathic arthritis. Arthritis Rheum 2009;61: 658–66.
35. Wallace CA, Giannini EH, Huang B, et al. American College of Rheumatology provisional criteria for defining clinical inactive disease in select categories of juvenile idiopathic arthritis. Arthritis Care Res (Hoboken) 2011;63(7):929–36.
36. Forrest CB, Bevans KB, Tucker C, et al. Commentary: the Patient-Reported Outcome Measurement Information System (PROMIS) for children and youth: application to pediatric psychology. J Pediatr Psychol 2012;37(6):614–21.
37. Cella D, Gershon R, Lai JS, et al. The future of outcomes measurement: item banking, tailored short-forms, and computerized adaptive assessment. Qual Life Res 2007;16:133–41.
38. Hullmann SE, Ryan JL, Ramsey RR, et al. Measures of general pediatric quality of life: Child Health Questionnaire (CHQ), DISABKIDS Chronic Generic Measure (DCGM), KINDL-R, Pediatric Quality of Life Inventory (PedsQL) 4.0 Generic Core Scales, and Quality of My Life Questionnaire (QoML). Arthritis Care Res (Hoboken) 2011;63(Suppl 11):S420–30.
39. Carle AC, Dewitt EM, Seid M. Measures of health status and quality of life in juvenile rheumatoid arthritis: Pediatric Quality of Life Inventory (PedsQL) Rheumatology Module 3.0, Juvenile Arthritis Quality of Life Questionnaire (JAQQ), Paediatric Rheumatology Quality of Life Scale (PRQL), and Childhood Arthritis Health Profile (CAHP). Arthritis Care Res (Hoboken) 2011;63(Suppl 11): S438–45.
40. Singh G, Athreya BH, Fries JF, et al. Measurement of health status in children with juvenile rheumatoid arthritis. Arthritis Rheum 1994;37:1761–9.
41. Filocamo G, Sztajnbok F, Cespedes-Cruz A, et al. Development and validation of a new short and simple measure of physical function for juvenile idiopathic arthritis. Arthritis Rheum 2007;57:913–20.
42. Klepper SE. Measures of pediatric function: Child Health Assessment Questionnaire (C-HAQ), Juvenile Arthritis Functional Assessment Scale (JAFAS), Pediatric Outcomes Data Collection Instrument (PODCI), and Activities Scale for Kids (ASK). Arthritis Care Res (Hoboken) 2011;63(Suppl 11):S371–82.
43. Jacobson CJ, Farrell JE, Kashikar-Zuck S, et al. Disclosure and self-report of emotional, social, and physical health in children and adolescents with chronic pain–a qualitative study of PROMIS pediatric measures. J Pediatr Psychol 2013;38(1):82–93.

44. Khanna D, Krishnan E, Dewitt EM, et al. Patient-Reported Outcomes Measurement Information System (PROMIS)–the future of measuring patient reported outcomes in rheumatology. Arthritis Care Res (Hoboken) 2011;63(S11):S486–90.
45. Katzan I, Speck M, Dopler C, et al. The Knowledge Program: an innovative, comprehensive electronic data capture system and warehouse. AMIA Annu Symp Proc 2011;2011:683–92.
46. Wagner LI, Spiegel D, Pearman T. Using the science of psychosocial care to implement the new American College of Surgeons Commission on Cancer distress screening standard. J Natl Compr Canc Netw 2013;11(2):214–21.
47. CAPRI – ReACCh Out. Available at: http://www.icaare.ca/. Accessed July 26, 2013.
48. CARRA. Available at: https://carranetwork.org. Accessed July 26, 2013.
49. PR-COIN. Available at: http://pr-coin.org. Accessed July 26, 2013.

Index

Note: Page numbers of article titles are in **boldface** type.

A

Abatacept
  for eye diseases, 817
  for juvenile dermatomyositis, 894
  for juvenile idiopathic arthritis, 756, 760–761
Acne, in SAPHO syndrome, 745
Activities Scale for Kids, 929
Adalimumab
  for eye diseases, 815–816
  for juvenile idiopathic arthritis, 755–759
Adrenocorticotropic hormone gel, for juvenile dermatomyositis, 892–893
Aicardi-Goutieres syndrome, 708
Alemtuzumab
  for eye diseases, 818
  for juvenile dermatomyositis, 895
American Heart Association, Kawasaki disease guidelines of, 862
American Recovery and Reinvestment Act of 2009, 922
American Scleroderma Stem Cell vs. Immune Suppression (ASSIST) trial, 917
American Uveitis Society, 814
Amyloidosis, in familial Mediterranean fever, 719
Amyopathic dermatomyositis, 879
Anakinra
  for cryopyrinopathies, 717
  for juvenile dermatomyositis, 894
  for juvenile idiopathic arthritis, 756, 759–760
Anemia, in Majeed syndrome, 742
Aneurysms
  in Kawasaki disease, 859–864
  in Takayasu arteritis, 869–870
Antibodies, in juvenile idiopathic inflammatory myopathies, 884–887
Anticoagulation, for Kawasaki disease, 862–864
Antineutrophil cytoplasmic autoantibodies, in vasculitis, 855–857
Aorta, Takayasu arteritis of, 865–870
Aphthous lesions, in Behçet syndrome, 808
Apremilast, for spondyloarthritis, 781
ARChiVe registry, 924–925
Arteritis, Takayasu, 865–870
Arthritis. *See also* Spondyloarthritis.
  juvenile idiopathic, **761–765**
  pediatric granulomatous, 708–709, 711, 721–722
  psoriatic, 778–780
  pyogenic sterile, 706, 721–722

Rheum Dis Clin N Am 39 (2013) 935–950
http://dx.doi.org/10.1016/S0889-857X(13)00083-5
0889-857X/13/$ – see front matter © 2013 Elsevier Inc. All rights reserved.

rheumatic.theclinics.com

United States Postal Service

Statement of Ownership, Management, and Circulation
(All Periodicals Publications Except Requestor Publications)

1. Publication Title
Rheumatic Disease Clinics of North America

2. Publication Number
0 0 6 - 2 7 2

3. Filing Date
9/14/13

4. Issue Frequency
Feb, May, Aug, Nov

5. Number of Issues Published Annually
4

6. Annual Subscription Price
$317.00

7. Complete Mailing Address of Known Office of Publication *(Not printer) (Street, city, county, state, and ZIP+4®)*

Elsevier Inc.
360 Park Avenue South
New York, NY 10010-1710

Contact Person
Stephen Bushing

Telephone *(Include area code)*
215-239-3688

8. Complete Mailing Address of Headquarters or General Business Office of Publisher *(Not printer)*

Elsevier Inc. 360 Park Avenue South, New York, NY 10010-1710

9. Full Names and Complete Mailing Addresses of Publisher, Editor, and Managing Editor *(Do not leave blank)*

Publisher *(Name and complete mailing address)*

Linda Belfus, Elsevier, Inc., 1600 John F. Kennedy Blvd. Suite 1800, Philadelphia, PA 19103-2899

Editor *(Name and complete mailing address)*

Pamela Hetherington, Elsevier, Inc., 1600 John F. Kennedy Blvd. Suite 1800, Philadelphia, PA 19103-2899

Managing Editor *(Name and complete mailing address)*

Adrianne Brigido, Elsevier, Inc., 1600 John F. Kennedy Blvd. Suite 1800, Philadelphia, PA 19103-2899

10. Owner *(Do not leave blank. If the publication is owned by a corporation, give the name and address of the corporation immediately followed by the names and addresses of all stockholders owning or holding 1 percent or more of the total amount of stock. If not owned by a corporation, give the names and addresses of the individual owners. If owned by a partnership or other unincorporated firm, give its name and address as well as those of each individual owner. If the publication is published by a nonprofit organization, give its name and address.)*

Full Name	Complete Mailing Address
Wholly owned subsidiary of	1600 John F. Kennedy Blvd., Ste. 1800
Reed/Elsevier, US holdings	Philadelphia, PA 19103-2899

11. Known Bondholders, Mortgagees, and Other Security Holders Owning or Holding 1 Percent or More of Total Amount of Bonds, Mortgages, or Other Securities. If none, check box ☐ None

Full Name	Complete Mailing Address
N/A	

12. Tax Status *(For completion by nonprofit organizations authorized to mail at nonprofit rates) (Check one)*
The purpose, function, and nonprofit status of this organization and the exempt status for federal income tax purposes:
☐ Has Not Changed During Preceding 12 Months
☐ Has Changed During Preceding 12 Months *(Publisher must submit explanation of change with this statement)*

PS Form 3526, September 2007 (Page 1 of 3 (Instructions Page 3)) PSN 7530-01-000-9931 **PRIVACY NOTICE:** See our Privacy policy in www.usps.com

---

13. Publication Title
Rheumatic Disease Clinics of North America

14. Issue Date for Circulation Data Below
August 2013

15. Extent and Nature of Circulation

			Average No. Copies Each Issue During Preceding 12 Months	No. Copies of Single Issue Published Nearest to Filing Date
a. Total Number of Copies *(Net press run)*			646	605
b. Paid Circulation (By Mail and Outside the Mail)	(1)	Mailed Outside-County Paid Subscriptions Stated on PS Form 3541. *(Include paid distribution above nominal rate, advertiser's proof copies, and exchange copies)*	288	257
	(2)	Mailed In-County Paid Subscriptions Stated on PS Form 3541 *(Include paid distribution above nominal rate, advertiser's proof copies, and exchange copies)*		
	(3)	Paid Distribution Outside the Mails Including Sales Through Dealers and Carriers, Street Vendors, Counter Sales, and Other Paid Distribution Outside USPS®	162	143
	(4)	Paid Distribution by Other Classes Mailed Through the USPS *(e.g. First-Class Mail®)*		
c. Total Paid Distribution *(Sum of 15b (1), (2), (3), and (4))*			450	400
d. Free or Nominal Rate Distribution (By Mail and Outside the Mail)	(1)	Free or Nominal Rate Outside-County Copies Included on PS Form 3541	60	105
	(2)	Free or Nominal Rate In-County Copies Included on PS Form 3541		
	(3)	Free or Nominal Rate Copies Mailed at Other Classes Through the USPS (e.g. First-Class Mail)		
	(4)	Free or Nominal Rate Distribution Outside the Mail (Carriers or other means)		
e. Total Free or Nominal Rate Distribution *(Sum of 15d (1), (2), (3) and (4))*			60	105
f. Total Distribution *(Sum of 15c and 15e)*			510	505
g. Copies not Distributed *(See instructions to publishers #4 (page #3))*			136	100
h. Total *(Sum of 15f and g)*			646	605
i. Percent Paid *(15c divided by 15f times 100)*			88.24%	79.21%

16. Publication of Statement of Ownership
If the publication is a general publication, publication of this statement is required. Will be printed in the **November 2013** issue of this publication. ☐ Publication not required

17. Signature and Title of Editor, Publisher, Business Manager, or Owner

Stephen R. Bushing

Stephen R. Bushing –Inventory Distribution Coordinator

Date September 14, 2013

I certify that all information furnished on this form is true and complete. I understand that anyone who furnishes false or misleading information on this form or who omits material or information requested on the form may be subject to criminal sanctions (including fines and imprisonment) and/or civil sanctions (including civil penalties).

PS Form 3526, September 2007 (Page 2 of 3)

Moving?

Make sure your subscription moves with you!

To notify us of your new address, find your **Clinics Account Number** (located on your mailing label above your name), and contact customer service at:

Email: journalscustomerservice-usa@elsevier.com

800-654-2452 (subscribers in the U.S. & Canada)
314-447-8871 (subscribers outside of the U.S. & Canada)

Fax number: 314-447-8029

Elsevier Health Sciences Division
Subscription Customer Service
3251 Riverport Lane
Maryland Heights, MO 63043

*To ensure uninterrupted delivery of your subscription, please notify us at least 4 weeks in advance of move.

Printed and bound by CPI Group (UK) Ltd, Croydon, CR0 4YY

03/10/2024

01040493-0008

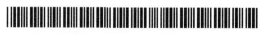